Conscious Caregiving

Plant Medicine, Nutrition, Mindful Practices to Give Ease

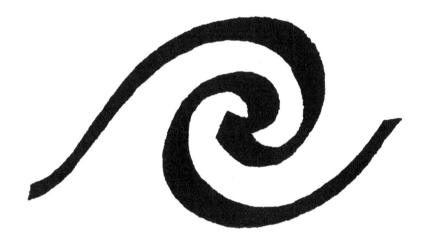

Carol Trasatto

herbalist

Greenwild Publishing

Conscious Caregiving

Plant Medicine, Nutrition,
Mindful Practices to Give Ease

Conscious Caregiving:

Plant Medicine, Nutrition, Mindful Practices to Give Ease

Booksellers and libraries may order via Ingramcontent.com.

Hardbound ISBN 978-0-9995787-0-4

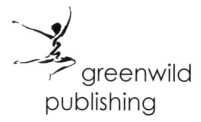

greenwild
publishing

120 State Ave NE #171 • Olympia WA 98501
Cascadia Bioregion

info@caroltrasatto.com • www.caroltrasatto.com

*Please note that the information offered herein is intended for educational and inspirational
purposes only. This is not an attempt to diagnose or prescribe for any health condition. Each
person has very specific individual needs regarding health and well-being. The author supports
self-empowerment and personal research. As part of that process she encourages active and
informed collaboration with a trusted healthcare practitioner when seeking to demystify
and address physical symptoms. Readers retain full responsibility
for their application of information presented in this book.*

Cover photograph: Jenu Prasad
Cover design: Carol Trasatto
with thanks to Debi Bodett 33 Image Design for her magic

To all who journey deeply
into the Mystery of Living and Dying with another soul —
May your footsteps be guided by Love and Compassion.

And may this honor the memory of Joni Pohlig, Night Magician,
who first led my own steps there.

"Through love, all pain is turned to medicine."

— *Rumi*

Contents

Navigating This Moment of Life

Engaging the Medical System

Presence / Surgery / Chemo & Radiation / Recovery

Nutrition / Liver Health

Adaptogens / Tonics / Nervines

More Tools for Support

Appendices

Introduction to the New Edition

Conscious Caregiving has been in print as a spiral-bound manual since 2004, with a major revision made in 2006. Previous to this, for many years, it was distributed through my classes and workshops in a much-abbreviated version. Through these iterations, it has already found its way into many homes and hospice situations. Now, I am extremely pleased to offer this fresh and greatly enhanced revision.

I have lived and worked as an herbalist for several decades now. I honor the natural world as my source of sustenance and renewal on all levels of being—and I celebrate the inherent capacity of our bodies to respond to the powers of nature. Over and over again, I have witnessed the blessing of skillfully chosen plants, as both food and medicine, in easing conditions that have caused suffering.

My professional life has been focused on promoting a holistic mind/body/spirit approach to wellness through teaching, writing, personal coaching, and as an herb buyer and educator for a community-treasured retail store/clinic in the Pacific Northwest. Clients, friends and family routinely commented on my own usually vibrant health.

Then, during 2009-2010, I embarked on my own life-changing journey—first the mystery space of unexplained symptoms, then traveling deep through the diagnosis of, treatment for, and recovery from an aggressive, pervasive non-Hodgkin's lymphoma. Not knowing the course my health journey would follow, one of the first things I did after receiving the diagnosis was to hand a copy of *Conscious Caregiving* to each of my closest friends who were companioning me.

During this profound healing process, I stayed deeply engaged with holistic healing as it applied in my own circumstances. I worked with herbal medicine, concentrated nutrition, prayer, meditation and energy work to complement the allopathic chemotherapy and biological treatments I underwent. From the inside out, I was able to fine-tune the many approaches I had worked with successfully with others for decades…and I generated new responses to discomforts and side-effects, as well. Now, healthy and vibrant once more, I am eager to share this expanded edition of *Conscious Caregiving*.

Being both a client of the medical oncology system as well as a partaker and practitioner of holistic medicine has given me a unique point of view through the process. At times, I found myself acting as a bridge person in educating oncology personnel as to the benefits of nutritional and herbal complementary support—for instance, how I was able to improve blood cell and platelet status with herbs, how I was able to gain weight while undergoing chemo, how I was able to prevent neuropathy, how I kept my bowels working daily, etc. Because of my background, I also was able to very precisely describe my experience of body and mind to my complementary team, which supported their work with me during treatments and consultations.

All through the intense process of discovery and treatment, I prayed that my experience would be of benefit not only to myself but also to others. This was a great comfort. I felt complete confidence in and gratefulness for the complementary approach I was taking, and knew there could be no other path for me. In this knowing, there was peace and focus to support the health of my being—even amidst the vast chaos and utter not-knowing that accompanies a life-threatening diagnosis.

I am currently working on a companion book, tentatively titled *Deep, Grateful Bow: Honoring Cancer as Fierce Teacher*. This work explores more of the inner process of my personal journey and details the healing practices that I personally engaged. For now, I have kept these two works separate, to allow the expanded *Conscious Caregiving* to continue to meet the needs of all who are drawn to it without additional delay. I have included a sample chapter from *Deep, Grateful Bow* at the back of this book. [If you resonate with my work, please visit my website at www.caroltrasatto.com and sign up to be informed about this and other offerings.]

Writing now, almost nine years after diagnosis, I remain in remission and have truly blossomed in health throughout recovery. I attribute my current health status to the holistic nature of the path that I took—incorporating all the ways of healing I needed to not only survive but thrive beyond cancer.

I fully embraced the intense allopathic treatment protocol, for without it I would not be alive today to write these words. As well, and as essential, I also fully embraced the potent healing medicines of attitude, language, discipline, inner reflection, spiritual practices, nutrient-dense daily foods, concentrated nutritional supplementation, herbal medicine, energy work, sound healing, movement, community, and deepening the practice of all that I knew to contribute toward health of mind and body. Finding ways to laugh heartily each and every day was crucial.

More than ever, I am honored and grateful to be able to offer you the document that you hold in your hands. There truly is a wealth of sound counsel in these pages, and I say that not to bring praise to myself. Our food and medicinal plants and our relationship with life and spirit have always been the most true medicine for our human selves, and I count myself blessed to be both a recipient and one transmitter of some of the ancient healing wisdom that has been passed along for countless generations. It is more clear to me than ever: Nature is our source, our substance, our inspiration. May each of us—blessed beings of nature—aid each other along the journey of life, doing whatever we can to give ease wherever there is suffering.

Blessed be,

Carol Trasatto

2018

Conscious Caregiving:

Plant Medicine, Nutrition, and Mindful Practices to Give Ease

"Indeed the tragedy is not that someday we must die,
but that so often during life we wish to remain numb."

— Stephen Levine

In the offering of care within a home environment, a multitude of situations arise which call for our attention as caregivers. At times, we may feel stretched beyond our capacities to cope. We may feel that each new day brings us to the edge and then beyond what we have known before. We find ourselves digging deep within for the strength to stay grounded and mindful as we watch our beloved transform before our eyes. In the midst of this, we are perhaps engaged on the most intimate physical levels of care—bathing, feeding, assisting with urination and defecation, administering enemas, soothing aching muscles, offering our bodies as comfort for grief or fear, and myriad other such callings. The needs change almost as surely as the moment remains fluid and vast. To offer such care in a way that does not impose our own will but instead follows the flow of our beloved's experience of sensation is a remarkable meditation. To do all this while caring well for ourselves requires even more concentration.

What I am calling "conscious caregiving," then, is two-fold. It is the very sensitive, meditative caring for a loved one undergoing physical and emotional and spiritual transformation, and it is also the very deliberate self-care that caregivers extend to themselves. To my mind, these two activities are inextricably interwoven and the quality of the one is dependent on the quality of the other. They are in dynamic interplay.

The ideas I touch on in the first part of the manual can benefit both caregiver and recipient, in that the frame of mind and spirit in which the work is approached is perhaps more important than the specific remedies given later to ease pain and discomfort. *Cultivating the Ground of Compassion* and *On Conscious Caregiving* offer ideas for setting the tone of the relationship; *Caregiver Self-Care Overview* suggests ways to maintain physical stamina, perspective, groundedness, energetic integrity, immunity, and emotional endurance; sections within *The Helping Repertoire* on **Consistency/Ritual**, **Energy Awareness**, and **Arranging the Healing Space** offer tips for establishing a rhythm to the days and a sacred feeling to the space. Working with the section on *Flower Essences*, either yourself alone or with your loved ones, can be a gentle way of allowing emotional material to surface in a safe context, especially for those who are not fluent in verbalizing their feelings.

The seeds of this compilation of material were sown almost 25 years ago in the living/dying process of my dear friend Joni as she dealt with advanced breast cancer. Joni honored me greatly by asking me to be her night nurse at the point when she had realized it was time to surrender her resistance and open to her dying—that subtle internal shift from seeking to regain health to allowing death its course. Although I had been working with plant medicine for years, I had never done such caregiving work before and the challenge was greater than any I had previously faced. But Joni and I and her partner Sara all drew on our inner resources to find our way through, collaboratively—each day, each moment new. Joni's ability to articulate the details of her full bodymind experience was remarkable and we all learned so much in those intense months that opened our view into infinite possibility. The energy of present moment revealed itself as both exhilarating and exhausting. In those intimate conversations in the middle of the night, Joni and I marveled that our souls' contract had led us to this rarefied experience. We prayed that her process and our remarkable dance together might hopefully benefit others in some way at some point in time.

Since that journey with Joni, I have had hundreds of opportunities as an herbal consultant to be of support to others in their caregiving roles as well as to offer direct care myself. Essentially, I view the work as meeting people where they are and going from there; about listening and tending with compassion and acceptance. There is always *some* approach, *some* option that will give ease in a situation without posing a threat to the recipient's comfort zone. I feel strongly that it is a form of violence to impose our beliefs or practices onto another, especially when they are vulnerable and depleted. But offering alternative ideas in a gentle, non-judgmental way so to relieve tension, contraction and constriction can be a blessing to all involved. Knowledge and skill is of little use without the capacity to improvise and adapt—and serve with lovingkindness.

This book *Conscious Caregiving* is not intended to provide everything you need to know to offer loving care at home—or for tending to your own needs, for that matter. At this writing, there is a wealth of material being published that offers many views into the process being addressed here. I strongly encourage you to review the annotated reading list toward the back of this manual to locate additional sources of guidance into what you are facing. There is much treasure there.

With this work you hold in your hands, my intention is to offer a detail-rich distillation, an accessible recipe book for the daily challenges you will be facing—either as a caregiver or as someone dealing with your own serious unwellness. I wanted to offer something that could be read at various levels and would be easy to reference in a moment of need. There is so much ease that can be given with such simple natural remedies and qualities of being. Other books to be found on the list of recommendations will further elaborate and explore the larger context in which these are utilized.

This is surely a work in progress, an offering to both caregivers and those in need of their heartfelt services. May it be of benefit in the journeys you undertake in these realms.

How to Use This Book

Although this edition of *Conscious Caregiving* is significantly expanded from previous versions, I strove to keep the format as straightforward and easily accessible as in the past. This format has proven itself "in the field," so to speak—referenced in the challenging moments that arise, day by day. Previous readers have thanked me for its simplicity, so that they could readily get to what they needed without sorting through extended narrative.

So, in opening this book for the first time at home, I suggest that you approach it in the following way, hopefully during quieter moments when you or your loved one is not in crisis mode. In that way, you will likely find what you are looking for more easily in such high-energy moments in future.

1. First, **familiarize yourself with the *Table of Contents***. Get a general overview of what is offered within. If the Table of Contents doesn't seem to mention a theme you are concerned with, be sure to check the **index** in the back.

2. **Read the introductory chapters**: particularly *Cultivating the Ground of Compassion, On Conscious Caregiving: Setting the Tone, Creating the Space,* and *Caregiver Self-Care Overview*.

3. Should you be tempted to simply dive in and employ some of the helping strategies suggested, please, please, **please read the introduction to *The Helping Repertoire*** before doing so. It is less than two pages long, yet offers key considerations to be aware of before you begin.

4. Then, **read through the italicized introductions** that preface each subject in ***The Healing Repertoire***. For instance, see what is said in general about nausea or constipation. Reading through these introductions will give you a deeper sense of what to look out for and provide a framework for understanding what may arise. Check out the details of those sections that are currently relevant or that you may anticipate.

The use of **boldface** within these sections in the ***Repertoire*** is used to help you find what you're looking for as efficiently as possible. There are numerous suggestions within each category—not to overwhelm you with choice but to provide multiple possibilities to lend relief in any given moment. Also, as circumstances change, new strategies may be tried. What works in one moment may not in the next—in fact, that is highly likely.

Notice that there is substantial **referencing within the body of text to related sections** or chapters to help expand on the conversation at hand.

5. Related to this, **note the topics discussed in the Appendices**. The aim is to provide enough background information to offer a working overview on the themes presented,

such as the lymphatic system or engaging pain or hydration/electrolytes or the relationship between stress and memory.

6. Included toward the back is a **glossary of herbal terms** [*The Language of Herbalism*] you may find within the book that may not be fully explained in the text. For example, the meaning of *actions*—such as astringent, cholagogue, or antimicrobial—which describe the healing attributes of a given plant are defined in the glossary.

7. The ***Recommended Reading*** section is annotated to help you discover other books that expand on the themes touched on here and to further support you on your journey. There is a blessed wealth of substantial support in print.

With this sort of review of the bones of the book, you should have a good sense of how to access what you are looking for when you need it. This book is not necessarily intended to be read cover to cover in sequence, although many readers have told me they've gratefully done so. It can easily be read in sections that speak to the needs most vividly presenting themselves. Again, please ***do*** read the introduction to ***The Helping Repertoire*** on page 31 before using any of the strategies for symptom relief contained within.

Overall, I would encourage you to simply go with the flow and follow the stream of your attention. May it lead you exactly where you need to go.

Cultivating the Ground of Compassion

As we begin this conversation, for both caregivers and those they serve, it seems extremely important to highlight the distinction between compassion and sympathy—the distinction between true, unconditional compassion and sympathetic attachment.

The difference between these two modes of being, of being *with*, is like night and day. One is deeply healing and the other a distortion that has a toxic quality to it.

Compassion, as discussed here, is a clean, clear energy. Compassion is a warm, attentive spaciousness in which needs may be met. When true compassion is present, nothing is needed from the person being helped other than for them to clearly express their needs as they arise. Nothing is needed from the helper other than willing presence, deep listening, and their commitment to take good care of themselves even as they give aid. No energy cords run between helper and helped, no identification with particular emotions or investment in some fixed dynamic of the relationship—in fact, in a truly compassionate dynamic, healing freely runs in all directions, within a vast field of loving presence.

Compassionate presence allows both caregiver and the person experiencing illness to deal with the unfolding reality of each moment in a very present-tense, forthright, kindhearted way. In compassionate presence, nothing need be turned away from.

In this way of relating, space is created for full focus on internal self-healing. The one experiencing illness is not burdened with making the caregiver feel better or feel needed. Within compassion, there is space for any and all emotions to arise, any and all needs to be recognized and articulated. Within compassion, there is no attachment to sorrow or grief or righteousness or roles. There is as much possibility for bliss and laughter as tears.

Sympathy, by definition, assumes a shared experience of feeling. However, sympathy, in excess approaching pity, can have more to do with the *caregiver's* inner milieu than the state of mind of the person facing illness. It may reflect more about their own fears and anxiety than anything else. Sympathy, in this way, can feel sticky and heavy—a projection of the sympathetic person onto the object of their sympathy. *"You must feel...."* or *"This is really a bummer..."* or *"How could this have happened to you?"* are neither helpful questions nor fruitful lines of discussion. They do not arise from a space of actual curiosity, but are more an assertion of belief from the one expressing them. This sort of sympathy contains a silent demand to confirm the truth of what is being said, to join the speaker in their own sorrow, disbelief, or distress.

The presence of such an overly sympathetic person can feel like a weight, a burden. It encourages the person dealing with illness to sink into a space of *"woe is me"* whether that is their default attitude in the moment or not. Such an expression of sympathy contains a silent energy cord [which some recipients will clearly feel as draining], energetically demanding that the receiver of sympathy acknowledge the truth of these projections and suffer with them in this sad, woeful space.

This way of being for the caregiver represents an over-identification with the pain present in the room. It does not arise from an open, curious space: How is this being in front of me dealing with this health circumstance in this moment? Anything other than living such an open question is not a true meeting of hearts; it is, instead, objectification. For the person they are tending, sympathy/pity can feel crushing, yucky, like a dampening down of the fire of one's internal self-healing spirit—and the focus they may have worked hard to achieve, that of fully accepting the circumstances they find themselves in with an intention to live each day as fully alive to its preciousness as possible.

Such sympathetic attachment does not promote the clear, fresh atmosphere that allows for the optimal health and well-being of *any and all* of those involved in a challenging circumstance—whether caregiver, the one being aided, family or friends.

What we are asked to do as helpers is quite straightforward. It does not involve depressing our own spirit in order to serve another. It involves honoring our own aliveness as we weave sacred space for the nurturance of aliveness in our companion. To do so is not a denial of death or pain, but an affirmation of the precious potential of each moment of now.

On Conscious Caregiving
Setting the Tone, Creating the Space

Sit

Hold a hand

Be a silent companion/witness

Listen

Be present

*"The most important therapeutic 'art' consists of being a fellow creature
with a human understanding of the body, soul and spirit."*

— **Tineke van Bentheim**

- Help initiate dialogue regarding honest communication and emotional authenticity. Make space for the whole of each other to be present.

- Meet your companion where they are. Examine your expectations. Dissolve your preconceptions. Become a spacious environment in which authenticity may arise.

- At any given moment in caring for another, discern what is at the forefront calling for attention—body, mind, or spirit?

- Relate to the person before you, not the disease.

- Cultivate patience, allowing a given process to unfold according to its own timing. Some sort of equilibrium or harmonious rhythm will eventually be regained.

- Co-create sacred and consistent rituals, both day and night—such as around eating, bathing, medication—allowing for some sense of predictability and control.

- Bring a focused attention to perceive each new situation from the point of view of the one who is ill. Attempt to modify the environment before it is requested.

- Perceive and honor the divinity of the being you have agreed to serve.

- Nurture the attitude that this being and this situation have much to teach you. Listen with all of your senses.

- Honor also the divine in your self—a willing vehicle for the healing balm of love, for the spaciousness of attentive presence.

- Dedicate this work to the highest good of all concerned, and undertake this service as a vigorous spiritual practice.

A Keynote of the Conversation

In no way do I wish to imply that there is a single way, a correct way to approach life-changing illness or the dying process. That attitude would undermine the goal of this work, which is to support our loved one in meeting the challenges presented by their changing bodies in such a way as to allow them the dignity of their own experience, their own journey; to help create the space for them to meet themselves as best as they are able—a space as free as possible from judgment, protocol, and preconceptions.

In his wonderful book *After the Ecstasy, the Laundry*, Jack Kornfield tells a story of Zen Buddhist teacher Dainan Katagiri Roshi as he was facing his own imminent death. Kornfield relates that when Katagiri Roshi was diagnosed with terminal cancer, many students gathered around to be of assistance. Along with love and respect they also experienced fear and confusion, trying to apprehend that their beloved teacher could be subject to such infirmity, as might any ordinary human being.

"One day he called the students to his bedside. 'I see you are watching me closely. You want to see how a Zen master dies. I'll show you.' He kicked his legs and flailed his arms with alarm, crying out, 'I don't want to die, I don't want to die!' Then he stopped and looked up at them. 'I don't know how I will die. Maybe I will die in fear or in pain. Remember, there is no right way.'"

Communication

Establishing and maintaining honest and effective communication between caregivers and the one receiving care can be one of the most challenging aspects of this dance—particularly when there is a long history of relationship dynamics. Entering this new chapter with awareness is crucial.

Suddenly, both parties may feel thrust into a deeply unsettling circumstance that tests the resiliency of the relationship—whether an intimate partnership, a familial connection, or a loving friendship. The quality of communication that existed before the crisis obviously influences what is brought to the moment of illness and caregiving, when previous roles may dramatically shift.

One or both parties may feel that any "safety" they felt in the relationship up to that point has been suddenly washed away, and there may be anger, resentment or anxiety—as a great flood of personal issues arise to be seen and dealt with. Alternately, material that once seemed to create stress or separation in the relationship may now be seen to be of no real substance—the essential core of the relationship, the love and appreciation, may flower. Obviously, there are as many permutations of what may present itself as there are iterations of individuals dancing in dyad.

It may be ideal if one or the other—the caregiver or the person to be aided—sets the tone for how they would prefer this chapter of life to be lived. This can require significant clarity and courage, particularly when there is long personal history at play.

All it takes is for one person to initiate the heartfelt conversation where together some foundational issues may be discussed—and for both people to be willing to speak from their most undefended, vulnerable hearts. Fears, anxieties, preferences, questions that are being held…Together, a framework of intention and personal needs can be articulated that can help smooth the path going forward as new challenges inevitably present themselves.

What am I most afraid of, given what I/you/we are facing here?

How would I like to be treated, given what I am feeling in this moment?

How will our power dynamic best work going forward? In what areas would I like to have some semblance of control in this otherwise mysterious journey through unfamiliar terrain?

What needs to change for this to work for us? What are the strengths we have together?

How can each of us best communicate our needs and boundaries as we go forward, knowing that these may change or vary in particular situations?

What are the needs we each know of now, today, in terms of how much companionship each of us might like or be able to offer—the balancing of availability/interaction and solitude/renewal?

These are just a few key questions to get you started. In a mutually supportive arrangement, perhaps, everyone involved would commit to speaking their truth in all situations in a clear, gentle, compassionate manner. To doing the personal work of recognizing the true need that is arising in any given moment and articulating it clearly and kindly. As humans pushed to our capacities during challenging times such as these we may sometimes fall short of our intentions. Yet, setting a foundation of openness and honesty can allow us to be more aware of what is unfolding and find our way back to the heart of the matter when we drift.

It will likely take many conversations, as day-to-day life progresses, to explore and communicate such needs and preferences. Initiating open conversation at the beginning of the process helps set the stage for the quality of communication and interaction that will follow.

For those who find they need third-party assistance to establish healthy communication, many medical clinics offer counseling services. Even if only one member of the relationship is willing to seek help, that act of reaching out can be an important step toward movement, should things feel stuck or sticky.

When cognitive function has been significantly impaired in the loved one, these matters obviously become more challenging. Even so, deep listening beyond the words or actions being expressed will help guide the helper in understanding what emotions may be at play, such as fear or anxiety or an echo of a past circumstance. Gentle, appropriate, loving touch remains one of the most powerful means of communicating to our loved one that they are not alone, that their experience is witnessed—and to help ground them in compassionate presence.

As we make our way through these journeys, we can find comfort and insight in the stories of others who have gone before. There are many fine books that can offer powerful personal experiences and wise counsel. Please review the annotated section titled *Caregiving and Cultivating Compassion* in the **Recommended Reading** chapter toward the back of this book.

Caregiver Self-Care Overview:
Taking Care of Thyself First of All

Caregiving is an intensely demanding calling. We are asked to assist and bear witness to another's experience of themselves during exquisitely difficult transformations. The questions faced are vast and the demand for physical, emotional and spiritual stamina is enormous.

How might the caregiver truly care for themselves in the process of giving ease to their beloved companion? Such self-care is crucial for the situation to unfold in the best possible manner. A caregiver who is not able to maintain their own health and wellness will be less than fully able to sustain the quality of mindfulness and endurance required.

The plant world is rich in energies that support our optimal experience of vitality and clarity. In addition, other practices may be of great benefit. As caregivers, we strive to give physical ease to our companions so that they may most skillfully work with the emotional and spiritual material that is arising into their awareness during this transition. And, of course, all caregivers who come with open hearts and minds will find similar material arising within themselves as well.

May these suggestions lead to respite during challenging times.

- **Use flower essences often**. They can help you work with the emotional material arising. See the following chapter for suggestions and details. Flower Essence Services [FES] offers two blends that are particularly relevant: *Compassionate Care Giver* and *Peace-Full*. See **Resources** section for information on FES.

- In tandem with nourishing food and adequate sleep, **support your adrenal glands** with daily herbal tonics as a first-line approach to dealing with stress and fatigue. Such herbs include: American and Asian ginsengs, eleuthero, codonopsis, he shou wu, stinging nettles, ashwagandha, holy basil. See the chapter *Adaptogenic and Tonic Plant Allies* for details and recipes. Also, please see entry on Chyawanprash in *Chemotherapy/Radiation Support*.

- Liberally enjoy **nerve tonics to allay stress**: Oatstraw, skullcap, chamomile, linden, rosemary, holy basil, and so on. Many of these herbs work well as simple teas. A blend of oatstraw, stinging nettles, and peppermint is a lovely, nourishing tea to soothe both 'frayed' nerve tissue and overworked adrenal glands. See the chapter on *Plants to Support the Nervous System* for more discussion of nervine herbs.

- **Sleep aids**: Homeopathic "Calms" or "Calms Forte" [Hylands brand]; teas, tinctures: skullcap, passionflower, valerian, hops, kava, ashwagandha, lavender, chamomile, etc. Once again, see *Plants to Support the Nervous System* and also the section on **Disturbed Sleep/Insomnia** in the *Helping Repertoire*.

- Favor **simple foods**, easy to digest: Millet, quinoa, miso soup, steamed veggies, green drinks. Avoid eating near sleep time. See *A Few Recipes for Gentle Foods*.

- **Distractions to provide rest**: Absorbing but light reading, soothing music, beautiful images. Making music, even if just banging rocks together or shaking gourds.

- **Find the humor**. Soften the belly, relax the shoulders—and allow yourself to laugh. Sometimes, it may take a vigorous walk, some stretching—or a growl or a wail or some other vocalization—to help open to this.

- **Movement**: Yoga, Qi gong, t'ai chi chuan, walking, deep breathing of fresh air. Walk barefoot if you can. Lay on the earth. These practices not only help you unwind, but they provide deep refreshment, renewal of vital force, and connection with that which supports your own sense of poise and groundedness.

- **Celebrate each challenge that you had the courage to meet**. Honor the obstacle encountered; honor yourself for opening to its teaching. This might become a daily ritual— as simple as a mental review at the end of the day, or a journal entry noting the highlights of your shift. Light a candle if you like, give thanks for guidance and support, see yourself growing and expanding to meet whatever appears on your path.

- **Read supportive, inspiring texts**: Stephen Levine, Sogyal Rinpoche, Elisabeth Kübler-Ross, etc. Explore: creating the space for someone to leave; essential *phowa* meditation [discussed in *Tibetan Book of Living and Dying*]; and so on. See the ***Recommended Reading*** chapter for many more suggestions.

- **Avoid environmental aromas**: Room fresheners, personal fragrances, shampoo or cream rinse aromas, laundry product scents, candles with artificial scents, etc.—or at least be highly conscious of them. Avoid *all* synthetic fragrances. Very ill individuals may find they are highly sensitized or intolerant of such permeating aromas and may feel sickened by them—even pure essential oils may prove intolerable.

- **Because of the caution mentioned above**, while essential oils are recommended in ***The Helping Repertoire*** where their considerable benefits must be noted, they are obviously not appropriate for all individuals or all situations. Numerous other options within each category of care may give ease without scenting the environment and causing a secondary challenge.

- **If smudging** to clear and harmonize energy surrounding a person or around the space, use a feather or salt or a bell or chime or rattle—instead of using potentially irritating smoke from burning plant material or incense.

- **Carry/wear a stone for grounding**, for alignment, for keeping the heart open in hell. Consider: rose quartz, garnet, ruby, carnelian, hematite, petrified wood, flourite, jade, bloodstone, aquamarine, smoky quartz, aventurine, peridot, or tourmaline. Rubellite in a lepidolite matrix is a lovely combination to lighten a space and keep it clear.

- **Write in a journal**. Make art. Let it out. What am I feeling? What is really going on for me? Be exquisitely honest. This is for you alone, bearing witness to yourself. Honor the process of being fully present in the now.

- **Chakra clearing/aura protection exercises**. Practice setting healthy boundaries in your encounters with others. See Donna Eden's *Energy Medicine* for exercises.

- **Get professional massage**; ask for touch. Massage your own feet and hands regularly. Use massage tools as appropriate to open your spine and refresh your feet. Stay well grounded in your own physicality.

- **Take long, relaxing soaks** in a setting where you won't be interrupted. Epsom salts added to the bath water help to relaxe tense muscles, aid deepened sleep, and help clear you from the day. Light candles. Make use of a sauna, if available.

- **Sleep in your own uncluttered space**: Make it as soothing, healing, comforting as possible. Candles, soft lighting, quiet music, lots of pillows, plants, fresh air. Allow yourself to feel embraced by unconditional love.

- **Find local resources**: Home health care nursing and household support, hospice volunteers—arrange for scheduled visits plus on-call counsel.

- Ask a friend(s) to help **create a circle of support**—errands, massage, hugs, time off, laundry, meal preparation (perhaps at another location so cooking smells won't bother), etc. See chapter on *Networking and Medical Fundraising*.

- **Ask for what you need** and apply discernment whether to accept what is offered. Support should be about true assistance for yourself and your loved one—not about accommodating others' emotional needs. If there are energetic "strings" attached to an offer of help, gracefully decline.

- **Do your own work diligently**: What is your relationship to Spirit, to life and death, to your own changing body, to your mind, to these feelings that arise? Cultivate mindfulness so that you are able to recognize your own emotional material and not project it onto your companions. See the *Recommended Reading* chapter for books to aid in your reflection.

- **Accept the experience as a meditation**. Do not attach to energies; observe them flowing through that which perceives and senses. Skillful teachers point our attention to the space or gap that exists before any emotion arises and blossoms. Within this gap lies undefined spaciousness—the potential to remain free of concept, interpretation, reference to the past, and the comforting taste of familiar emotions. The more we are able to breathe into the gap rather than allow our perceptions to be colored with habitual tendencies of mind, the more we are able to rest in peace and lightness within whatever circumstances arise.

Cultivated both within and without,

rhythm supports the healing process—

helping to restore order to a disordered system.

Flower Essences:
Emotional & Spiritual Support for All Involved

Flower essences are vibrational remedies that can support the integrated health of body, mind and spirit. They possess no aromas (unlike essential oils). They are made during meditation with the plant at its peak of bloom in its natural habitat. The healing essence of the flower is imparted into the vehicle of water, which is a proven medium for retaining such vibrational imprints.[‡] These "mother" essences, as they are known, are then carefully preserved with the addition of brandy and later further diluted for use.

The vibrations of each flower are transmitted into the energetic fields of those working with them, helping the individual(s) to entrain with the plant's healing energy. The flower essences do not suppress the emotional material, such as grief or despair, but rather assist in allowing the deeper nature of the emotion to be felt and recognized so that it may be gently allowed and utilized in the process of transformation. The following are essences I have found particularly beneficial in my work; there are many others to discover.

Applications: Flower essences can be added as desired to drinking water, dropped directly onto the tongue, added to bath water, used to anoint head/heart/forehead/wrists, added into a healing cream, diffused into a room by placing in a glass bowl filled with pure water into which a quartz crystal has been placed. Follow your intuition as to appropriate use. Two to four drops are usually considered a dose. If circumstances allow, speaking aloud or calling to mind the gift of each plant when working with these seems to amplify the benefits.

Grief—

- **Borage**: Optimism and courage; uplifting the heart to face the challenges presented.

- **Wild rose**: Indicated for resignation or lack of hope, which can deplete one's vitality; especially useful for long-term illness, protracted convalescence, and so on.

- **Dandelion**: When grief and intensity express as physical tension, held in the muscles. Helps encourage the physical body to remain soft and relaxed.

- **Bleeding heart**: For releasing attachment to this lifetime, to the beloved, to the relationship; indicated when there is over-connection with "other" and anguish associated with a sense of separation. Supports healthy, unconditional loving founded on a well-nourished sense of self.

- **Fuschia**: Supports the ability to express powerful emotions; encourages genuine emotional vitality, presence and authenticity.

- **Yerba Santa**: Releasing constricted feelings in the chest, especially grief and sadness. Helps deepen the breath, thus opening and lightening the heart.

Anger—

- **Scarlet monkeyflower**: Supports emotional honesty, directness. Sheds light on shadow material—the fear of anger and other intense "dense" emotions—so that these can be acknowledged and accepted within the wholeness of being.

- **Willow**: For those who feel victimized by life circumstances, bitter and resentful—and who become contracted and inflexible in response, emotionally and/or physically.

Suffering, pain—

- **Love-Lies-Bleeding**: Supports moving beyond an experience of isolated personal pain or anguish to a more witnessing, compassionate, universal awareness of suffering as inherent in human experience.

- **Penstemon**: Helping to move beyond feelings of life's unfairness or being persecuted to a space of courage, resilience, perseverance, and trust in an overlighting power and expanded meaning of the journey.

- **Pink Monkeyflower**: Allowing feelings to flow through the heartmind more fluidly.

Obsessive thinking—

- **White chestnut bud**: Extreme mental agitation, repetitive thoughts, obsessive anxiety; experiencing the mental landscape as message loops that replay endlessly.

Acceptance—

- **Black-eyed Susan**: Fear of powerful, perhaps dense emotions coming to surface.

- **Sage**: Helps calm the heart and spirit, clarify the mind, and access inner wisdom. Encourages peaceful acceptance and perception of higher meaning in life events.

Making peace—

- **Holly**: To resolve feelings of isolation or anger; opens the way to an experience of divine love and inclusive compassion and mercy that, first of all, embraces oneself.

- **Sweet chestnut**: An ally when things seem bleakest. Supports expanded sense of courage when anguish is encountered in meeting personal "edge." This courage arises from surrendering, opening to the transformational power of allowing what is to be.

- *See also* ***Surrender***.

Patience—

- **Impatiens**: Helps one to quiet the mind, still the attention, appreciate and open to the delicate preciousness of each unfolding moment.

Surrender—

- **Angel's trumpet**: Supports a conscious surrender to the mystery of death, whether for the person crossing the threshold or for those who bear witness. Indicated for releasing fear, attachment, and opening the heart to the spiritual guidance and divine embrace available in such moments. Lovely used for an anointing ritual at bedtime.

- **Sagebrush**: Opening into freedom, spaciousness, awareness; help in discerning the essential Self within and beyond that which is associated with the outer persona.

Courage—

- **Aspen**: Courageously facing the unknown; confronting fears with confidence in the abiding presence of spirit and trust in whatever arises as a perfect aspect of the whole.

- **Borage**: Optimism and courage; uplifting the heart to face challenges.

- **Fawn lily**: Strength and fortitude to openly give oneself and one's gifts to the world, to others, despite a reflexive desire to retreat.

- **Poison oak**: Fear of intimate contact, anxiety around emotional vulnerability. Helps transform sense of protective armoring into open-heartedness.

Disturbed dreams / Night fears—

- **St. Johnswort**: Provides sense of protection and groundedness when one feels psychically and physically vulnerable or over-expanded. Offers a sense of shielding and illumination in transition states.

- **Mugwort**: Assists in navigating the dream realms to diminish any sense of overwhelm. Enhances perception and insight. Helps in harmonizing the relationship between waking and dreamtime consciousness.

- **Chaparral**: Helps cleanse the psyche of its stores of chaotic, disturbing, or violent images and impressions from previous exposure to media or actual life events.

Trauma—

- **Five-Flower Formula / Rescue Remedy**: A classic, broadly applicable emergency remedy. Helps stabilize, organize and integrate body, mind, spirit during times of extreme stress and disorientation, pain or other trauma, chaos or confusion.

- **Star of Bethlehem**: Indicated when shock or trauma from the present or the past has numbed awareness and deadened connection with one's experience of Spirit in the Now. One of the components of the Five-Flower Formula/Rescue Remedy.

Healthy boundaries / Sensitivity—

- **Golden yarrow**: To address tension in solar plexus, oversensitivity around others.

- **Pink yarrow**: Promotes appropriate emotional boundaries for those who tend to be overly absorbent of the emotions of others. Supports sustainable compassion toward others, grounded in a loving awareness of one's own emotional presence.

- **Yarrow Special Formula**: Protective remedy for the subtle body; indicated during exposure to invasive electromagnetic fields such as X-rays, magnetic resonance imaging, radiation therapy, medical equipment, microwave radiation, and so on.

- **Yellow star tulip**: To develop empathic, compassionate recognition and understanding of the needs of others.

- **Mountain pennyroyal**: Strength and clarity of mind; cleanses negative thoughts.

Protection—

- **Angelica**: Moving through unknown terrain by aligning with the supportive presence and guidance offered by the spiritual realms. Lovely before sleep or meditation.

- **Angel's Trumpet**: Surrendering to the protection of spiritual guardians in the face of profound transformation. Releasing resistance and fear, and opening in trust.

Despair—

- **Chrysanthemum**: For those who overly identify with the physical body and the personality, fearing illness and death as disruption or annihilation of the self. Helps to shift awareness to the impermanence and transitory nature of the material realm and the immanence of our essential spirit.

- **Olive**: Indicated for those who have reached a state of utter exhaustion, weariness, physical or emotional collapse. Opens the consciousness to the perfusion of spirit in matter—offering a renewed experience of life force, rejuvenating bodymind.

Synthesis—

- **1,000-petal lotus**: Supports meditative insight and synthesis; helps integrate spiritual awareness throughout the energy centers in a balanced, dynamic way.

Overall Helper—

- **Self-Heal**: To help recover from illness or any trauma. To invigorate the awareness, inner resources and confidence that may lead to the deepest possible healing.

To further explore these and other essences, please see the *Flower Essence Repertory: A Comprehensive Guide to North American and English Flower Essences for Emotional and Spiritual Well-Being* by Patricia Kaminsky and Richard Katz [Nevada City, CA: The Flower Essence Society, Earth-Spirit Inc, 1994]. Please see more information about FES and their offerings in *Resources/The Suppliers* section toward the back of this book.

[‡] See *Sensitive Chaos: The Creation of Flowing Forms in Water and Air* by Theodor Schwenk [East Sussex, England: Rudolf Steiner Press, 1996 edition]

The Helping Repertoire

My heartfelt intent is for this book to assist in giving ease—during disease process or recovery—for both the caregiver and the one receiving care. One may also be one's own caregiver, and I particularly honor those who must go it alone. For all, may this section be much like the phone call to a trusted helpmate in the middle of the night, offering a calm, loving voice and some suggestions for addressing experiences that tend to arise.

Having said that, several points must be made absolutely clear before you begin—

- It is very important to **know when to report bodymind sensations, experiences and conditions** that arise to your medical care team. These discomforts and changes may simply be side effects that are expected or predictable with particular treatments or medications—or they might be signs that something is deeply amiss and intervention needs to happen quickly. It is essential to **ask your professional care team what to look out for, what needs to be reported, and to whom such experiences should be reported.** Keep this information in a readily visible location—and make sure all household members and helpers are aware.

- As a culture, we are still learning about the consequences of **use of herbs and concentrated nutritional supplements taken concurrently with specific medications, chemotherapy agents, radiation, and other powerful treatments**. Though herbs have been used to promote healing for thousands of years around the world, this mixing of modalities is still relatively new territory. It is exciting ground that holds much promise for extraordinary complementary care. Yet, there can also be undesirable or unpredictable consequences.

  Please do not fear the plants, which are ultimately the source of all food and medicine, but do practice informed discernment. In some cases, taking herbs or nutrients in tandem with a particular allopathic therapy may be seen to actually increase that therapy's healing benefit. However, the dynamic at play is to be examined on a case-by-case basis. **Please consult with your physician, pharmacist, or other knowledgeable healthcare practitioner as to potential contraindications or clinical benefit in your particular circumstance**. The extensive and highly detailed reference *Herb, Nutrient, and Drug Interactions: Clinical Implications and Therapeutic Strategies* by Stargrove, *et al* [2008] is also an excellent resource for all in seeking to understand the potential benefits as well as potential risks of combining particular medications/treatments with herbs or nutritional supplements.

- While the recommendations that follow in this repertory are based on several decades of professional—and personal—practice and study, as well as both ancient tradition and modern insights, **the responsibility resides in the reader for actual application of a given suggestion in their particular circumstance**. I have attempted to provide enough information and a varied selection of suggested strategies to guide the caregiver toward some relevant remediation that might offer relief in a given moment. What works for one might not work for another—and what works in one moment may not work the next moment. Only the reader and their health support team know their particular situation and backstory—and undertake the ultimate responsibility for their use of this information. In particular, "typical dose" recommendations in the holistic health arena are generally geared for an adult weighing 150 pounds—elders, children, and those with heightened sensitivity to substances may require significantly reduced dosing. Please refer to the extensive, annotated **Recommended Reading** chapter—particularly the section on *Natural Therapeutics and Wellness Support*—for more detailed information that may help guide your choices.

Please note: All medicinal herbs and foodstuffs recommended in the following sections should ideally be organically cultivated or ethically gathered from clean, wild places; oils, extracts and other preparations should be produced without the use of toxic solvents. All suppliers are not equally mindful about these considerations. Be sure to verify sources as best as you are able. Numerous reputable growers, suppliers, medicine makers, and manufacturers are listed in the **Resources** section at the end of this book.

Consistency / Ritual / Rhythm

Rhythm supports the healing process. Life on planet Earth is expressed through rhythm, cycles, pulses, and tides. The procession of the planets around the sun, the turning of the seasons, the cycle of night and day, the rhythms of the seas, the hormonal ebbs and flows, the pulse of our hypothalamus, the harmonies of endocrine function, the drumming of our heart. It can be asserted that all disharmony that occurs within the bodymind is somehow related to disruption of an overlighting health-coordinating rhythm and order.

That being said, from a holistic point of view we can address disharmony and dis-ease and unwellness by doing what we can to re-establish rhythm and order and harmony. We can work with plant medicine to restore and maintain homeostasis, as with the adaptogenic and tonic plants discussed later in this book. But perhaps the very first place to begin is to re-align with rhythms and cycles by the way we craft routines day-to-day. This is especially pertinent for someone whose usual life and patterns have been disrupted by illness. Creating new daily rituals and routines is a way to bring grounding and a sense of predictability to an unsettling and uncertain period.

The suggestions that follow directly—as well as those in the sections beyond—may be of benefit in bringing rhythm to the fulfillment of daily needs.

- First and foremost, creating structure to the day—to whatever degree is possible—benefits *both* caregiver and the one receiving care. **For the caregiver**, especially, this will help them to maintain their efforts in a more grounded and sustainable way. In particular, knowing when relief persons will be present is a huge advantage in being able to pace one's energy.

- **Alternate activities with rest** periods throughout the day, as the flow of each day will allow.

- **Create predictability around mealtime patterns**, especially if person needs grounding or some sense of control.
    - ◆ If bedridden, attend to toilet requirements and hygiene first.
    - ◆ Limit food selection. Keep it simple, with clear expectations and communication.
    - ◆ Provide adequate warmth and physical support while eating.
    - ◆ Familiar/favorite cups, bowls, glasses can add pleasure and comfort to each meal.

- **Systematize and organize mouth/teeth hygiene**: Assemble tray with glass of water, spit bowl, small towel, brush, toothpaste or powder, tongue scraper, mouthwash.

- **Wash your own hands thoroughly and frequently** to help limit the spread of germs—not only for your own benefit but also for the benefit of the person you are tending and other household members.

- Routinely provide a **healing herb-based lip salve** or straight vitamin E oil.

- **Allow bathing to help frame the day**. For instance, if aroma is tolerated, give a stimulating rosemary sponge, foot, or full bath in the morning and a relaxing lavender version in the evening. Prepare a strong tea or infusion with the herbs or utilize their concentrated essential oils. To disperse oils in water, mix a few drops first with a bit of liquid soap. Sage tea also makes a lovely antiseptic liquid for bathing.

- **Smooth wrinkles from sheets while person is up**, or during transition moments.

- **Announce what you're about to do** if moving into their personal space, rearranging person on the bed, straightening sheets, and so on.

- Arrange for and **protect private time for your loved one** during day—after mid-day meal, etc. Visits and good intentions of others can be wearying.

- **Nurture deep sleep**, for both tender and tended:
    - ◆ **Refresh the atmosphere of the sleeping area** while performing pre-bedtime rituals such as bathing and dental hygiene. Open a window and clear stale air. Some will want to close the window during sleep; others may prefer it opened, even just a crack.

    - ◆ Clear the mind of the day's cares. Conduct a **thankfulness review** before sleep.

    - ◆ **Refreshing bathing** of some sort to relax body and mind.

    - ◆ **Herbal tea to support relaxation and sleep**. Sedative herbs include passionflower, hops, valerian, linden, chamomile, skullcap—alone or in various combinations. See *Plants to Support the Nervous System* for more information.

    - ◆ Create **bedtime protection/prayer ritual** especially if fear of nightmares or repetitive anxious thoughts or anticipation of pain tend to prevent restful sleep.

◆ Provide **calming soft music or ambient sounds**. Alternately, soft earplugs may help create a sense of secure calm surroundings. See *Recommended Listening*.

◆ **Darken the sleeping space** by drawing shades or curtains. Alternately, soft dark eyeshades may block out ambient light sufficiently.

◆ **Avoid exposure to artificial light** in the evening as much as possible to promote normal biological [circadian] rhythms. This means dimming or eliminating ambient light, avoiding computer and television screens, etc. Nightlights may even be disturbing to some. Darkness promotes natural secretion of rhythm-regulating hormones which, in turn, promote restorative sleep.

Energy Awareness

This awareness—and its mindful practice—is the foundation of any and all other helping interventions. Of itself, it is a profoundly healing act—the awareness that the quality of our presence impacts the space around us and those we encounter, whether they be awake or asleep, conscious or unconscious. Our mood, our voice, our tone, our attitudes, our language, the fluidity or roughness of our bodily movements are tangible. We leave a trail of vibrational echoes in our wake, day in and day out. What quality of vibration shall this be?

• Unwellness or dying can radically heighten sensitivity—to taste, smell, touch, sound, vibration. **Heighten your own capacity to be sensitive** and create a clear, sacred space in which your companion may be at peace.

• **Ground and clear yourself** before entering loved one's space. Pause, breathe, feel your feet on the floor and your body supported by the earth. Imagine a waterfall flowing over you, cleansing and refreshing. Slow down your movements. Focus your attention. Bring an undistracted mind.

• **Ventilate** and bring fresh air into the space as appropriate.

• The person dealing with unwellness may want to limit exposure to certain people, conversation, language, media, music that seem particularly agitating or distressing. Allow them to be the master of their domain in this regard, without judgment or resistance. This may be one of the only arenas in which they may feel any semblance of "control." See the appendix entry *Reflections on Environmental Influences* for more on this topic.

Arranging the Healing Space

Mindfulness in arranging the healing space can make a significant difference on multiple levels to all concerned. Each potential space will present its own assortment of benefits and challenges, but attempt to take into consideration as many of the following factors as possible. Co-create the space with the involvement of your loved one in a way that quietly confirms the message of love and respect your attentive presence brings. Constructed with such focused intention, the space itself will echo with compassion and sanctity.

- **Locate the bed in a private place** in the home, if possible—convenient for caregiving and hygiene yet affording a sense of retreat. Utilize portable screens if necessary to make the space feel safe and intimate.

- **Situate bed away from walls** on three sides to provide ease of access for caregivers.

- **Can the bed face a window**? Can green living things be in view? Is light better coming in from the side?

- **Cleanse the room physically and energetically** before proceeding with intentional placement and arrangement. Use only plant-based cleaning products that are unscented or scented only lightly with beneficial essential oils. Use burning herbs or, preferably, soundwaves to remove stale energy and bring refreshment—a bell, a rattle, a drum, a wind instrument, chanting or toning; even rhythmic clapping will do.

- **Clear the space of clutter** and relocate any objects that do not—in this fresh moment—offer visual or sentimental pleasure, or otherwise provide convenience, ease or support.

- **Carefully select pictures for display** on walls according to what brings comfort, pleasure, or inspiration. Rotate a small selection of images as desired.

- Provide **shades or curtains on windows** to moderate light. This improves quality of daytime sleep and offers more privacy, intimacy and feeling of protection at night.

- Bedside table(s) for **convenient access to often-used items**: Lamp, lip balm, lozenges, lidded water vessel, notebook and pen, tissues, telephone, music, book, bell.

- **Walker/stool/appropriately sized chair** to help with various bedside and bathroom positions and safety, as necessary.

- **Remedy bothersome aromas, repetitive noises** (ticking clock, squeaky hinges, etc.).

- Maintain a **warm, comfortable ambient temperature** in which the body can relax.

- If loved one is bedridden, **loosen blankets** at foot of bed to give toes room to roam.

Therapeutic Touch

Therapeutic touch in general describes a whole range of hands-on approaches, any of which can give great ease. Compassionate touch has been shown to offer amazing benefit—it calms, soothes, grounds, reassures, re-connects, rejuvenates. It may be as little as holding a hand, palming the shoulders, slowly rubbing the scalp or forehead, gently massaging the feet, stroking the back—or as much as a tender full body massage.

Therapeutic Touch also describes a particular approach to energy work, usually one-on-one. After sharing meditative silence and asking silently to be a suitable vehicle for whatever healing is needed, the practitioner assesses the recipient's energy field to note patterns of disturbance, overactivity, underactivity, and so on. Assessment is done without judging these patterns as good or bad. This is followed by a treatment in which the practitioner gently passes their hands over and through the receiver's field—just above the body—carefully working so as to smooth and harmonize the overall energy. It is done slowly, with full attention and deliberateness.

Therapeutic Touch is a learned technique although variations of compassionate touch and energy work have been practiced intuitively through the ages. What is required to practice such work in a good way is humility, compassion, patience, inner quiet, listening with all of one's being, tenderness, and non-attachment to outcome.

- **Especially beneficial before sleep** time to settle and clear from the day.

- **Set a healing tone**: lower the lights, light some candles, adjust ambient temperature…

- A session can be accompanied with **soothing music** to amplify the effect. See the chapter on ***Recommended Listening*** for suggestions.

- As adjunct, **keep soothing inspirational reading material at hand**, something the person really resonates with—use this to help calm fears, release nightmares, etc.

Foot Massage / Hand Massage

The feet and hands provide communication with all areas of the body through reflex action—touching or stroking them can profoundly influence physical or emotional sensations. In addition, massaging these extremities can feel less potentially invasive than touch on other areas of the body. It is such a simple yet powerful act to hold a hand or place a palm under a loved one's foot to offer a sense of ground and support. It is a safe and wonderful way to make contact. Of course, always first ask permission or communicate your intentions before extending touch of any kind.

- First and foremost: **Caregivers, remember that you can gently massage your *own* hands and feet** as often as you can find the time. Doing so while sitting vigil or keeping a loved one company may prove ideal moments. Compassionate self-massage of hands or feet can be a lovely act of tending to oneself.

- Caregiver: Keep **fingernails** short and clean.

- Be gentle! **Do not overly stimulate** tender points. Provide long, slow, flat strokes or simply hold hands or feet.

- **Stabilizing**—Can relieve nausea and unsettled feelings.

- **Grounding, comforting**—Especially to one bound to bed.

- **Calming**—Can lull recipient into peaceful sleep.

- Daily massage, by self or another, **can improve circulation** and ease drug- or disease-induced numbness of hands or feet. Other suggestions for **Neuropathy** follow in a section of its own.

Body Massage

If loved one is receptive, obtain the regular services of a licensed massage therapist—or follow your own leadings as willing caregiver. As mentioned above, be certain to honor the boundaries and preferences of the one who will receive the treatment. Seek professional advice if uncertain about the appropriateness of massage for the particular health circumstances the recipient is dealing with.

- First and foremost: **Caregivers should arrange for regular massage or energy work for themselves**. Find a therapist who is willing to make home visits, if needed, or arrange for caregiving backup from your support network so that you can visit a massage clinic. Self-care is the key to healthful caregiving that can sustain the tests of time. You can only give of yourself in a balanced, centered way when you yourself attend to renewal and restoration.

- As caregiver, **focus on calming and grounding yourself** before tending to another. See previous section on **Energy Awareness**. Always bring a relaxed, centered presence to any extended session of touch.

- **Offer casual, superficial touch**, at the very least, in daily comings and goings—hand placed on upper back, shoulders, arm, etc. Loving touch is healing medicine, appropriately applied.

- With permission, very gently **holding or massaging the forehead and scalp** can feel wonderfully intimate and soothing.

- **Allow touch to be grounding, calming**—use long, slow strokes or little movement at all. No poking or prodding unless requested.

- Massage **helps with skin tone and itching** (apply salve or lotion if acceptable). See section on **Pruritis/Itching** for specific suggestions.

- **Healing plant oils**: Calendula oil/salve or jojoba oil is very healing to the skin.

- **Helps to increase circulation** and prevent bedsores—when person senses a hot spot or a red spot appears, massage it often (every couple of hours, if possible). See following section.

Bedsores [Pressure Sores] / Skin Ulcerations

Pressure sores are also known as bedsores or decubitus ulcers. They result from intense pressure on skin over a short period of time or minimal pressure exerted over an extended period. Spending long periods in bed is an obvious risk factor—especially when resting in a single position or with skin pressed against wrinkles or folds in the bedding. These sores can also occur from long sitting.

Additionally, the pressure of medical tubing against skin of the mouth or elsewhere can also cause them to develop. One must do everything possible to prevent or delay such skin damage. Development of these sores is a factor in increased mortality among movement-challenged populations, as breakdown of the skin can lead to infection and underlying tissue destruction.

In addition to pressure, other factors contribute to skin breakdown. Friction or shearing can occur when the skin rubs against another surface or two layers of skin slide against each other—as when a person slides up/down in bed or is pulled up without the use of a dedicated sheet on the bed or slides up or down in a chair. Excessive moisture—as from excessive perspiration, urinary or fecal incontinence, or oozing wounds—softens the skin and impairs its integrity.

Other risk factors include poor nutritional status, low body weight, anemia, infections, edema, blood sugar disorders, peripheral vascular conditions, smoking, steroid use, and more.

*See the section above, **Body Massage**, for other physical touch considerations. Consult with home nursing professionals for additional prevention and treatment strategies.*

- **Especially sensitive spots** are those points where bone is just below the skin—outer ear, back of head, along the spine, shoulders, ribs, elbows, buttocks, hips, knees, heels, ankles.

- **Reddened areas** may be detected at these sensitive spots. If the reddened area blanches when touched and then rebounds to redness, it is a sign that this area must be tended to. This stage is generally reversible. Even a shallow skin ulcer may be reversible, though the breakdown process needs to be seriously addressed.

- **Movement is prophylactic**—walking; rotating positions on bed at regular intervals; subtle, small shifts when sitting, if possible; caregiver gently turning ankles and wrists, bending and stretching limbs, etc.

- **Provide fresh sheets often**, and make sure they are fully dry and well-smoothed on mattress. Use scent-free, allergen-free natural ingredient-based laundry products.

- **Avoid eating in bed** if at all possible. Errant food particles can become irritants.

- Support **meticulous skin care**: Keep skin dry and clean. Use very little soap while bathing (glycerine-based may be best). Dry skin thoroughly yet gently (hair dryer can be used). Massage healing salve into potential hot spots, especially elbows, heels, and buttocks. Dust arrowroot powder into moist skin folds to dry and lubricate. Manage incontinence effectively—develop a plan with home healthcare professional.

- As required, use **sheepskin fleece** as bed pad or place locally under feet, heels, buttocks, etc. (direct skin-to-fleece contact). If necessary, moleskin patches can be used to prevent sores; trained home healthcare providers can advise.

- Intake of **astragalus root**, a premier immune-enhancing herb that has been used for thousands of years in Chinese herbal medicine, has been shown to lessen incidence of bedsores. One of its classic therapeutic actions is to promote the discharge of pus and generate flesh. Preferably, astragalus [*Astragalus membranaceus*] can be taken as powder in smoothies or capsules, or chopped roots may be simmered and used as beverage or soup stock. It is also available in tincture form and as a 5:1 extract powder. See section on *Adaptogenic and Tonic Plant Allies* for more details.

- **Essential oils**: Add a few drops of either myrrh or helichrysum essential oil to a base oil or lotion for massage of tender spots—to promote healing and prevent infection.

- **Oozing wounds**: **Myrrh gum powder** or myrrh in combination with **goldenseal, Oregon grape,** and/or *Echinacea* **spp.** root powders can be dusted onto oozy wounds. Antimicrobial, astringent, anti-inflammatory, wound healing. **Slippery elm** powder can also be added for additional soothing and vulnerary support.

- **Propolis** salve or powdered resin applied as needed. Propolis, the name given to tree resins collected by honeybees and incorporated into their hives, is antiseptic and has an anesthetizing and anti-inflammatory effect on tissue. *Please note*: Use cautiously if prone to allergy or hypersensitivity to bee stings, bee products, or tree resins.

- **Turmeric**: as salve or as powder mixed with raw honey—or applied directly, dusted onto oozy wounds. [Can also be added to other powders noted above.] Prepared from the rhizome of *Curcuma longa*. Anti-inflammatory, antimicrobial, wound healing. *Please note*: A natural dye, the pigments in turmeric can stain skin, clothing, bed linens. Take care to use with appropriate dressing or with dark clothing.

- **Horsetail** [*Equistum arvense*]: Salty/bitter/sweet, cool. The green vegetative shoot of this ancient plant is a mineralizing tonic, rich in silica—rebuilder to connective tissue throughout the body, including that within the skin. Antioxidant, anti-inflammatory. Diuretic, astringent, wound healing. Can be both used as a beverage or as topical wash or compress to strengthen the skin and promote healing. **Formats**: Decoction or commercial products made from water extracts. To decoct, simmer ¼-½ cup horsetail in 1 quart water for 20 minutes.

- **Nutrient support**: Maintaining blood sugar balance throughout the day, sufficient folic acid and B vitamins, vitamin C, bioflavonoids, etc. Coenzyme Q_{10} [now preferred as the more absorbable Ubiquinol] has been shown to support cellular energy and tissue health.

- See these sections for additional support in promoting more robust nutrition and immunity: **Simple Nutrition, Building the Blood, Lack of Appetite/Weight Loss, Nausea, Mouth Sores, Loss of Taste/Smell** as well as the chapters *Recipes for Gentle Foods, Natural Strategies for Tube Feeding*, etc.

- ***Baptisia tinctoria*** [Wild Indigo]. Strong alterative, antimicrobial, lymphagogue, bitter, choleretic, cholagogue. Laxative and cathartic. Indicated in septic conditions accompanied by ulceration and tissue degeneration with enfeebled circulation; fetid discharges; low, sluggish fevers, typhoid; fullness of tissue, with dusky, leaden, purplish or livid discoloration [especially face]; malodorous stools resembling prune juice. It has been used for gangrene, ulceration of nipples, mammary glands, cervix. According to Harvey Wickes Felter MD, Eclectic physician of the 19th century, "Baptisia is not, as a rule, a remedy in acute diseases showing great activity, but rather for disorders showing marked capillary enfeeblement and tendency to ulceration—in fact, a condition of atony. It is contraindicated …in capillary stasis." **Can be used at home as homeopathic remedy**. *Cautions*: Large doses of the material medicine, such as in tinctures, can be toxic—resulting in nausea, vomiting, diarrhea, tachycardia, respiratory paralysis. Use material preparations of Baptisia *only* under the guidance of a qualified health care practitioner. Avoid during pregnancy.

Melancholy / Anxiety

*Whole books have thankfully been written to explore the physical and spiritual considerations in addressing these mind states that are sure to arise in all who are human, let alone those facing challenging illness. The **Recommended Reading** chapter of this book describes a number of those that may be especially helpful. Meditation, music and movement can all be supportive and are highlighted below. Meanwhile, the plant kingdom provides profound assistance in calming the mental process and stabilizing the bodymind.*

*A calm mind, relaxed body and bright spirit benefits immunity and the functioning of all systems—and liberates the life force toward healing. It is impossible to say enough about the myriad blessings the greenworld provides in this regard. Below is an outline guide to some of the resources that are available in lieu of turning to pharmaceutical relief as one's first or only recourse. Please know that there is a wealth of depth and nuance to be explored within this category, for all concerned. Please see the appendix **On Depression: Finding Our Way Home** for additional considerations.*

- **Flower essences** to address emotional and spiritual dimensions: Taken internally, used as a spray, added to bath, or used for anointing. See the earlier chapter on *Flower Essences* for a selection of common issues.

- **Soothing, uplifting essential oils**, if scent is tolerated. What soothes may be very personal. Some common favorites: lavender, chamomile, bergamot, *Melissa*, rose, rosemary, rosewood, sandalwood [from sustainable sources only], spruce, tangerine. Can be inhaled directly, diffused into a space, applied to body [diluted in lotion or body oil], added to laundry, added to baths [a few drops mixed with bit of liquid soap to diffuse it through the bathwater], and so on. Choose pure essential oils, *never* synthetic fragrances. Essential oils distilled from organically or biodynamically grown plants are superior to ones produced from plants grown with chemicals.

- **Customized herbal formula** designed by a well-trained herbalist, naturopath, or Ayurvedic or Traditional Chinese Medicine practitioner. Homeopathy and homeopathic remedies offer another realm to explore.

- See chapters on ***Plants to Support the Nervous System*** and ***Adaptogenic and Tonic Plant Allies*** for guidance to self-assess relevant herbal support. Adaptogens and nervines go well hand-in-hand, together supporting a more poised, relaxed response to stress at both the endocrine and nerve tissue levels. Suggested combinations and uses in food are included in these sections.

- **Honokiol**: An isolated extract from the bark of several species of the **magnolia** tree [*Magnolia* spp.] available in capsule form. Calming, relaxing, strongly antioxidant, seen to support cellular health through multiple mechanisms. As of this writing, honokiol has been found to have antiangiogenic, anti-inflammatory, and antitumor properties against multiple malignancies in preclinical models.[1,2]

- **Lemon balm** [*Melissa officinalis*] infusion sweetened with honey is a classic brew, gentle enough for anyone over two years old [tea *without* honey is also delicious and suitable for all ages]. Relaxing, uplifting nervine, carminative, antiviral. Lemon balm extract—tincture, glycerite or capsules—can be especially helpful if stress chronically tends to manifest as outbreaks of *herpes* lesions. See chapter ***Plants to Support the Nervous System*** for more details.

- **Holy Basil** [*Ocimum sanctum*]: Anti-anxiety, adrenal tonic/adaptogen, anti-inflammatory, radioprotective, and much more. Shown to normalize cortisol secretion in the presence of stress. Taken as tea or extract. See chapters on ***Adaptogenic and Tonic Plant Allies*** and ***Plants to Support the Nervous System***.

- **L-Theanine**: Amino acid present in green tea [*Camellia sinensis*] that is calming to the mind and nervous system. Shown to reduce anxiety, stabilize mood, improve concentration, and enhance sleep. Taken as extract in capsules or tablets.

- **Medical *Cannabis***: Calming, pain relieving, sedative, anti-nausea, promotes mood elevation, more. *Cannabis sativa* and *C. indica* are legally available for approved medical use in some jurisdictions. Whole books have been written on the history and use of *Cannabis* as a medicinal herb. In particular, recent results of studies using non-psychoactive CBD-rich strains [cannabidiol] are opening up exciting additional possibilities for therapeutic use, including direct antitumoral effects and as anticancer adjunct to conventional chemical therapies. Consult with your healthcare provider if you think medical *Cannabis* is indicated for your situation.

- **Humorous or inspirational books, stories, films, cards and images**. Recorded books can be downloaded from many library systems.

- **Guided meditation**: Professional recordings or can be simply read or recorded by caregiver. See *Recommended Listening* and *Recommended Reading* for suggestions.

- **Yantra or mandala meditation**: An ancient practice of meditatively gazing on a pattern based on sacred geometric principles. Yantras visually represent divine or universal energies. The Sri [Shri] Yantra is considered the mother of all yantras. Yantra gazing can be a way to enter into meditation. Calms, settles and centers; helps concentrate one's inner focus. Many religions have some version of this practice.

- **Soothing music.** Playing or listening to **Tibetan singing bowls** or **crystal bowls** is deeply harmonizing to body, mind and spirit. These are remarkable instruments of healing. Ideal to choose one or more that resonate with the individual who will be using it, although there are some high-quality recordings that create a healing sonic space. Additionally, there are numerous **musical offerings recorded by trained sound healers**. See *Recommended Listening* for suggestions.

- **Soothing water/sweat therapies**, always as personally appropriate. Warm full-body baths, saunas, foot or hand baths all relax the body and thus help calm the mind. Adding epsom salts [magnesium sulfate] to the bath increases muscular relaxation [use with care with cardiovascular issues; consult with physician as to situational appropriateness]. Relaxing essential oils can also be used with these water therapies [e.g. lavender, rose, chamomile, basil, cardamom, bergamot, neroli, jasmine, patchouli, sustainably sourced sandalwood…]

- **Regular whole body massage, foot massage, or energy work.** Can promote profound sense of lightening and release, while enhancing a sense of groundedness and embodiment. See **Therapeutic Touch**, **Foot/Hand Massage**, **Body Massage**.

- **Moving and opening the body.** Again, gentle practices such as yoga, t'ai chi chuan, qi gong, and stretching help unclench bodymind holdings and help shift emotional states—as well as more vigorous activities [as appropriate] such as dance, shaking of arms and legs, hand drumming. See *Resources* chapter for home support.

Disturbed Sleep / Insomnia

Sleep can be disturbed for any number of reasons: Anxiety, worry, depression, pain, need to empty bladder, need for fluids, hormonal and blood sugar dynamics, digestive issues, caffeine or alcohol consumption, liver or gall bladder issues, cardiovascular issues, disease process, side effect of treatments and pharmaceuticals, noise or light, warm bedroom, stale air, and so on. It's best to address possible environmental and dietary considerations first, then go from there.

Adequate sleep can obviously be difficult for both caregiver and the one dealing with illness; caregivers should commit to do all they can to promote restful sleep for themselves. The period of sleep is a crucial cycle within the body's natural biorhythms for detoxification, renewal, repair, reset.

- Insomnia or disturbed sleep can also arise from a sort of **hyper-vigilance related to trauma** one has experienced through surgery, difficult and prolonged treatments, accidental injury, loss of function, or intense disease process. It may be as if the bodymind remains alert to ward off such trauma from occurring again. This hyper-vigilance may be conscious or unconscious, vivid or subtle. Many of the following suggestions may prove helpful, but working directly with this cellular memory and attendant anxiety—emotional, physical, spiritual—seems essential. While personal awareness and meditative practices may create the space for healing this echoing wound, assistance from others is often deeply beneficial to further resolution. The caregiver may be the one to help the person suffering from this sort of insomnia to connect the dots. Bodymind services such as counseling, healing ceremony, skillful energy work, types of somatic release massage therapy may each offer support.

- **Sleep in a relatively cool, darkened, quiet space** if at all possible. Employ light-blocking window covering, eyeshades, earplugs as needed.

- **Refresh the atmosphere of the sleeping area** while performing pre-bedtime rituals such as bathing and dental hygiene. Open a window and clear stale air. Some will want to close the window during sleep; others may prefer it opened, even just a crack.

- Review section on **Consistency/Ritual/Rhythm**. Wake, eat and retire to bed with as much consistency as possible from day to day. Movement, rest, hygiene and visitation periods can also be planned in a rhythmic way. Entrain the body with the day/night, light/darkness cycle and the inner circadian biorhythms. Provide predictable and sufficient nutrition and water throughout the day.

- **Move the body during the day** to whatever degree is appropriate for one's health condition. Stress is held in the muscles and a clenched body may not easily relax into sleep. Stretching, t'ai chi, qi gong, massage, walking, bicycling or dancing help release this pent-up energy—choose forms of movement appropriate to given individual's situation. Avoid stimulating sorts of exercise directly before bedtime.

- **Avoid beverages close to desired sleep time** if you tend to awaken during the night from the need to empty the bladder. Be sure to hydrate well during daylight hours.

- **Avoid bright room lights and blue light from computer**, phone and tablet screens for at least one hour before desired bedtime. Dim ambient lighting in the evening.

- If reading in bed, **choose a focused-beam, book-reading lamp** instead of a bright light-diffusing fixture, to limit stimulation from the illumination.

- **Vibrational hygiene**: Refrain from disturbing images, or stimulating/agitating music, reading or conversations in the hours preceding bed. Choose quiet, calm activities. See the appendix entry ***Reflections on Environmental Influences*** for more on this.

- **Meditation, prayer, deep breathing, gentle cat-like stretches**, and/or **chanting** or **toning** can help clear the bodymind from the day's concerns.

- Particularly **for caregivers**, if energy levels allow—and you're not headed immediately to bed—**make time for gentle exercise** at the end of your shift: yoga, a short walk, meditative dance. Significantly helps to release tension.

- Keeping a journal by one's bed is a useful tool, not only to record dreams or insights, but also to use just before bedtime. **Record the day's blessings and/or concerns or things you wish to remember the following day**. This practice helps release them from body and mind—or at least turn down the volume of the thoughtstream.

- Morning focus: "I am grateful for this day, this opportunity to experience Life in its fullness." Nighttime focus: **"Tomorrow is another day, fresh with possibility."**

- At any time of day, **employ calming ambient music, soothing chant** or **guided meditation** to help downshift the system toward rest, relaxation, and sleep. Playing a **singing bowl** [or listening to recorded singing bowl tones] can do likewise. See chapter on *Recommended Listening* for some suggestions.

- Reserve **caffeine-containing beverages** for morning only or, ideally, eliminate them altogether. If caffeine is absolutely desired, choose organically grown green teas over coffee or black tea, if possible. The caffeine contained in green tea is lower in content and milder in activity. Green tea also contains L-theanine, discussed below.

- **L-Theanine**: Amino acid present in green tea [*Camellia sinensis*] that is calming to the mind and nervous system. Shown to reduce anxiety, stabilize mood, improve concentration, and enhance sleep. Can be taken as directed throughout day or reserved for evening use. Ingested as extract in capsules or tablets.

- **Avoid complex or difficult to digest foods at dinnertime**. Keep it light and simple, and try to eat early enough to allow efficient food processing before sleep—finish eating before 7pm or earlier if possible. Support digestion with a bit of naturally fermented condiment such as kraut, supplemental digestive enzymes, or an herbal bitter aperitif.

- If food is still not digesting properly, try one or more of the following **digestion-enhancing herbs**:

  - Peppermint leaf tea.
  - Chamomile flower tea.
  - Hops, a sedative bitter, can be added to either peppermint or chamomile tea.
  - Cardamom seed tea.
  - Rosemary leaf tea.
  - Ginger root tea or light decoction.
  - Dandelion root decoction [alone or with some cinnamon chips]
  - Chewing on some fennel or nigella [black cumin] seeds.

- Enteric-coated peppermint essential oil capsules.
- Classic Chinese patent medicines such as Curing Pills or Calm Stomach.
- See sections on **Nausea** and **Hydration** for additional details.

- Proprietary homeopathic formula **Calms Forte** provides a popular combination of botanical remedies and mineral salts. *Note*: Homeopathic remedies are taken at least 15 minutes away from either food or drink.

- Either **abstain from alcohol** completely or limit to small amount of wine with meal.

- Consume a preparation of **sedative herbs** after dinner and within 30 minutes of retiring to the bedroom: Select from among hops, passionflower, valerian, linden, chamomile, skullcap, California poppy, kava, magnolia bark…. Synergy among herbs can often heighten sedative activity, e.g. kava + passionflower, hops + chamomile, and so on. See *Plants to Support the Nervous System* for details on these plants.

- **Medical *Cannabis***: Calming, pain relieving, sedative, anti-nausea, promotes mood elevation, more. *Cannabis sativa* and *C. indica* are legally available for approved medical use in some jurisdictions. Consult with your healthcare provider if you think medical *Cannabis* is indicated for your situation.

- Ingesting **adaptogenic plants** during the day can help keep the mindbody system calmer and thus more primed for restorative sleep, through an array of actions: Holy basil, ashwagandha, eleuthero, schisandra, and so on. Numerous plants tonify the adrenal glands and help stabilize blood sugar regulation; some benefit the liver. See chapter on *Adaptogenic and Tonic Plant Allies* for descriptions of such plants.

- Review the chapters on *Food Considerations for Liver Health* and *Plant Allies for Liver Support* if one is awakening consistently between 1 and 3 a.m. or otherwise feels that liver issues are associated with sleep concerns. In addition, review the entry on schisandra in the *Adaptogenic and Tonic Plant Allies* chapter. In the body's circadian biorhythms, the gall bladder is particularly active from 11 p.m. to 1 a.m. and liver detoxification activity peaks between 1 and 3 a.m.

- **Evening bathing**: A relaxing bath or sponge bath [especially rinsing face, hands and feet] cleanses the skin of the day's elimination and helps to calm the body. Teas made from calming herbs such as lavender, chamomile, linden, or rose petals are lovely as bathing water. Epsom salts [magnesium sulfate] added to bath water help relax sore or tense muscles [use with care with cardiovascular issues]. Rose water or lavender hydrosol can also be sprayed onto face and skin if bathing is not possible.

- **Natural fiber** sheets, blankets, pillows, and sleepwear allow the body to breathe.

- **Warm cold feet**. Low-cut cotton sport-type socks are ideal for warming the feet while allowing them to breathe freely—and are easy to remove, if needed.

- **Consult with prescribing physician** and/or pharmacist regarding possible pharmaceutical or physiological factors at play in insomnia or disturbed sleep. Modify what can be modified.

Fatigue

Fatigue, like insomnia, can be a consequence of any number of factors—nutritional deficiencies, pain, disease process, sleep disturbance, lack of movement or exercise, constipation, emotional distress or despondency, spiritual exhaustion, dehydration, lowered red blood cell counts, and side effects of medical treatments or drugs. This is best addressed together with a holistic health practitioner who can help perceive the big picture and make personalized recommendations. That said, some of the observations shared below may be relevant.

- Please also refer to the sections on **Pain**, **Disturbed Sleep**, **Melancholy/Anxiety**, **Building the Blood**. These are key factors to address, if present.

- **Hydration**: Ensure that daily intake of water is sufficient. Are you drinking beverages that dehydrate tissues, such as coffee or alcohol? See section on **Hydration** below and the article on *Water, Hydration, Electrolytes* in the Appendices.

- **Review dietary choices**, making sure they include sufficient protein, complex carbohydrates, and vibrant fruits and vegetables. What might be improved? If on some sort of limited dietary regimen—even if for therapeutic purposes—make sure it contains adequate calories, protein, fiber, and healthy fats. Revise as necessary.

- **Explore digestion and assimilation** of foods. In the short term, try high-quality digestive enzymes with meals, as needed, to ensure proper nutrient absorption— evaluate as to whether these seem to be improving overall sense of wellness. Alternately, or additionally, consult with knowledgeable holistic health practitioner to explore this further and assess what herbs or other nutrients might also be of benefit to enhance digestive process at a deeper level.

- Consider increasing blood-building foods. See section on **Building the Blood**.

- Aging, disease process, and some therapeutic agents can be associated with **decreased energy production** at the level of cellular mitochondria. Supplements such as CoQ_{10} and Ubiquinol [active form of CoQ_{10}] help catalyze energy production within the cells, as well as providing other health-promoting activity.

- **Adaptogenic plants** such as *Panax ginseng, Panax quinquifolius, Rhodiola rosacea, Eleutherococcus senticosus, ashwagandha, schisandra, cordyceps* mushroom and others can promote a heightened sense of sustained physical endurance when taken for a course. Please see the chapter on *Adaptogenic and Tonic Plant Allies* to get a sense of which plants or medicinal mushrooms might best match your circumstance.

- **Rosemary** [*Rosmarinus officinalis*]: leaf. Anti-inflammatory, muscle relaxing, circulatory stimulating, rejuvenative. Rosemary awakens, warms and brings light to our beings. See entries in **Plant Allies for Liver Support** and **Plants to Support the Nervous System** for additional indications. **Formats**: Tea, tincture, extract, in food. Strong water infusion or essential oil diluted into a bit of liquid soap may be added to baths to both relax and revive aching, tense or tired muscles. The essential oil may also be added to massage oil or lotion. *Caution*: Avoid using at night as its circulatory stimulating properties may delay sleep.

- Starting each morning with even 15 minutes of **meditation,** or settling into it as needed throughout the day, can clear the bodymind of mental and bodily static that drains energy. Staying focused on the present moment and noticing what arises within it can expand our sense of time, vitality, and fulfillment.

- Be sure to allow some **quiet, solo time** in the course of the day, no matter how much your presence may be desired by others. You deserve to recharge. It is essential. This is not selfish or self-centered; it is simply taking responsibility for your health and well-being and supporting your own resiliency.

- Include **some focus each day that deepens the breath and promotes oxygenation**. Depending on one's circumstance, this can range from vigorous exercise, to walking, to stretching or yoga, to t'ai chi chuan or Qi gong, to pranayama, to simple mindful meditation focused on the breath. Singing, chanting, or toning can also be refreshing. Choose what is suitable and do it daily.

- Spend some time each day either in **direct contact with nature** or looking out into some favored green space. If you are able, walk or rest in the greenworld; if you are not mobile, drink in the healing emanations from where you are. Wild nature is vibrant with life force.

- **Reflect on the integrity of your energetic boundaries**. Do you take on the emotions, concerns, or needs of others in a way that saps your own energy reserves? What do you need to do to be less absorbent? What cords need to be cut and how? Remember to put the proverbial oxygen mask on your own face first before assisting others. This is key for both caregivers and those needing care.

- Improve night-time vibrational hygiene and allow for **adequate, restorative sleep** time. See previous section on **Disturbed Sleep/Insomnia** and the appendix entry *Reflections on Environmental Influences*.

- **Medical *Cannabis***: Calming, pain relieving, sedative, anti-nausea, promotes mood elevation, more. *Cannabis sativa* and *C. indica* are legally available for approved medical use in some jurisdictions. Can be ingested via medicated butter, vaporization, foods, or liquid or encapsulated extracts for this purpose. Consult with your healthcare provider if you think medical *Cannabis* is indicated for your situation.

Hot Water Bottle

Sometimes, it's the simplest things that mean the most.

- Both for simple comfort and to warm areas where circulation has diminished.

- Wrap hot water bottle in cozy flannel pillowcase.

- Placed over the bladder, a hot water bottle may assist a bedridden person in successfully voiding into bedpan.

- Used to enhance the warmth of a castor oil pack and deepen its action, a hot water bottle may help to promote bowel movement. See instructions for preparing a castor oil pack in the section on **Constipation**.

Hydration

Water is life's essential elixir. It gives rise to life. It sustains, heals, cleanses, restores, refreshes. It is essential for a host of metabolic processes. Water is the one nutrient we cannot live without. We can deprive ourselves of other nutritive substances and still manage to function, even if sub-optimally. But without water, our body systems shut down completely in a matter of days, the exact length of time dependent on other factors such as environment, body temperature, whether food is eaten, etc. Water accounts for approximately 50-60% of an adult's body weight, relative to the percentages of fat and muscle—and more than 75% of our brains.[3]

*The most obvious physical signs of dehydration, or depletion of bodily fluid, are scant or darkened urine, parched lips, dry mucous membranes, light-headedness. Sufficient hydration benefits all bodily functions and may improve irritating skin sensations. The appendix contains a discussion of this issue: **Water, Hydration, and Electrolytes**. Please also see the following section on **Simple Nutrition** for some considerations as to the ailing person's right to refuse fluid or food.*

- First and foremost: **It is essential that caregivers remain well-hydrated**, as part of their foundational self-care. It is so easy to forget this, in the course of appointments, household chores, meal prep, tending to others. Carry a water bottle around with you on errands and stage one somewhere obvious in the home so that you can track the volume of fluid you are ingesting during the course of each day.

- **Aim daily for eight ounces of water for every 20 pounds of body weight**. Warm or room temperature water may be more welcome than cold.

- **Dilute herbal teas** (e.g. raspberry leaf or ginger root—to ease nausea).

- **Plain water with a splash of organic pomegranate juice**. Pomegranate adds a refreshing flavor and beautiful color to the water as well as providing a host of health benefits. Rich in antioxidants, pomegranate is being explored for its potential in preventing cancer and cardiovascular disease, in particular.

- **Agar-agar jello**—make with organic non-citrus fruit juice (grape, cherry, apple, pomegranate, etc.).

  To prepare: Add 2 tablespoons agar flakes to 3 cups juice. Bring to a boil. Simmer and stir until agar fully dissolves, about five minutes. Pour into custard cups or glass pan. Refrigerate. The amount of juice can be adjusted, depending on the firmness desired.

- **Organic coconut water!** Clean, natural, delicious way to replace essential electrolytes. Available plain or flavored with lemon, lime, etc.—in liquid or powdered form. Powder from organic coconuts is easy to carry and add to water bottle as needed or desired. Coconut water is great to sip during and after chemotherapy sessions—much preferable to commercial sports beverages that are often recommended.

- **Chipped ice cubes** to be sucked (frozen mild ginger tea or raspberry/thimbleberry tea may help with nausea as well).

- **Kudzu** broth with a little umeboshi plum for nausea, flatulence, reflux, and general gastric upset (caregiver, too, may benefit from this). A true blessing when needed.

  To prepare: Add 1 heaping tablespoon kudzu starch to 1 cup cool water. Cook over medium heat, stirring constantly. When it turns from milky to translucent, cool slightly and serve. Flavor with a bit of umeboshi plum paste for salty taste and additional benefit—though not essential if flavor is unpalatable. Eat calmly, sip by sip.

- **Miso soup**. The lighter the miso, the sweeter and milder it tends to be. Darker miso is more salty and sharper tasting. Soothing, alkalinizing, source of natural ferment; supplies beneficial microorganisms to the gut. Stir in 1-3 teaspoons to a bowl or cup of soup, broth, or hot water just before eating; cooking destroys its gastrointestinal benefits. Keep miso refrigerated between uses.

- **Simple vegetable broths**: Yams, celery, carrots, greens, kombu, turkey tail mushrooms, shiitake, onions [if tolerated] simmered in water....Strain or blend before serving. Though best fresh, broth can be frozen in portions for later use. See the chapter *A Few Recipes for Gentle Foods*.

Simple Nutrition

So many issues come forward at almost any stage of living or dying with food and eating as the catalyst. My belief is that food may be provided and eating encouraged but never forced. I believe that on one level or another our appetites guide us in choosing whether to continue nourishing our physical aliveness — or not — in a given moment. There is something sacred about trusting the higher wisdom of those promptings. In some cultures, consciously abstaining from food and drink is part of a respected personal choice toward encouraging the end of physical life.

*When someone **wishes** to eat, however, and has trouble keeping food down or digesting well, the following suggestions may be of benefit. These foods are simple, soothing and nourishing. Please also review the earlier section on **<u>Consistency/Ritual/Rhythm</u>** for thoughts on the fuller context of nourishment. See the chapter **A Few Recipes for Gentle Foods** for additional ideas.*

- First and foremost: **It is essential that caregivers eat regular meals** throughout the day as part of their foundational self-care. It becomes very easy to forget about one's own needs when caring for another. The more rhythm you can establish for yourself, the better you will sustain the rigors of caregiving. Emphasize fresh fruits and vegetables and easily digested proteins. Try to eat in a quiet space if at all possible, a place where you can focus as much as you can simply on the fact of eating, on the beauty of your own health, on your gratefulness for this great life.

- If a **circle of support for food preparation or meal delivery** has been established, be sure to ask for foods for yourself and/or your family beyond the specific needs of the one receiving care. The support required, ultimately, is for all of you.

- **Miso soup** (simple broth made with carrots, onion and perhaps sea vegetables for those who can tolerate them). Miso is a traditional fermented salty soybean condiment that is rich in live microbial cultures that are beneficial to gut health. Miso is added to each bowl or mug at the table to preserve its benefits, never cooked. See previous section on **<u>Hydration</u>** for more.

- **Vegetable broths** and **congee**. See the chapter *A Few Recipes for Gentle Foods* for details on how to prepare.

- **Bone broths**. Mineral-rich, fortifying, they strengthen the marrow. See the chapter *A Few Recipes for Gentle Foods*.

- **Cauliflower/coconut milk puree**. Soothing, satisfying. Contributes good fats, calories, anti-cancer and antiviral nutrients. See *A Few Recipes for Gentle Foods*.

- Freshly pressed **organic vegetable juice**, diluted with water and thoroughly mixed with saliva before swallowing. Use with discretion and always diluted, to avoid overwhelming the system with plant sugars. To avoid that, focus on juicing greens, celery, ginger, turmeric, a little beet, a little carrot…

- **Slippery elm porridge** [*Ulmus* spp.]. A traditional country food prepared from the fluffy inner bark of this tree, used to soothe and heal the throat and gut while delivering nutrition.

  To prepare: Place 1 tablespoon slippery elm powder into a small cup or bowl. Slowly add water to make a porridge consistency. Can add honey or maple syrup for more flavor. Eat slowly.

- **Smoothies** with nourishing powders added. Consider micro-filtered isolated whey protein powder, adaptogenic/tonic herbs as appropriate to build vital force: stinging nettles, ashwagandha, eleuthero, astragalus, and so on. See chapter discussing *Adaptogenic and Tonic Plant Allies* in order to select the most appropriate plant powders. See chapter featuring *Power Smoothie Recipe* for a fuller discussion of additional ingredient options, including information on calories and protein content.

> *To make a basic smoothie: In a blender, combine—2 cups water; ½-1 cup fresh or frozen blueberries and/or raspberries; 1-2 tablespoons freshly ground flax seeds [or blend of chia, flax, sprouted seeds, etc.]; 1 scoop micro-filtered whey protein-isolate powder or eggwhite protein; 1-2 tablespoons stinging nettle powder, alfalfa or barley grass juice powder; 1-2 teaspoons ashwagandha or eleuthero root powder, other powdered nutrients as desired [see* **Adaptogenic and Tonic Plant Allies** *for ideas]; warming ginger powder or cinnamon powder or vanilla extract to taste. Blend all but the protein powder together; add the whey, then briefly pulse to mix. Drink promptly after blending, as the flax or chia seeds will thicken the drink over time.*

- Steel-cut **oatmeal** or **multi-grain "Moosh."**

> *To make Moosh, select from among a variety of organic whole grains—millet, brown rice, quinoa, oats, barley, amaranth, buckwheat [small proportion of total], whatever suits your dietary needs. Quinoa, amaranth, buckwheat, millet, and both cultivated brown and wild rice tend to be the best-tolerated grains.*
>
> *Grind each grain to a powder. Mix approximately equal portions together in a bowl [use less of strong-tasting buckwheat]. Transfer to a well-sealed jar and store in the refrigerator. As needed, scoop out ¼ cup of the mix and stir into 1 cup boiling water. Lower heat and cook until water is absorbed, stirring to prevent lumping. Deelish.*

Building the Blood

Stem cells within the bone marrow called hematopoietic cells produce the living cells which circulate in the blood: red blood cells [RBC], white blood cells [WBC], platelets. These blood factors circulate within a liquid matrix called plasma. Normally, plasma constitutes about 55% of total volume of whole blood, red blood cells about 45%, white blood cells and platelets together account for less than 1%.

The blood as a whole serves several crucial roles in maintaining health and aliveness. It is a distribution vehicle for nutrients, oxygen, hormones, and metabolic waste. It helps regulate inner temperature, acid/alkaline balance, and sufficient fluid volume within our bodies. The blood also provides protection and defense functions: promoting clotting to prevent excessive blood loss as well as supporting the circulation of immune cells to defend against pathogens, etc.

Certain medical treatments can have the consequence of suppressing bone marrow production of these blood factors, which then negatively impacts immunity [WBCs], proper blood clotting [platelets], and the capacity of the blood to supply sufficient oxygen to the tissues [RBCs]. Abnormal quantity, size and shape of blood constituents are all important diagnostic indicators and should be monitored carefully when following a person dealing with serious disease or medical treatments which can impact normal body chemistry and organ function.

*It is important to know what one is dealing with. Various forms of anemia [there are at least 400 medically defined types] can arise as a consequence of **many** different causes: hereditary factors; bone marrow issues; pharmaceutical side effects, such as from chemotherapy; nutritional deficiencies; digestive insufficiency; and as a corollary to numerous disease processes. Anemia can manifest experientially as fatigue, rapid heartbeat, shortness of breath, dizziness, difficulty in concentration, lack of appetite, pale skin, leg cramps, and so on. Particular types of anemia have specific presenting symptoms. Be sure to consult a physician promptly if you suspect you may have anemia.*

Meanwhile, there are numerous basic approaches that can be taken to support optimum bone marrow function and blood cell production and dynamics. As always, understanding the full scope of what you or your loved one is dealing with is a key step in making the most applicable health-supportive choices. Consult a holistic practitioner to help you navigate your allopathic diagnosis and treatment recommendations.

- If issues are based on nutritional capacity or deficiency, consider **increasing digestive fire** by ingesting pre-meal bitters or digestive enzymes along with the meal. See the section on **Loss of Appetite / Weight Loss** for more details.

- **Assess vitamin B$_{12}$ and folic acid sufficiency**. Increase daily intake as indicated. B vitamins, essential to healthy blood factors, are especially needed during times of metabolic stress; food intake often needs to be supplemented during such times. Food sources include: Dark leafy greens, seaweeds, nutritional yeast, whole grains.

- **Bone broths** are essentially decoctions of animal bones and cartilage, in which the abundant nutrients they contain extract into the cooking water over time. They are an ancient means for getting the most out of animal foods. Minerals, collagen, and many corollary nutrients become available as the animal parts soften or disappear into the broth through sufficient cooking; desired vegetables and herbs are generally added toward the end of cooking. Imbibed on a regular basis, these readily available nutrients particularly help to maintain and nourish the bones and essential structure of the body. See *A Few Recipes for Gentle Foods*.

- **Astragalus root** [*Astragalus membranaceus*]: root. Slightly warm, mildly sweet. Adaptogen, immuno-stimulant, pectoral, anti-pyretic, antibacterial, antiviral, anti-inflammatory, diuretic. An ancient remedy, astragalus has been recognized as a superb and potent immune system tonic by modern researchers—found to be a tonic to bone marrow. Invigorates Qi [the vital force often damaged by chemotherapy and radiation treatments], builds stamina, strengthens superficial resistance, promotes tissue regeneration/generates flesh, reduces inflammation. It is also a digestive tonic that can promote the digestion and assimilation of food. Indications: Wasting or exhausting diseases, fatigue, colds, poor digestion and metabolism, weakness, chronically weak lungs with shortness of breath, prolapsed organs, spontaneous sweating, nephritis, tumors, adjunct to chemotherapy and radiation. Astragalus has been used for thousands of years to fortify the body as a whole. **Formats**: Decoction as beverage and as broth base in soups and grains, tincture, powdered root as food, in capsules. A concentrated 5:1 extract powder is available and can easily be added into smoothies, if indicated. *Cautions*: Discontinue use during hot, acute conditions.

- What is termed Blood, in the Chinese medicine way of knowing, includes the status of the vital force or Qi. In addition to astragalus, **other blood-building herbs used in Chinese botanical medicine** include: Panax ginseng root [*Panax ginseng*], codonopsis root [*C. pilosula*], prepared rehmannia root [*R. glutinosa*], atractylodis root [*A. lancea*], dong quai root [*Angelica sinensis*], white peony root [*Paeonia lactiflora*], he shou wu root [*Polygonum multiflorum*] and others. These are selected and combined in formulations by practitioners according to the constitution and presenting symptoms of each client. Know that there is much out there that may be of benefit and seek professional counsel accordingly.

- **Marrow Plus** [Health Concerns] or **ImmuneCare I** [Natura Health Products]: These outstanding products deserve mention by name. Both of these proprietary, practitioner-grade formulas are based on similar traditional principles of supporting bone marrow production of immune cells and blood factors. Either of these formulations can be especially beneficial taken concurrently with chemotherapy and are often recommended as adjunct support. They both contain *Spatholobus aka Milletia, Astragalus membranaceus, Polygonum multiflorum, Rehmannia, Lycium* fruit, *Angelica sinensis*. The formulations vary from there, each with additional tonifying and synergistic plant ingredients. Consult with a knowledgeable practitioner to assess which might be best for a given constitution and health status.

- **Yellow dock or broad-leaved dock** [*Rumex* spp.]: root. One of its traditional uses is to improve impaired iron absorption. Additionally, you will see this common weed mentioned in various places throughout this repertoire—particularly as a digestive bitter and cholagogue, improving bile secretion and thereby waste excretion. Easiest to administer as tincture of fresh root. *Caution*: Use all *Rumex* plants carefully if there is a history of kidney stones—as roots and leaves contain calcium oxalate.

- **Chlorophyll-rich herbs and foods.** Within our bodies, chlorophyll serves as a building block for production of healthy red blood cells, especially when taken with iron-rich foods or food-sourced iron supplements. Great sources include stinging nettles, dandelion leaves, alfalfa leaves, dark leafy greens of all types, single-celled algae such as chlorella….Chlorophyll concentrates are also available, both as liquid or in gelcaps [see ***Resources***].

Lack of Appetite / Weight Loss

Gaining weight and muscle mass can be the most immediately important job and necessity for someone dealing with debilitating illness such as cancer or AIDS. The disease process is catabolic, destroying tissue such as muscle in its wake. Promoting health means promoting the body's building, anabolic processes—that by which it repairs and constructs itself. Normal aging also tips metabolism more toward catabolism.

Essentially, surviving allopathic cancer treatments and much disease process itself comes down to eating more protein than you ever thought possible and eating lots of beneficial fats. The ideal diet going through chemotherapy treatment is focused on maintaining body mass and keeping red blood cells and platelets at safe levels (with white blood cells in health-protective range as well, of course). The following details some specific aids I have found helpful through the years.

Again, the individual's wishes regarding continuing sustenance should obviously play an important role here and must be respected.

- **Herbal bitters taken as aperitif** before meals to stimulate appetite and improve digestion and assimilation: alcohol extract of gentian root, dandelion root, Oregon grape root, yellow dock, yarrow, ginger rhizome, orange peel, hops or other such digestive stimulants. Used as single plants or in combinations. Typical dose is one dropperful in a little water taken 15-20 minutes before eating food.

- **Vitamin B$_{12}$**: Essential in many physiological processes, vitamin B$_{12}$ is sometimes administered intramuscularly to improve digestive function in deficient patients. Consult with your healthcare practitioner as to its relevance in your situation.

- **Medical *Cannabis***: Well-known plant medicine for sharpening the appetite. Calming, pain relieving, sedative, anti-nausea, promotes mood elevation, more. *Cannabis sativa* and *C. indica* are legally available for approved medical use in some jurisdictions. Can be ingested via medicated butter, vaporization, or extracts for this purpose; also incorporated into foods. Consult with your healthcare provider if you think medical *Cannabis* is indicated for your situation.

- **Cinnamon tea** [*Cinnamomum verum*]: Pleasant, familiar taste as simple tea or lightly simmered to stimulate appetite. The scent and taste is often associated in memory with warm emotions and pleasurable foods. Aromatic, carminative, antispasmodic, antibacterial, antifungal, astringent, demulcent.

- **Digestive enzymes** taken with meals can improve appetite and digestion. Bromelain, green papaya, mixed enzyme blends containing amylase, protease, lactase, lipase, cellulase, etc. See **Resources** chapter for some reputable sources.

- Supplemental **zinc** can be of benefit to improve appetite. See **Loss of Taste/Smell** which follows for more details.

- **Flaxseed oil** added into foods, if oil is tolerated. Make sure the oil has a somewhat buttery nut-like flavor; if extremely bitter or with a pronounced bitter edge, the oil has turned rancid and should not be used. Flaxseed oil should always be refrigerated and never heated in any way in order to preserve its integrity. One-to-two tablespoons per day is considered a maximum daily dose. Easy and delicious to add some into a smoothie or onto protein-rich quinoa or vegetables.

- **Organic coconut flesh and oil**. Great, satisfying source of beneficial fats and flavor. Add to smoothies or nibble pieces as a snack. Available powdered, shredded, flaked, pureed, and whole, of course. Coconut "manna" or "butter" is a unique, spreadable whole food product made from organic coconut flesh and oil. Absolutely delicious. Alternately, **coconut milk-based frozen dessert** is a wonderful low-sugar food—both as a soothing treat on its own or as an amendment to smoothie, making it more like a "shake." In addition to supplying needed calories and good fats, coconut contains antiviral, anti-yeast constituents such as lauric acid.

- **Organic, non-hydrogenated nut and seed butters** in moderation. Avoid peanut butter—contains methylxanthines which have been found to promote cyst and possibly tumor growth. Almond or sunflower butter are delicious added to smoothies or eaten by the spoonful; tahini [hulled sesame butter] is wonderful drizzled on grains and vegetables; zinc-rich, green pumpkin seed butter is perfect in all these ways and more. These supply protein, good fats, minerals, and concentrated calories.

- **Schmoo**. A delicious, nutty-tasting, spreadable combination of tahini and miso. Stores well in a closed container in the refrigerator. Can be diluted as desired to use as a dressing for quinoa, moosh, or vegetables.

  > *To make schmoo*: Into a small bowl, place some organic raw tahini. The exact amount is not critical, but try starting with about half a cup. Very gradually mix in small amounts of mellow white miso. The mixture will thicken as you do so. Taste after each addition. Stop when the mixture suits your taste and the blend is still spreadable in consistency. Schmoo can be used, as is, as a simple spread or a portion may be blended with water to use as a pourable dressing for salads, vegetables, grains, whatever. The base itself has a long shelf life when refrigerated. Various seasonings may be added when a portion is used, such as chopped chives, fresh or dried minced garlic, chopped fresh parsley, chopped fresh ginger, and so on.

- **Ghee** made from organic butter. Ghee is clarified butter; the milk proteins that naturally exist in butter can challenge some constitutions and are removed through gently heating and then straining the butter. Ghee is the finished product. It is a delicious way to add calories and flavor to foods. Eggs scrambled in ghee are soothing and satisfying. In Ayurvedic tradition, this ancient food is considered to impart the essence of motherly love and strengthen our core. Ghee is an extremely stable food—and can be stored without refrigeration.

- The beautiful **avocado**—organically grown, of course—provides delicious, satisfying calories and texture to the diet. Avocado is a rich source of minerals, fiber, vitamin K, folate, and beneficial fats—and is moderately anti-inflammatory. Eat it by the spoonful right out of the skin, mash it onto the occasional brown rice cake or into dips for veggies, cube it into quinoa and salads, puree it into dressings. Additional inspiration: One cup of mashed avocado provides 4.5 grams of protein and 384 calories. Maintain a bowl on the kitchen counter with avocados in various stages of ripening. Check them daily for readiness and use promptly: Always retain the seed-half of a cut avocado if only using a portion at a sitting. Adding lemon juice to prepared avocado-based foods also prolongs their color and freshness. See *A Few Recipes for Gentle Foods* for a Cacao-Avocado pudding.

- **Fish oil**. The omega-3 fatty acids in fish oil are not only anti-inflammatory, but these and other nutrients in fish oil have been found to help to preserve and build lean body mass. Essential fatty acids are added to enteral nutrition formulas, for those who cannot or should not take food through normal eating; marine oils are often part of recommended supplementation following recovery from bariatric surgery as well.

- **Royal jelly**, the substance worker bees feed to one of their number to create a new queen, is an amazing food for building muscle and strength. It is a very concentrated food and is often sold mixed in honey. A better choice for those monitoring sugar intake might be freeze-dried royal jelly available in capsules that can be swallowed as is or opened and added into foods. Can be added to herbal fudge [see *Recipes Using Adaptogenic and Tonic Plants*], mixed into seed/nut butters, or used in smoothies.

- **Protein-rich smoothies**, especially using microfiltered, isolated whey protein. Whey protein powder, especially prepared in this manner, is one of the best supplemental sources of protein available. It is readily metabolized in the body and is a rich source of the amino acid L-glutamine, critical to cellular health and overall protein synthesis. Ashwagandha root powder makes a fine addition to help build flesh. See previous section, **Simple Nutrition,** and the *Power Smoothie Recipe* for recipes; see the chapter on *Adaptogenic and Tonic Plant Allies* for more information on ashwagandha and other herbal powders to consider.

- **Herbal fudge** [see *Recipes Using Adaptogenic and Tonic Plants*] is a delicious source of calories, a yummy delivery system for beneficial plant powders, and solid nutrition for those who can allow some honey in their diet. Another easy-to-make food that stores well in the refrigerator.

- Freshly pressed **organic vegetable juice**, diluted with water and thoroughly mixed with saliva before swallowing. Use with discretion and always diluted, to avoid overwhelming the system with plant sugars. To avoid that, focus on juicing greens, celery, ginger, turmeric, a little beet, some carrot…

- Alternately, take advantage of the wide array of **organic vegetable and fruit powders** available in the marketplace to help increase overall nutrition when the need is high and appetite is low. These can **easily be added to smoothies, juice, yogurt, other foods, or plain water** in some cases. Choose powders made from organically cultivated plants, ideally freshly freeze-dried after harvest or juicing. These should seem to "come alive" when added to liquids. Choices out there include numerous formulations of mixed greens (and algaes such as chlorella), seaweeds, super fruits— as well as individual plants: kale, stinging nettles, celery, tart cherries, blueberries, raspberries, mixed berry blends, beets, broccoli and broccoli sprouts, alfalfa, pomegranate, turmeric, cultured cabbage…See the section on *Resources* for some suggested high quality products.

- Simply prepared **organic eggs from free-range hens**. Source of high-quality protein and vitamin D. Consult with your practitioner to see if eggs are an appropriate food in your situation. See *A Few Recipes for Gentle Foods* for some ideas to keep things interesting.

- **L-glutamine**: An amino acid existing naturally in the body, L-glutamine is a building block for proteins, produced in the muscles and distributed where needed by the blood. It is a factor in many metabolic processes including wound repair. L-glutamine can be supplemented if needed—during situations of nutritional deficiency, metabolic stress, muscle wasting [cancer, AIDS, etc.], tissue injury [surgery, radiation, etc.] particularly if the digestive/intestinal membranes have been compromised. Shown to improve gut health, immune function, and enhance wound healing. Whey protein and cabbage juice are rich sources of L-glutamine. Isolated glutamine powders are also available and are easily added to smoothies. Other food sources include miso, legumes, beef, chicken, fish, and dairy products.

- To set the stage for a meal, **try lighting a candle** made of natural wax. If tolerated, the candle may be scented with pure essential oil that the challenged person finds soothing, calming or uplifting. Consider peppermint, ginger, lemongrass or citrus essential oils. This can help relax the belly and mind, define the mealtime as a break from worry, and create a sacred space within which food may be eaten. See **Loss of Taste/Smell** for other candle considerations.

- Please see the chapter *Natural Strategies for Tube Feeding* if difficulties in chewing or swallowing have presented. The ideas offered there may be of use.

Loss of Taste / Smell

As with dry mouth and mouth sores, this loss of sensory awareness can be caused by chemical, pharmaceutical or radiation therapy—perhaps just when you most need to maintain appetite and a desire for food. Fortunately, there are some strategies that might improve this situation. If touch remains sensitive, eating with the hands may help.

- Ginger has been shown to be protective against radiation-induced taste aversion in laboratory studies. An alcohol/water extract of ginger was used in the research. Ginger's strong antioxidant action was seen to be key to its radioprotective activity.[4,5]

- A sufficient level of the trace mineral **zinc** is required to help maintain an adequate sense of taste and smell. Also, low levels of zinc are associated with lowered immune function. Zinc is also needed for proper wound healing, blood sugar balance, and a host of enzymatic activities. Low zinc levels in the blood, in tandem with relatively high serum copper levels, are often observed in people dealing with cancer. Zinc is poorly stored in the body and needs to be replenished through daily diet or supplementation. **Food sources** rich in zinc include fish and eggs, beans [soak first], mushrooms, quinoa, seeds, and some nuts. **Zinc lozenges** deliver the nutrient directly to the oral cavity. **Supplemental zinc** is most absorbable in aspartate, citrate, chelated, and picolinate forms but the most preferable is a food-based supplement produced from nutritional yeast and other whole foods. Simple blood tests can check for zinc status and help guide any long-term supplemental use, if appropriate.

- If iodine is an appropriate nutrient for a given individual, bring **seaweed** onto the table as a salty condiment. Powders or flakes may be sprinkled onto foods instead of salt to help awaken the taste buds and also help offset taste changes. Powdered kelps, especially in combinations, or dulse flakes alone are good ones to try. Be sure to choose organically certified seaweeds or at least sea vegetables that have been harvested from uncontaminated northern waters by responsible harvesters. See *Resource* section in back for list of suppliers.

- If natural fragrances are tolerated, **try lighting a scented candle** during mealtime. Some essential oils possess calming or uplifting properties that can help settle the bodymind and make it more receptive to food. Clean, pure aromas can sometimes improve taste sensation. Suggested scents include: ginger, clary sage, lemongrass, etc. Here, I am speaking *only* of healthy candles, made from beeswax, soy or sustainably sourced palm oils and scented with aromatherapy-grade pure essential oils distilled from plants. Synthetic fragrances, petroleum-based waxes, and lead wicks are to be strictly avoided, as they may promote long-term health consequences when inhaled.

Chasing Medication

- Pharmaceutical drugs such as liquid morphine, if taken by mouth, can be very bitter and unpleasant to ingest. Chase with shot of organic grape or pomegranate juice and/or dilute as desired to mask the taste. Be sure to follow drug instructions as to waiting period before eating or drinking.

- Note on morphine: Can stimulate very vivid and/or disturbing dreams.

- If drugs create unpleasant sensations, ask medical prescriber to evaluate dose and available delivery formats. Explore appropriateness of crafting suppositories at home [see section on **Suppositories** for instructions] or ask pharmacist to supply in suppository or other format.

- These days, dermal patches and IV-drip lines deliver steady doses of pain-relieving meds such as Fentanyl: Do not casually combine pharmaceutical drugs that bind to opioid receptors in the brain and central nervous system with sedating herbal substances to avoid unpredictable synergistic effects. Discuss specific situation with pharmacist, naturopathic physician or clinical herbalist for guidance.

Nausea

At some point in their lives, it is likely that almost everyone has had the unpleasant sensations associated with nausea, a state that may or may not proceed vomiting. Nausea can be a consequence of disease process or associated with therapeutic interventions such as anesthesia, pain relief, chemotherapy, or radiation. Pharmaceutical drugs may be prescribed to address persistent nausea but have their own side effects. And even with these, an underlying ocean of unsettledness can often be perceived. Short of the pharmaceutical path—or in addition to it—the following simple suggestions may offer another level of relief. Also see **Plants to Support the Nervous System**.

- **Kudzu root starch**: Starch extracted from the root of *Pueraria montana var. lobata* is demulcent and profoundly soothing, helping to soothe the digestive tract, clear gas from the system and calm the stomach. Use alone or mix with a little umeboshi plum for nausea, flatulence, general gastric upset.

  To prepare kudzu broth: Add 1 heaping tablespoon kudzu to 1 cup cool water. Cook over medium heat, stirring constantly. When broth turns from milky to translucent, cool slightly and serve. Flavor with a bit of umeboshi plum paste for salty taste and additional benefit—though not essential if ume flavor is unpalatable. Eat calmly, sip by sip.

- Sipping **red raspberry leaf** tea or sucking raspberry tea ice chips.

  To prepare tea: Steep 1 teaspoon to 1 tablespoon red raspberry leaf in 1 cup boiled water. Steep 10-20 minutes or more. Make a bigger batch if intending to freeze as cubes.

- **Ginger** rhizome. Could sip warm ginger tea, suck ginger tea ice chips, suck slices of crystallized ginger, sip a naturally sweetened commercial ginger brew/ale.

  To make tea, combine 1 teaspoon chopped dry ginger rhizome plus ½ teaspoon licorice root or crushed fennel seed for every 1 cup water. Gently simmer 10-20 minutes. If the dried ginger root seems too sharp, steep a couple of slices of fresh ginger rhizome in boiled water with the licorice or fennel instead.

- Other herbal teas: **Peppermint, fennel, chamomile, lemon balm**.

  To prepare, steep 1-2 teaspoon of one of the herbs in 1 cup boiled water for 5-10 minutes. Sip slowly and calmly.

- **Cardamom seed** [*Elettaria cardamomum*]: Settles the stomach plus inhibits growth of yeast, fungi, and bacteria.

  To prepare cardamom tea: Combine ½ teaspoon dry seed with 1 cup boiled water. Steep, covered, for 30 minutes. Use half cup at a time.

- A commercially available children's remedy for colic can be of benefit. **"Gripe Water"** is traditionally composed of fennel seed, dill, ginger, and sodium bicarbonate. Read labels carefully—avoid all products that contain carcinogenic parabens as preservatives.

- **Wrist bands** designed to apply consistent pressure on the acupressure point Nei-kuan. Position pressure about three-fingers' width from wrist flexure, in the middle of the inner wrist between the tendons. This can also be done manually, of course, but the bands require less attention and energy.

- **Acupuncture** and **ear beads.** Can help reduce anxiety and calm the stomach. Visit your acupuncturist for treatments as needed.

- **Grounding**: Caregiver applies gentle support to the soles of the recipient's feet with the flat palms of their hands. Experiment with the degree of pressure required to help move the energy of the body gently downward and ground it through the feet.

- **Medical *Cannabis***: Calming, pain relieving, sedative, anti-nausea, promotes mood elevation, more. *Cannabis sativa* and *C. indica* are legally available for approved medical use in some jurisdictions. Can be ingested via medicated butter, vaporization, or extracts for this purpose. Consult with your healthcare provider if you think medical *Cannabis* is indicated for your situation.

- **Homeopathic *Ipecacuanha***: incessant nausea; vomiting does not relieve it; it persists whether the stomach is empty or not. ***Gelsemium***: vomiting related to fear. *Note*: Homeopathic remedies are taken at least 15 minutes away from either food or drink.

- **Biofeedback**: Personal biofeedback devices can be attached to the earlobe help guide the user into a calm, meditative state.

- Follow any episode of vomiting with a **baking soda/salt mouth rinse** to remove gastric acids from teeth and to soothe irritated mucous membranes.

    Baking soda rinse: Combine ¼ teaspoon baking soda and 1/8 teaspoon sea salt in 1 cup warm water. Mix well until powders dissolve. Rinse mouth gently; do not swallow. Follow with plain water rinse. **Use as needed***.*

Dizziness

This may occur for any number of reasons, including the sheer intensity of the health reality one is facing. Many therapeutic agents such as chemotherapy or other pharmaceuticals can unsettle one's sense of balance and center. Though there may be many likely suspects contributing to dizziness or vertigo, be sure to let a healthcare provider know this being experienced—it may be a symptom pointing to a circumstance that needs to be addressed medically, such as anemia, blood sugar vagaries, blood pressure abnormalities, and more.

- **Hydrate**! Insufficient water intake can contribute to this sensation, which can be considered a powerful reminder to drink more fluid. Coconut water can help provide proper electrolyte balance. Each day, aim for eight ounces of water for every 20 pounds of body weight.

- **Reflect on the day**: When was the last time nutritious food was eaten? Water drunk? Fresh air breathed? Are the shoulders and neck tense, the spine in alignment?

- Review the suggestions listed under **Nausea** as the need to settle the stomach may be another contributing factor. Resting while having the feet held by a silent companion can be helpful during a heightened episode.

- When standing or walking, **feel your connection with the earth** through the soles of your feet. Gently draw energy from the stable root of that connection, up through your legs, your trunk, out through your arms, hands and top of your head. Use awareness of your natural, unforced breath as you do this—feel the energy filling and stabilizing your being. Walk or move from this awareness.

- **Allow yourself to slow down**. Stay focused on the present moment, the task immediately before you. Assume the attitude that there is no rush or pressure weighing on you. Find the pace of walking or shifting positions or accomplishing the task that allows you to move gently from your center. Softly exaggerate your movements, to whatever degree allows the lightheadedness to settle down.

- Practice some basic **t'ai chi chuan** movements or **gentle yoga postures**, if you are familiar with these meditative practices or can follow along with recorded visual instruction. Silent practice or entrainment with a muted video would likely be most soothing. See *Resources* for online demonstrations.

- If no other obvious cause, try applying **lavender essential oil** to the temples.

- **To increase blood flow and, therefore, oxygen circulation**: Rosemary tea can be added to foot or full-body bath; a few drops of rosemary essential oil may be added to massage oil or body lotion. Best to avoid using rosemary at night; for some, the increased sense of circulation can delay sleep.

- **Ginger root** [*Zingiber officinale*]: May help quell any accompanying nausea. Can be taken as tea, decoction, in capsules, as food, as aromatherapy. See the section on **Nausea** for additional suggestions.

Body Odors

To the casual reader this may seem a superficial topic in a book of this nature. But for anyone who has dealt with life-threatening disease process, either as the one experiencing it directly or as a caregiver, there is little need for explanation. Tissue necrosis and discharge can become a vivid part of the challenge of coping, for all involved.

The smell from tissue breaking down can provoke psychological and emotional challenges, providing constant reminder that the body in question is undergoing huge stress. It can also make it difficult for the caregiver while offering basic hygiene assistance and tending to other needs, a strong reminder that their loved one is deeply unwell or dying. While accepting the reality of tissue decay is of a piece with accepting what is presenting in the moment, still, it can be a challenging sensory experience for all concerned. The suggestions below may be of benefit in mitigating this circumstance.

In addition, general body odor, the breath, urine and stools can also be intense during illness and treatments. This can result from multiple factors, particularly if the person is less active than usual. Consider: heightened anxiety, irregular or incomplete hygiene, digestive challenges, detoxification issues, constipation, and so on.

Remember that since antiquity our ancestors have used aromatic herbs and medicated unguents both to prevent tissue degradation by bacteria and to override the odors of the sickroom. Whether dealing with burns, cancerous or gangrenous wounds, or the consequences of incontinence, nature offers options. Again, begin slowly with any and all scents as the person being given care may have strong preferences and aversions—and do remember that these preferences and aversions may change over time.

- First and foremost, **caregivers should renew themselves regularly**—taking time throughout the day to simply step outside and breathe deeply of fresh air. Take care to do this in a low-key way that does not bring shame or emotional distress to the one you are caring for.

- **Ensure sufficient hydration** to allow the body's systems of waste processing and elimination to function optimally. This is a keynote. Aim for eight ounces for every 20 pounds of body weight. Warm or room-temperature water may be more welcome than cold. Warm broths seasoned with parsley can also be helpful.

- **Sage tea as wash** [*Salvia officinalis*]: Cool or gently warmed, to use in sponge bathing. Antiseptic, antibacterial, astringent.

- **Antiseptic essential oils**, as tolerated. For example, eucalyptus, tea tree, thyme, lavender, fir, pine, spruce, rosemary, etc. May be infused into the environment via essential oil diffuser, vaporizer, or hand-spraying; can be added to liquid soap during bathing, used in foot baths, added to body lotion or creams, applied as deodorant, etc.

- Light a **non-toxic candle scented with pure aromatherapy-quality essential oils**: During mealtimes, sponge baths, visits from friends and family, massage or energy work sessions, and at other times as desired. Choose candles crafted from beeswax, soy wax, or sustainable palm wax fitted with lead-free wicks.

- **Patchouli essential oil** [*Pogostemon patchouli*]: This earthy aroma can be very useful in underarm, inner thigh or foot applications. Extend in oil, salve or lotion.

- Similarly applied, **essential oils** of chamomile, lemongrass, lavender, nutmeg, clary sage or ginger may be of benefit. Extend in oil, salve or lotion.

- **Tend to wounds**, areas being drained, and other tissue suppuration **on a regular basis**, renewing dressings promptly. As appropriate, activated charcoal poultices on superficial wounds can be deodorizing as well as drawing. Follow instructions from nursing advisers in given situation. If you are the caregiver, quietly step outside for some deep, calming, refreshing breaths after completing a wound-tending session.

- **Create a healing, aromatic balm.** Using wound-healing calendula or St. Johnswort infused oil, cream or salve as the base, add various combinations of essential oils to small test quantities until the most desirable single scent or blend is achieved. Try thyme, lavender, tea tree, patchouli, or eucalyptus. Even if the finished product cannot be applied directly to the wound, try applying it to perimeter.

- **Raw honey**, a potent antimicrobial and wound-healing agent, can serve to deodorize putrid wounds when applied directly as a dressing. Honey has been used since ancient times in wound management and has shown direct activity against a wide spectrum of microbes, including those that have become resistant to pharmaceutical antibiotics. Nature's perfect wound dressing. Consult with nursing advisers as to appropriateness in your particular situation if you have concerns or questions.

- **Keep bed linens, towels, and clothing as fresh as possible**. Add lavender essential oil to the laundry soap if that scent is agreeable.

- **Chose natural fibers** for all bed linens, towels and clothing to allow the body to breathe freely. This may also lessen any sensation of itching in sensitive skin.

- **L-glutamine** consumption has been shown to promote general wound healing. Glutamine, an amino acid, is a component of whey protein powder and can also be supplemented on its own. Cabbage juice is also a rich source of glutamine. Please see the section **Lack of Appetite / Weight Loss** for more information on L-glutamine.

- **Zinc supplementation** may be of benefit to help promote wound and general skin healing. Please see the section on **Loss of Taste/Smell** for more information.

- **Ostomy patients**, in particular: Talk with your medical adviser about adding drops of **liquid chlorophyll** to your drinking water. As with eating parsley, though perhaps more convenient, chlorophyll concentrates have been known to freshen the breath as well as the odor of stool. Use typically darkens the stool. See *Resources* for suggestions on high-quality products.

- **Beneficial bacterial cultures**: Probiotics, miso, yogurt or kefir, naturally cultured foods or juice from kraut, etc. can benefit breath by benefiting healthy intestinal microbiota, particularly following a course of pharmaceutical antibiotic treatment.

- **Stinging nettles** [*Urtica dioica*]: Rich source of chlorophyll; alkalinizing. As tea, infusion or leaf powder added to smoothie or other food.

- Include **herbal mouth rinse as part of daily routine**. See section on **Dental Hygiene** for suggestions.

- As indicated, see section on **Constipation** and chapters *Food Considerations for Liver Health* and *Plant Allies for Liver Support* for additional ideas to support efficient detoxification and elimination of metabolic waste.

Suppositories: Possible Applications

Suppositories provide an alternative format for administering some therapeutic substances. It is useful to recall this option during problem-solving sessions, such as when there exists difficulty in swallowing or there is frustration with pills. Caution: The pharmacology of drug-delivery is a complex field; delivery methods are specific to each substance under consideration as well as therapeutic goal. Do not assume suppositories are an appropriate route; always discuss alternative delivery formats with a pharmacist.

- **Some drugs can be administered this way**: to bypass a sensitive palette; to outmaneuver nausea; if recipient can't swallow, etc. Some drugs can be prescribed in this format; others can be transformed into suppositories in the compounding pharmacy. **Very important**: Do not attempt home preparations with drugs that are tightly dosed for safe and effective use—Consult with your pharmacist as to appropriateness with drug in question and to obtain effective product.

- **Morphine**, with its bitter taste, can be prepared as a bolus for rectal or vaginal insertion. Drips or patches of pain-relieving drugs are other common solutions used in current medical practice. Discuss options with physician or pharmacist.

- **Some medicinal herbs** can also be administered in this manner.

  To make suppositories: Professional suppository molds can be purchased through full-service pharmacies or pharmacy supply companies. First, stabilize molds in a baking dish or other supportive surface. Next, melt the cocoa butter in the top of a double boiler. While it is melting, add desired dose of herb [liquid or powdered extract] into each chamber. When the cocoa butter is liquid, remove from heat. Before it cools, carefully pour the melted butter into the molds. Allow them to harden. When suppositories are solidified, remove from molds. Store in an airtight, dated, well-labeled jar in the refrigerator or other cool spot—out of the reach of children.

Chapped Lips

Lips can become dry and eventually peel or crack if not attended to regularly. If dry, chapped lips are associated with dry skin generally, first explore whether sufficient water is being consumed and whether healthful fats are part of the daily diet.

- **B complex vitamins** may be indicated, particularly if the corners of the mouth are raw. Sublingual and liquid forms are available if swallowing pills is problematic.

- **Zinc** supports tissue healing. See section on **Loss of Taste/Smell** below for more discussion.

- **Herb-based lip balms**: The best are made from herbs infused into and blended with quality oils, thickened with beeswax or cocoa butter. Look for natural ingredients such as calendula, chamomile, rose, jojoba oil, shea butter, coconut oil, etc., either unscented or flavored with pure plant essential oils. These tend to help the skin heal, not just offer moistening.

- **Hyaluronic acid**: As liquid directly applied with cotton swab or in lip balm form. See subsequent section on **Dry Mouth** for details.

Dry Mouth

Known in medical parlance as xerostomia, dry mouth occurs from an insufficiency of salivary secretions. This may be caused through the aging process or as a side effect of drug ingestion or radiation therapies. It can be experienced as an unpleasant sensation and also can compromise overall oral health.

- Root or leaf of **marshmallow** [*Althea officinalis*] or **common mallow** [*Malva* spp.]. Soothes and moistens mucous membranes. Ideally, prepare as a cold infusion, to extract more of the mucilage—then sip throughout the day. If this preparation feels too daunting, choose marshmallow *leaf* and use as a simple tea prepared with mildly warm water.

  To make a cold infusion of the root or leaves, fill a small muslin sack half full with the herb. Suspend the bag just over the lip of a quart jar and fill the jar with room-temperature water. Screw the lid on over the sack's drawstring. Steep for at least one hour to overnight. [Refrigerate if leaving overnight.] Remove sack from infusion. For immune-compromised patients, heat ½-1 cup of the brew as needed to reduce potential pathogens before serving—or simply use alternate strategies.

- **Slippery elm bark** [*Ulmus* spp.]. Like marshmallow, very soothing to mucous membranes. Readily available lozenges are gently mucilaginous and may be sucked on throughout the day as needed—but this does require some saliva to work. Alternately, sprays containing slippery elm are available or the plain powdered bark can be made into a soothing gruel that is eaten by the spoonful.

  To make slippery elm gruel, place about 1-2 tablespoons into a tiny bowl or tea cup. Gradually, stir in room-temperature water until the consistency is something like a watery paste. A small bit of honey may be added, both for sweeter taste and to contribute natural antimicrobial benefits. Eat slowly, using the tongue to swish each spoonful around the mouth before swallowing.

- Mix equal parts **coconut oil** and **vegetable glycerine**. Swish around mouth as needed.

- Stimulating tincture of **prickly ash bark** [*Zanthoxylum clava-herculis, Z. americanum*] or **spilanthes** [*Spilanthes acmela, S. oleraea*] to perk up the salivary glands and promote gum health: 10-20 drops in a little water 3-6 times per day, used as a rinse held in the mouth for about a full minute before spitting. In addition to stimulating circulation, topical use of both spilanthes and prickly ash acts as a local anesthetic, and is anti-inflammatory and antimicrobial. Chewing on a small piece of peeled **fresh organically grown ginger** can offer similar benefits, if tolerable and condition-appropriate.

- **Acupuncture treatment**, given concurrently with radiation therapy for head and neck cancer, has been shown to reduce xerostomia, according to clinical research.[6]

- **Hyaluronic acid [HA]**, aka hyaluronan. HA is a ubiquitous natural substance found throughout the body, especially concentrated in the eyes, joints, and skin. A thick, sticky substance, HA is the primary agent responsible for the viscosity and lubricating qualities of synovial fluid, and for years its benefits in joint health have been appreciated and explored. It is also being used currently, via various means of administration, to support eye, skin and gum health. HA has different roles depending on tissue location. Used topically, it can be soothing, moistening and healing when directly applied to gums and the lining of the mouth.[7] Lozenges are also available.

Dental Hygiene

If at all possible, visit the dentist for routine teeth cleaning at least two weeks before start of any therapeutic regimen that may impact oral health. If appropriate, consider a course of herbal antimicrobial therapy following this visit to minimize bacterial impact on a compromised system.

During chemotherapy or radiation it may be advised to avoid flossing, so as not to damage gum tissue made more sensitive by these therapies. Adhering to this, of course, creates a challenge in terms of keeping the mouth and teeth healthy. [It must be mentioned that those who are working with complementary nutrients that support gum health may not encounter this issue and may find they are able to floss as normal, using floss designed for sensitive gums.] One's regular dentist can provide pastes and rinses specifically intended to help with this circumstance. Here, a few alternatives from the herbal world are offered:

- **Tongue cleaning**: Particularly after morning brushing, use a stainless steel tongue cleaner to gently scrape any bacterial "fur" from the tongue surface. Work carefully from back to front several times to accomplish this; rinse the cleaning tool as needed. Rinse mouth well afterwards, with plain water or with any of the following suggested substances. Tongue cleaning is an ancient Ayurvedic practice.

- **Herbal mouth rinses** manufactured by reputable companies such as HerbPharm, Wise Woman Herbals, The Herbalist, Herbalist & Alchemist, Gaia Herbs, BioForce, etc. These formulas contain various combinations of plants traditionally used for mouth care—plants that are antimicrobial, astringent, pain-relieving, and stimulating to circulation within gum tissue. Such allies include spilanthes, propolis, goldenseal, myrrh, cloves, peppermint, cinnamon, rosemary, thyme, witch hazel, red root [*Ceonothus* spp.] and others.

    To use commercial herbal mouth rinse: After gently cleaning the teeth and gums, rinse well with water. Dilute a dropperful of herbal rinse in a small amount of water and swish in mouth for a full minute. Spit out when done.

- **Triphala as mouth rinse**. It has been shown that rinsing with a solution of this ancient Ayurvedic blend of three highly esteemed healing fruits inhibits plaque formation, similar in effect to chlorhexidine.[8,9]

    To use Triphala rinse: Combine a half-teaspoon of organic Triphala powder in half a cup of warm water. Stir well. Swish thoroughly around mouth and gums for at least one minute. Spit it out. If working on a specific oral problem such as gingivitis or Streptococcus mutans [an organism linked to tooth decay], use twice as much Triphala powder in the rinse.

- **Infusion of green or black tea** [*Camillia sinensis*]. Rich in polyphenols, fluoride, and much more. Raw leaves and water extractions from the tea plant have been shown to help promote oral health—calming gum inflammation, lessening tooth decay, possibly preventing oral cancers. Using brewed green [or black] tea as a rinse following brushing and flossing may benefit oral health. One study showed that holding either brewed tea or green tea leaves in the mouth for 2-5 minutes, acted upon by saliva, released the beneficial constituents into the oral cavity.[10]

- **Tea made from culinary herbs**: Sage, thyme, rosemary, oregano, marjoram. Taken from garden or pantry, these plants—rich in essential oils—offer antimicrobial and anti-inflammatory benefits. Use cooled tea that has steeped, covered, for about 10 minutes as mouth rinse and gargle. A small amount of pure sea salt may be added for additional tissue-soothing benefit, if desired.

- Make a **strong infusion of astringent plants** you find growing around you—members of the *Rubus* clan [leaves of blackberry, raspberry, thimbleberry, salmonberry, etc.], other members of the rose family [rose petals or leaves of avens, lady's mantle, hawthorn, strawberry], leaves of many trees [alder, poplar, oak, hazel, etc.]. Infuse in recently boiled water for up to one hour. A small amount of pure sea salt may be added to the rinse for additional tissue-soothing benefit, if desired.

- Strong infusion of **rosehips** [*Rosa* spp.] used as gargle to ease sore throat or as rinse for tender mouth and gums. Astringent, cooling, and rich in collagen-supporting vitamin C.

- **Baking soda/salt mouth rinses**: To soothe irritated mucous membranes.

    Baking soda rinse #1: Combine ¼ teaspoon baking soda and 1/8 teaspoon sea salt in 1 cup warm water. Mix well until powders dissolve. Rinse mouth gently; do not swallow. Follow with plain water rinse. **Use as needed** *throughout day.* **Also use after any episode of vomiting** *to rinse gastric acids from teeth.*

    Baking soda rinse #2: Add 1 teaspoon baking soda to 1 cup warm water. Mix well until baking soda dissolves. Swish and spit. **Use before and after each meal to help minimize mucositis**, *inflamed mucous membranes.*

- **To help resolve thick saliva/mucus:**

    Baking soda rinse #3: Combine ½ teaspoon sea salt and 2 tablespoons baking soda in 4 cups warm water. Mix well until powders dissolve. Swish and spit.

    Yerba santa leaf infusion [Eriodictyon californicum]: Combine 2 teaspoons or so of this resinous expectorant herb with 2 cups of boiled water. Steep for up to 30 minutes. Drink in small amounts throughout the day.

    Zinc lozenges taken as desired.

- Use a **probiotic** product containing various strains of *Lactobacillus, Bifidobacteria,* etc. to help keep populations of beneficial/damaging bacteria in balance. Some products are specially formulated to replenish strains of beneficial bacteria native to the mouth. Use according to product label instructions—or use either a diluted liquid or a capsule's contents added to water as a mouth rinse. See ***Resources*** for suppliers.

- Some formulations offer **enzymes specifically useful for dissolving excess mucus**. See chapter on ***Resources*** for suppliers.

Mouth Sores [Mucositis] / Raw Mouth

*Like dry mouth, these painful manifestations are also often a consequence of chemical or radiation therapy. Aphthous ulcers, or canker sores, can also manifest with abnormally high stress levels. You may find one or more of the suggestions below to offer relief. As the quality of the tissue changes, new strategies may be tried. Using L-glutamine regularly as well as sucking on ice or popsicles during administration of some chemo agents may prevent mouth sores from occurring in the first place. Each person and each therapeutic protocol makes for a unique combination of factors. Thus, the assortment of remedies offered below. Also, check the previous section **Dental Hygiene** for additional suggestions.*

*To protect a sensitive inner mouth, smoothies and freshly juiced or pureed vegetables may be vehicles to support nutrition if such continuing sustenance is desired and mouth sores discourage eating. See the section on **Simple Foods** for more ideas. Additionally, please review the chapter **Strategies for Tube Feeding [Enteral Nutrition]** if the condition of mouth and throat requires that intervention.*

- The essential amino acid **L-lysine**, a nutritional factor in collagen production and wound healing, may help prevent or lessen the severity of mouth sores when supplemented internally— including ulcerations caused by chemotherapy or radiation treatments. Fish, dairy products, and nutritional yeast are good food sources. Focus on legumes and fruits and vegetables to help ensure adequate lysine in the diet.

- **Mouth rinse prepared from turmeric rhizome** has been clinically demonstrated to significantly delay and reduce radiation-induced oral mucositis in cancer patients receiving head/neck treatments, compared with cohort using povidone-iodine gargle.[11]

    To prepare turmeric mouth rinse: Place ¼ teaspoon turmeric powder into a cup and gradually mix in ¼ cup warm water. Use as mouth rinse after cleaning teeth or at any time during day to prevent or relieve inflammation. Be aware of its staining pigments.

- **Zinc lozenges**. Zinc is a factor in wound healing and immunity.

- See suggestions on **marshmallow root cold infusion** and **slippery elm** in the previous **Dry Mouth** section. Alternately, ice cubes or popsicles made from marshmallow infusion can be used, both to soothe sores already present and to prevent them from arising in the first place. Some chemotherapy agents are known to provoke mouth sores—sucking on ice or popsicles while the medicines are being infused into the body can limit or prevent mouth tissue problems. Ask the oncology nurse managing the infusion to alert you when to use ice.

- **Aloe vera gel or juice**, from the gelatinous inner leaf of homegrown plants or sourced commercially from organically cultivated plants prepared without preservatives. Soothing and pain relieving, anti-inflammatory and wound-healing.

- **Propolis** tincture or spray [diluted], or lozenges may be applied directly several times per day. Propolis, the name given to tree resins collected by honeybees and incorporated into their hives, is an antiseptic substance that has an anesthetizing and anti-inflammatory effect on the tissue it contacts. *Please note*: Use with caution if prone to allergy or hypersensitivity to bee stings, bee products, or tree resins.

- **Licorice root** powder alone or mixed with honey and applied to raw area—or **DGL tabs** [deglycyrrhizinated licorice] dissolved in mouth several times per day. A thick, tar-like **solid extract** of licorice root may also be directly applied to sores.

- **AlkaThymol**, a patent remedy long recommended to promote oral health, can be used as an alkalinizing, antiseptic mouth rinse. Use full strength for this purpose. Once manufactured by the pharmaceutical company Parke-Davis [now owned by Pfizer], it is currently available in natural health stores, produced by Heritage Products.

- **Warm miso broth** can feel wonderfully soothing to irritated mouth tissue. Simply add a dollop of traditionally prepared, organic miso paste to a cup or bowl of freshly boiled water. Stir well to infuse. Sip slowly. Swish some around the mouth as well, if desired. Miso is a traditional fermented salty soybean condiment that is rich in live microbial cultures that are beneficial to digestive tract health. The lighter the miso, the sweeter and milder it tends to be. Darker miso is more salty and sharper tasting.

- Use a **probiotic** product containing various strains of *Lactobacillus, Bifidobacteria*, etc.—either a diluted liquid or a capsule's contents added to water—as a mouth rinse. Alternately, sugar-free lozenges that contain probiotic strains native to the oral cavity are available. These are slowly dissolved in the mouth after brushing. Diluted unsweetened organic yogurt can also be used for this purpose.

- **Spilanthes** [*Spilanthes acmela, S. oleraea*] to perk up the salivary glands and promote gum and mouth health: 10-20 drops in a little water 3-6 times per day, used as a rinse held in the mouth for about a full minute before spitting. In addition to stimulating circulation, topical use of spilanthes acts as a local anesthetic, and is anti-inflammatory and antimicrobial.

- **Calendula succus** added to water as rinse. Anti-fungal and antibacterial, calendula [*Calendula officinalis*] promotes skin healing and lessens inflammation. A succus is a preparation made by juicing a suitable fresh plant and adding about 25% alcohol to prevent spoilage [that is, 3 parts juice by volume to 1 part grain alcohol by volume].

- **L-glutamine** consumption as well as use as a rinse has been shown to lessen mouth sores in those undergoing chemotherapy. Glutamine, an amino acid, is a component of whey protein powder and can also be supplemented on its own. Please see the section on **Lack of Appetite / Weight Loss** for more information. L-glutamine powder may also be used mixed with saline solution and swished in mouth several times a day.

- **Kava** [*Piper methysticum*]: Preparations from root. Mucous membrane analgesic, among other applications. Can be swished in mouth to ease inflammation and pain. Use water-based extractions or low-alcohol tincture diluted into water for this purpose. *Cautions*: Please see entry in ***Plants to Support the Nervous System***.

  To make simple preparation: *Soak 1 tablespoon kava root powder in 1 cup room-temperature water for 30 minutes. Stir frequently. Add 1 tablespoon non-GMO lecithin and blend in blender. Strain and use liquid as mouth swish.*

- **Cleavers** [*Gallium* spp.] and/or **chickweed** [*Stellaria media*]: Soothing and wound healing. In season, fresh succulent plants may be juiced and frozen in ice trays. Sucking these cubes, or chips from them, may be soothing and healing to raw or ulcerated mouth tissue.

- Strong infusion of **rosehips** [*Rosa* spp.] used as gargle to ease sore throat or as rinse for tender mouth and gums. Astringent, cooling, and rich in vitamin C.

- Strong infusion of **raspberry leaves** [*Rubus idaeus*] used as gargle or as rinse. Astringent, antioxidant, nutrient dense [e.g., calcium, iron, magnesium, manganese, selenium, vitamins A and C…]

- **Hyaluronic acid** [HA], aka hyaluronan. HA is a ubiquitous natural substance found throughout the body, especially concentrated in the eyes, joints, and skin. A thick, sticky substance, HA is the primary agent responsible for the viscosity and lubricating qualities of synovial fluid, and for years its benefits in joint health have been appreciated and explored. It is also being used currently, via various means of administration, to support eye, skin and gum health. HA has different roles depending on tissue location—Used topically, it can be soothing, moistening and healing when directly applied to gums and the lining of the mouth.[12] Lozenges are also available.

- **Neem oil** [*Azadirachta indica*]: extracted from leaf and seed. Astringent, antibacterial, antifungal, insecticidal, anthelmintic. Neem is an Ayurvedic remedy for many internal and external applications. The oil is traditionally applied to the skin to treat stiff joints, wounds and ulcerations [including in the mouth], boils, ringworm, eczema, urticaria, scabies, lice, leprosy, sprains, etc. Has pronounced aroma and taste.

- **Folic acid**, part of the B vitamin complex, may have a role to play in promoting healing. See **Building the Blood** for information on sources. The B vitamin complex as a whole is essential to support a bodymind undergoing chronic stress.

- **Red root** [*Ceanothus americanus*]: root bark. Astringent, antimicrobial. Used as a mouth-rinse—as a water-based decoction or as liquid extract diluted in water—red root may be useful in addressing canker sores and/or gum inflammation.

- **Rosemary** [*Rosmarinus officinalis*]: leaf. Antiseptic, astringent, antimicrobial, anti-inflammatory. Tea or tincture diluted into warm water may be used as a mouth-rinse.

- **Sage** [*Salvia officinalis*]: leaf. Antimicrobial, antiseptic to mucosa, mildly astringent, anti-inflammatory. Tea or tincture diluted into warm water used as a mouth-rinse.

- **Silver hydrosol**, broadly antimicrobial, may be used as mouth rinse or spray.

Yeast Infections / Thrush

Overgrowth of Candida albicans can present as "yeast infection" anywhere on the body; when localized in the mouth, it is called thrush. These conditions can be challenging to clear in an immune-compromised individual. Ingestion of simple carbohydrates such as sugars contributes to a hospitable internal environment, both through their direct biochemical contribution and through suppression of immune function. Eliminate these as much as possible. See the book **The Body Ecology Diet** *listed in the* **Recommended Reading** *chapter for a detailed discussion of dietary considerations. Meanwhile, the following suggestions offer a place to begin.*

- See previous section on **Mouth Sores** for additional applicable suggestions.

- **Probiotic supplementation** to enhance populations of beneficial intestinal organisms. Choose a brand containing multiple species of bacteria: for example *Lactobacillus rhamnosus, L. acidophilus, L. plantarum, L. salivarius, Bifidobacterium breve, B. infantis, B. longum, B. bifidum, B. lactis*, etc. Take internally and use as mouth rinse also, if desired. See note above under **Mouth Sores**.

- A non-glycemic sugar known as **fructoogliosaccharide (FOS)** can be taken in supplemental form to enhance the benefit and activity of the probiotics. It is sometimes included in probiotic formulations. FOS is said to provide readily available food for the beneficial flora and thereby helps their numbers to flourish while not feeding "bad" gut bacteria. FOS, as inulin, is naturally found in plants such as Jerusalem artichoke, jicama, burdock root, dandelion root, chicory, artichoke, asparagus and more—sourcing directly from foods is ideal.

- **Traditionally cultured foods** may be of benefit in re-establishing proper microbial balance in the body, if tolerated by the individual. Kraut, miso, and unsweetened yogurt are some of these foods. The key is that these foods be naturally fermented, containing live cultures. For thrush, warm miso soup or diluted yogurt can be swished around the mouth. Again, please refer to the book *The Body Ecology Diet* for more information.

- Numerous natural substances possess broad antimicrobial properties. Consider extracts of **Oregon grape root** [*Mahonia* spp.], **usnea lichen** [*Usnea* spp.], **propolis resin**, **spilanthes herb** [*Spilanthes acmela, S. oleracea*]—used singularly or in combination. A typical starting dose for internal use might be one dropperful in a little water three to six times per day.

- **Pau d'arco** [*Tabebuia impetiginosa*]: This South American tree's inner bark possesses antifungal/anti-yeast properties, plus antibacterial, antiviral, astringent, anti-inflammatory activity. Also traditionally used as anticancer herb. Use as mouth rinse as needed—or drink as tea for systemic issues.

  To use: Dilute tincture in water or prepare as light decoction, simmering 2-3 teaspoons in 2 cups of water for about 15 minutes and dividing this brew into two to three doses during the day.

- **Cardamom seed** [*Elettaria cardamomum*]: Inhibits growth of yeast, fungi, bacteria.

  To prepare: Combine ½ teaspoon dry seed with 1 cup boiled water. Steep, covered, for 30 minutes. Use amount as needed for mouth rinse, other direct application, or as tea.

- **Thyme** [*Thymus vulgarus*]: Inhibits growth of yeast, fungi, bacteria, viruses.

  To prepare: Combine 1 teaspoon dry leaf with 1 cup boiled water. Steep, covered, for 20 minutes. Drink as tea two to three times per day, use as skin wash, or use as needed for mouth rinse. Prepare freshly each time.

- **Organic apple cider vinegar** wash for yeasty skin or mouth.

  To use: Combine 1 pint of warm water and 1 tablespoon of organic apple cider vinegar. Swish around the mouth and gums for a full minute. Can also apply as needed to affected skin. This can also be administered as a douche, as appropriate.

- **Baking soda** wash for yeasty skin or mouth.

  To prepare baking soda rinse: Add 1 teaspoon baking soda to 1 cup warm water. Mix well until powder dissolves. Swish around the mouth for a full minute and spit.

- **Essential oils**, 1-2 drops—mixed in a tiny bit of honey and water, blended into yogurt, or added to the cider vinegar wash above—can be swished around the mouth. They may be used individually or in combinations. **Rosewood** [*Aniba rosaeodora*], **tea tree** [*Melaleuca alternifolia*], **myrrh** [*Commiphora myrrha*], **rosemary** [*Rosmarinus officinalis*], **lavender** [*Lavandula* spp.], **patchouli** [*Pogostemon patchouli*] essential oils are among those indicated. Rosewood is antiseptic, antifungal, antiviral, calming; tea tree is antiseptic, antifungal, vulnerary; myrrh is anti-inflammatory, antiseptic, antifungal, vulnerary, astringent; rosemary is antiseptic, stimulating to circulation, uplifting; lavender is antiseptic, calming, uplifting; patchouli is antifungal and calming.

- Like thyme above, the leaves of **rosemary** and **sage** are broadly antimicrobial, including antifungal, as well as anti-inflammatory and astringent. Tea or tincture diluted into warm water may be used as a rinse, compress, or footbath.

Herpes Eruptions

The stress of unwellness itself or the responsibility of caregiving can provoke an outbreak of Herpes simplex sores on the lips, around the mouth, etc. The same stress can result in a Herpes outbreak in the nose, in the genital area or a Herpes zoster manifestation on the trunk of the body [shingles]. Shingles is addressed in its own section later; the other Herpes manifestations can be addressed with the suggestions below.

- Take the initial signs of pending outbreak as **a signal to rest**. Call upon others in the extended circle of support to pitch in with tasks that need to be done and cannot be deferred. See section on **Disturbed Sleep/Insomnia** for additional support.

- **Apply ice** to area at first sensation of tingling or heat. Repeat as often as possible to quiet down the nerve. Combine each application of ice with an opportunity to pause, rest and relax.

- Increase **water** consumption.

- **Avoid or limit L-arginine-rich foods** such as: nuts; sesame and sunflower seeds; peas and lentils; oats, corn, buckwheat and barley; chocolate; coconut. Excessive levels of the amino acid L-arginine in the diet [especially relative to L-lysine] can promote eruption of *Herpes simplex* lesions…

- **Consider taking L-lysine** internally, particularly if the diet has been heavy with nuts, seeds, grains. The amino acid L-lysine helps balance L-arginine dominance and helps to inhibit the *Herpes* virus—may help to prevent outbreak or shorten duration of lesions. Supports proper wound healing. A dose of 1,500-3,000 mg divided through the day is typically recommended for this purpose. Fish, dairy products, and nutritional yeast are good food sources. Focus on legumes and fruits and vegetables to help ensure adequate lysine in the diet.

- **Boost dietary nutrition** to promote wound healing, particularly vitamins A [as beta-carotene], B-complex, C and E, zinc, lysine. See section on **Shingles/Herpes Zoster** for food sources of these nutrients. Perhaps it goes without saying that the following foods should *always* be avoided in the promotion of optimal health: **Avoid** simple sugars, white flour products, refined foods of all kinds, transfatty acids [hydrogenated or partially hydrogenated fats].

- **Lemon balm** [*Melissa officinalis*]: Calming, antiviral [against *Herpes*], antibacterial, antispasmodic, mildly astringent, mildly choleretic. Taken internally as extract, strong tea or decoction [to concentrate the tannins]. Can also be applied topically to lesion in compress or salve/ointment form. Applied directly, a mashed fresh leaf, diluted **Melissa essential oil**, as well as **rose essential oil**, can speed remission. The essential oils may be extended in a small amount of oil—jojoba, grapeseed oil, etc.

- **St. Johnswort** [*Hypericum perforatum*]: fresh flowering tops and leaves. Helpful antiviral nerve tonic to forestall or shorten herpes outbreaks. Nerve tissue restorative, anxiolytic, sedative, anti-inflammatory, astringent, anti-microbial, vulnerary. Used topically as infused oil or in salve; taken internally as tincture, extract in capsules, or *Hypericum* as homeopathic remedy. **Cautions**: Please see entry in *Plants to Support the Nervous System* for issues potentially pertaining to internal use.

- To ease pain, prevent itching, inhibit viral replication, and promote healing, **topically apply one or more of the following**, as needed: licorice root solid extract or powder, lysine in gel or salve, propolis resin in gel or salve, St. Johnswort infused oil or salve, zinc oxide cream [diaper rash creams, etc.], dragon's blood aka Sangre de drago [*Croton lechleri*], neem oil. All have a role to play. In addition to the supplemental use of lysine previously mentioned, propolis, licorice, zinc and dragon's blood **may also be used internally**. *Please note*: Use propolis with caution if prone to allergy or hypersensitivity to bee stings, bee products, or tree resins.

- **Additional antiviral essential oils** specifically active against *Herpes simplex*: Bergamot, *Eucalyptus globulus*, hyssop, tea tree, niaouli, *Melissa*, basil, geranium, sweet marjoram, rosemary, peppermint, clove bud. Myrrh essential oil also offers antiviral and anti-inflammatory benefits. Extend in a bit of oil or cream as indicated per essential oil.

- **Vitamin E oil** can be applied topically to prevent scarring and ease pain. As mentioned above, it may also be taken internally to promote wound healing.

- **To prevent recurrence**, embark on a course of deep renewal with adaptogenic botanical tonics—to boost immunity and lessen physiological reactivity to stress. See the chapter on ***Adaptogenic and Tonic Plant Allies*** or work with a practitioner to determine which plants are most relevant for your circumstances.

Diarrhea

Loose or watery stool can result from causes including: anxiety or overexcitement; allergic reactions; pharmaceutical side effect; food contamination; intestinal infection, infestation, or other disruption of gut ecology. Acute diarrhea typically resolves within a few days; should the condition persist, it may be a signal that something more chronic or entrenched needs to be addressed. Always seek professional assistance if there is pus, mucus or blood in the stools, if fever is present, if it persists for more than 24 hours [infant], or if the person becomes dehydrated.

- **Restore fluid and electrolyte balance**: Teas; broth (miso paste added into warm water as broth); seaweed-rich soup; fresh lemon juice in water; coconut water. See appendix ***Water and Electrolytes*** and the chapter ***A Few Recipes for Gentle Foods***.

- **Astringent teas**, drunk freely: Blackberry leaf, red raspberry leaf, thimbleberry leaf, yarrow leaf and flowers, lady's mantle, avens, roots of wild geranium, and so on. Plain **black tea** is a global standby, without milk or sweetener for this purpose.

- **Blackberry root bark** [*Rubus* spp.] tincture. Strongly astringent. Start with one full dropper as a dose, repeated as needed. Add to ginger tea to prevent griping.

    Dire-Aid Tea: *Equal parts chopped blackberry root, oak bark, cinnamon chips. Add ¼+ cup of the blend to 1 quart water. Bring to a boil, then simmer 10-15 minutes. Let stand, covered, for another 30+ minutes before straining. Drink 1-4 ounces at a time, as needed.*

- **Betonite clay**, food grade. Add ½ to 2 teaspoons to 1 cup of water. Let stand one hour or overnight. Drink once per day until resolution.

- **For diarrhea caused by microbial infection or parasitic presence**: Antimicrobial herbs such as garlic, usnea lichen, propolis, Oregon grape root [all berberine-containing plants], andrographis; antiparasite, vermifuge plants such as elecampane, cloves, wormwood, black walnut green hull, garlic, neem, andrographis, quassia bark, medical *Cannabis*... Foundational immune support is also indicated. See entry on L-glutamine in this section. Please see section on **Drug-Resistant Bacterial Infections [MRSA, VRSA, C. diff.]** for other considerations. *Note*: Use propolis with caution if prone to allergy or hypersensitivity to bee stings, bee products, or tree resins.

- *Clostridium difficile [C. diff.]* **infection**: A healthcare-associated bacterial infection. Some 14,000 deaths in the United States are caused by this infection each year, according to the Center for Disease Control [CDC] in 2013. Symptoms include: watery diarrhea, fever, loss of appetite, nausea, abdominal pain. Older adults and others with immune-compromised circumstances are most at risk, particularly following courses of prescribed antibiotic medicines and exposure to medical settings. According to the CDC, *C. diff.* spores can be found on bed linens, bed rails, bathroom fixtures, medical equipment, etc. It can be passed from person to person, including from medical personnel to patients. Consult the webpage www.CDC.gov for more information. **Suggested approach**: Clean your own hands after all medical visits, using hot water and soap and/or essential oil based antimicrobial sprays. For temporary symptom relief, explore suggestions in this section and seek medical help if *C. diff.* is suspected. Consider supplementing with *Saccharomyces boulardii*, a non-pathogenic yeast that has been prescribed for at least 30 years both to prevent and to treat diarrheal diseases caused by bacteria. Additional studies have been recommended by researchers looking into its specific efficacy with *C. diff.*[13] In my experience, *Saccharomyces boulardii* has a profoundly useful role to play, especially in combination with other probiotic strains. It may be taken concurrently with antibiotic medications.

- **Simple broth** (from non-gas-producing vegetables such as potatoes, celery, carrots) plus white rice. See *A Few Recipes for Gentle Foods*. Add traditionally cultured **miso paste** as appropriate, to replenish electrolytes and supply live microbial cultures that are beneficial to digestive tract health. The lighter the miso, the sweeter and milder it tends to be. Darker miso is more salty and sharper tasting. It is always added directly into the cup or bowl, never cooked, to preserve its full range of benefits.

- **White rice eaten with a pinch of salt** is another traditional food remedy wherever rice is a staple food.

- **Probiotics supplementation** twice a day, preferably on an empty stomach. Choose a formulation that combines numerous strains of beneficial flora: *Lactobaccilus acidophilus, L. rhamnosus, L. plantarum, Bifidobacteria longum, Streptococcus thermophilus*, etc. Take away from any antibiotic medications for best results.

- **L-glutamine**: An amino acid existing naturally in the body, L-glutamine is a building block for proteins, produced in the muscles and distributed where needed by the blood. It is a factor in many metabolic processes including repair of the mucosal lining of the gut. Cabbage juice, a source of glutamine, has a proven record of enhancing healing of peptic ulcers. L-glutamine can be supplemented if needed—during situations of nutritional deficiency, metabolic stress, muscle wasting/cachexia [cancer, HIV/AIDS, etc.], tissue injury [surgery, radiation, chemotherapy, etc.], enteric infection—particularly if the digestive/intestinal membranes have been compromised. Shown to improve gut health and immune function. Whey protein is a rich source of L-glutamine; isolated glutamine powders are also available. Both are easily added to smoothies.

- **Carob bean powder** [*Ceratonia siliqua*]: Demulcent, anti-diarrheal. Absorbs fluids, so be mindful of ingesting sufficient water. Do not take if there is bowel obstruction. Take at least one hour away from any vital oral medication.

- **To ease cramping**: Ginger, cinnamon, peppermint, chamomile, or wild yam root taken internally as hot water extractions or as water/alcohol or encapsulated extracts. Enteric-coated peppermint essential oil is also available, for direct delivery to lower bowel. A hot water bottle placed on the abdomen can also be soothing.

Constipation

Constipation can occur as a side effect of certain medications, lack of movement or exercise, insufficient intake of fiber-rich foods or water, liver/gallbladder dysfunction, etc. Prolonged constipation can cause physical discomfort and emotional edginess.

Try these remediations in the following order: Movement, dietary/hydration changes, massage, castor oil packs with heat, laxative foods/teas, enemas.

Please note that agents strong enough to assertively empty the bowel, such as cascara sagrada, senna, high doses of vitamin C, and such are generally contraindicated during pregnancy as they might stimulate uterine contractions.

- Ensure **sufficient water intake.** At least 48-60 ounces per day is the minimum required to replenish what is lost through perspiration, respiration, urination, etc. A useful rule of thumb is a minimum of eight ounces of water for each 20 pounds of body weight; for example, at least 56 ounces of water for a person weighing 140 pounds [$140 \div 20 = 7 \times 8 = 56$].

- **Lemon juice in warm water**, especially first thing in the morning on an empty stomach. Try the juice of half a lemon to 1 cup of water.

- Ensure **sufficient beneficial oils** in the daily diet: Fish, flaxseed, olive, coconut…

- **Avoid highly refined foods** [white rice, white flour…] and dense animal proteins and include **more fiber-rich foods**, such as whole grains, berries, vegetables—to whatever degree possible.

- **Abdominal massage**, preferably in a rolling, rhythmic clockwise direction.

- **Castor oil pack** applied to lower abdomen to stimulate peristalsis.

  To prepare a castor oil pack: Fold undyed cotton or wool flannel 2–4 thicknesses to cover an 8–12" area. Soak flannel with unrefined cold-pressed castor oil. Carefully press flannel out so that the cloth is just wet but not dripping. Place in baking pan and gently heat at lowest setting of oven until cloth is warm. While cloth is warming, bring a pot of water almost to boiling.

  Apply the warm cloth to the area of the body to be treated. Cover flannel with plastic or waxed paper, and top this with a carefully filled hot water bottle [as warm as is comfortably bearable] wrapped in a small towel or flannel pillowcase. Relax and breathe deeply.

  Leave pack on for 40-60 minutes. Refresh the water bottle with hot water, if needed. After the session is completed, wash the oil off your body with warm water and baking soda (1 teaspoon to 1 pint water). Store oily flannel cloth in covered pan or container for future use (in refrigerator, if possible). After 20–30 uses, thoroughly cleanse the flannel and reuse as needed.

- **Laxative foods**: Dried prunes or figs, soaked overnight; flaxseeds, chia seeds mixed with water. Drink any remaining soak water as well. As an alternative, after soaking the fruit, a "pudding" can be made by blending 2 parts prunes with 1 part figs—this can be eaten a teaspoonful at a time throughout the day.

- **Prune juice** taken in small amount before breakfast or in evening, either taken straight or diluted in warm or room-temperature water.

- **Triphala**: A classic intestinal tonic of Ayurveda, Triphala is composed of three fruits: amalaki [*Phyllanthus emblica*], haritaki [*Terminalia chebula*], bibhitaki [*Terminalia belerica*]. Considered in Ayurveda to be both a rejuvenative and detoxifying agent. Gently reinvigorates bowel function, while delivering antioxidant and anti-carcinogenic compounds such as ellagic acid to the system. Available in capsules or tablets—or as traditional powder, which is added to water and drunk. **Licorice root powder or tea** can be taken with the blend if more moistening of the bowel is needed.

  To prepare Triphala powder: Add ¼-½ teaspoon Triphala powder to 1 cup warm water. Stir well, then drink. Triphala may be used alone or with the addition of 1 teaspoon of either ground organic flax seed or chia seed for their bulking properties. Licorice root powder [¼-½ teaspoon] may be added to help moisten the bowel.

- **Amalaki / Amla** [*Phyllanthus emblica*] fruit, one of the three ingredients in the Ayurvedic rasayana tonic **Triphala**, is sometimes used alone. It is strongly antioxidant, rich in ascorbic acid, gallic acid, and ellagic acid. Amla fruit has also been shown to be immunomodulating, antimicrobial, liver protective, anti-carcinogenic, and more.

- **Vitamin C / ascorbic acid**: High doses stimulate peristalsis of lower bowel and promote evacuation. This dosage level, which varies by individual, is referred to as "bowel tolerance."

- **Magnesium**: Classic relief for constipation and hardened stools. Typically, 400-800 mg. is recommended.

- **Beverage teas to relieve constipation**: Drink at bedtime to promote morning evacuation. These teas are listed in *descending order from the most strongly motivating at the top to the most gentle at the bottom.* If at all possible, start with the gentlest ones toward the end. These options can also be used in enema solution, per instructions that follow this list.

   ◆ **Senna + Cinnamon** tea. **Senna** leaf [*Cassia senna*]: Laxative, bitter. Plus **Cinnamon** bark [*Cinnamomum verum*]: Carminative, antispasmodic, astringent, antibacterial, antifungal, demulcent. The addition of cinnamon helps prevent abdominal griping. *Cautions*: Appropriate for short-term use only; prolonged consumption of senna can lead to electrolyte imbalance, particularly potassium. Avoid using senna in intestinal obstruction or inflammation, abdominal pain of unknown origin, or for longer than eight consecutive days.

   To make tea: Combine ¼ - ½ teaspoon senna leaves + ½ teaspoon cinnamon bark [finely cut]. Steep in 1 cup boiled water for 10 minutes. Start with ¼ cup of the tea at a time.

   ◆ **Cascara sagrada + Fennel** tea. **Cascara sagrada** aged bark [*Frangula purshiana*]: Laxative, antibacterial. Plus **Fennel** seed [*Foeniculum vulgare*]: Carminative, antispasmodic, expectorant, antimicrobial. *Cautions*: Appropriate for short-term use only. Avoid using cascara in pregnancy, lactation, intestinal obstruction or inflammation, abdominal pain of unknown origin, for longer than eight consecutive days, and in children younger than 12.

   To make tea: Mix 1-2 teaspoon cascara sagrada bark with 1 teaspoon fennel seed. Steep in 1 cup boiled water for 10 minutes. Start with ¼ cup of the tea at a time.

   ◆ **Red alder** bark [*Alnus rubra*]: tea or tincture. Alterative, chologogue, mild laxative, antibacterial. Particularly indicated in constipation with clay-colored stools. For tincture, add 20-40 drops in a cup of warm water.

   To prepare tea: Add 1 teaspoon red alder bark for each cup of water used. Bring to a boil and simmer 10-15 minutes. Remove from heat and steep another 30 minutes. Drink in half-cup doses up to 3 times per day. If the bowels become unformed, reduce intake.

   ◆ **Yellow dock aged root** [*Rumex crispus*] tincture. Alterative, chologogue, mild laxative, astringent, antibacterial. Especially indicated with fat present in the stool. *Caution*: Roots contain calcium oxalate; use cautiously if history of kidney stones.

   To prepare: Add 1 dropperful to 1 cup warm water. Can also be added to burdock and dandelion root decoction noted below. Alternately, all three plants can be used in tincture form and added to warm water on daily preventive basis or as needed.

♦ **Burdock** and **dandelion root** decoction or tinctures. Two of my favorite allies for keeping the bowels moving. **Burdock** root [*Arctium* spp.]: Mild alterative, choleretic. **Dandelion** root [*Taraxacum officinale*]: Bitter tonic, cholagogue, choleretic, mild laxative [aperient], diuretic. Both burdock and dandelion roots contain inulin, a prebiotic that enhances the proliferation of beneficial flora in the gut; eat as food or prepare as water extract [decoction] for this benefit.

To make decoction: Combine 2 teaspoons of each chopped root to each 1 cup water and simmer for 20 minutes or more. Start with ½ cup of the brew at a time.

♦ **Fenugreek seed** tea [*Trigonella foenum-graecum*]: Demulcent, emollient, stomachic, expectorant. A moistening laxative. *Cautions*: Avoid during pregnancy unless under supervision of qualified healthcare practitioner. Mucilage may slow the absorption of orally administered drugs—take drugs one hour prior to consumption or several hours after.

To make decoction: Simmer 2 teaspoons seed in 1 cup water for 10 minutes.

♦ **Licorice root** decoction or tea [*Glycyrrhiza* spp.]: Anti-inflammatory, antispasmodic, demulcent, expectorant, antioxidant, antimicrobial. A gentle, moistening laxative. *Cautions*: Avoid prolonged use or during pregnancy unless under supervision of qualified healthcare practitioner. Avoid in hypertension, liver disorders, edema, kidney or cardiovascular disease.

*For decoction: Simmer 2 teaspoons chopped root in 1 cup water for 10 minutes. **For tea** of finely chopped root: Infuse root with freshly boiled water for 10-15 minutes.*

• **Enemas**: Prepare warm water or a laxative tea [above] for rectal insertion.

To administer enema: Cool boiled water or hot tea for 10 minutes. Use ½ cup tea per each quart of body-temperature water. Carefully fill enema bag. Hold bag 2-3 feet above rectum. Retain liquid for 10-20 minutes, if possible, before evacuating.

• **Antispasmodic herbs** can be taken internally for cramping, and/or applied topically. Some examples include: tinctures of cramp bark [*Viburnum opulus*], valerian root [*Valeriana* spp.], butterbur/Western coltsfoot [*Petasites* spp.], Jamaican dogwood [*Piscidia piscipula*]. Apply tinctures to the skin undiluted like liniment or mixed into a cream or lotion. Gentle heat may be applied as well. *Caution*: Use *Petasites* internally with caution as it contains potentially toxic pyrrolizidine alkaloids [PAs]. PA-free products are available. Numerous cautions apply to internal use of *Piscidia*.

• **Culinary antispasmodics** include fennel seed [*Foeniculum vulgare*], cinnamon bark [*Cinnamomum verum*], peppermint leaf [*Mentha piperita*]—nibbled or used in tea. Enteric-coated peppermint oil capsules are specific for intestinal cramping.

Hemorrhoids / Anal Fissures

Hemorrhoids are varicosities that protrude into the interior of the rectum and/or from the exterior of the rectum. They may present no symptoms, but typically manifest with intermittent bleeding after defecation [shown on stool or toilet paper], itching, pain, and either lingering or diminishing discomfort. Hemorrhoids arise from increased pressure in the area in question—which can be caused by numerous factors including: prolonged standing or sitting; straining due to constipation, diarrhea, coughing, or vomiting; general loss of muscle tone; rectal surgery or episiotomy, etc. Please note that other contributing factors can include cardiovascular or liver disease, and infection.

*An **anal fissure** is a slit-like separation in the anal mucosa that becomes very painful during bowel movements, and can trigger painful sphincter spasms. They can arise from multiple causes: as a wound resulting from strain-related chronic constipation, from congenital anal deformity, or be related to internal bowel disease or carcinoma.*

***Medical assessment is strongly recommended** in all such cases of rectal/anal pain to determine proper treatment paths. Essentially, the palliative caregiving goals are: to ease pain, tone tissue, lessen swelling and circulatory congestion, and regulate and ease bowel function.*

- **Ensure sufficient water consumption** throughout the day, to keep the bowels moving easily and prevent the need for straining.

- Constipation and the strain to evacuate hard, dry stool can add pressure to the venous connective tissue. See the section on **Constipation** for recommendations to ease bowel movements. Low-fiber diets and dehydration are obvious contributing factors.

- **Witch hazel** [*Hamamelis virginiana*]: Long-famed in topical preparations to ease these conditions and other varicosities. Astringent, anti-inflammatory, wound-healing, blood staunching [topically applied]. Witch hazel extract is a well-known cooling liquid. Witch hazel leaves can be made into strong tea and used as a wash or compress—or compounded into salves and creams. Pads may be soaked with witch hazel and applied directly. Commercial preparations are widely available.

- Other relevant **herbal astringents and anti-inflammatories**: Yarrow, calendula, chamomile, lady's mantle, self-heal, alder, oak, avens, bistort, etc. can be of great benefit to cool and tone inflamed tissue. Infusions can be used as **compresses**, sitz baths, or perineal sprays. Oil infusions of many of these are made into **salves or suppositories** for direct application. Combining soothing, demulcent herbs with the strong astringents makes for a more comfortable experience. Commercial preparations are available in herb shops and natural health stores; see the ***Resources*** section as well. **Sitz baths** by their very nature—particularly alternating soaks in warm and cool water—help to increase circulation. A sitz-bath variation is to spray heated water [safe temperature] onto the perineal area, alternating with sprays of cold water—repeating several times.

  ***To make an herbal sitz bath**, combine 4 parts of yarrow leaves and flowers, 4 parts either comfrey or marshmallow/mallow leaves, and 2 parts calendula blossoms. Put ½ cup of this mixture into a canning jar or pot; add 1 quart boiled water and steep for 30-60 minutes or so. Strain into tub or basin and add fresh warm water. Sea salt may be added. Stir well—and sit.*

To make simple suppositories for hemorrhoids or anal fissures: Combine 1 part yarrow leaf/flower powder with 2 parts comfrey leaf or root powder. Mix together well. Melt ¼-½ cup cocoa butter in the top of a double boiler. Gradually add some of the powdered mix and stir well to combine. Continue adding the powders until the blend is thickened yet still pourable. Pour into suppository molds and allow to harden. Remove from molds and refrigerate suppositories in well-labeled canning jar. Use as needed.

- **Potato poultices** are a traditional country treatment. A slice of organically cultivated, peeled raw potato is gently inserted between the buttocks.

- **Comfrey leaf** [*Symphytum officinale*]: Tea of the leaves can be used as a compress or in sitz bath, especially for anal fissures.

- Use **baby wipes** from natural health suppliers to wipe after each bowel movement. Much more soothing and gentle to irritated bottoms than regular toilet paper.

- **Diaper cream containing zinc oxide** may provide relief applied topically.

- Alternately, after bowel movements, gently **wash with herbal infusion** of chamomile flowers, yarrow leaves and flowers, and peppermint leaves. Anti-inflammatory, astringent, cooling. Avoid peppermint if tissue is extremely raw.

- **Vitamin E**, taken internally and/or applied externally to support the healing process. The viscous oil can be applied as often as desired.

- Internally, increasing the amount of **vitamin C and flavonoid-rich foods** in the diet helps to promote integrity of venous tissue, thus aiding in prevention and treatment. Supplementing with the flavonoid **rutin** is often prescribed in naturopathic practice.

- **Internal ingestion of astringent plants** may be of benefit as well, particularly yarrow, calendula, self heal, and any of the rose family astringents, such as rose, lady's mantle, avens, red raspberry leaves, blackberry leaves, thimbleberry leaves, and so on. Avoid internal use of astringents if constipated.

- If possible, **elevate feet for 10-15 minutes** against chair or wall a few times each day while reclining in a comfortable horizontal position on the floor.

Gas / Flatulence

Gassiness can be quite an uncomfortable sensation following a meal. Relief may be found by expelling out one end or the other, but this can prove challenging for companions.

What causes flatulence is a complicated conversation, beyond the scope of this section. In addition to the considerations mentioned here are potential lactose intolerance or gluten sensitivity, gall bladder issues, use of some pharmaceutical medicines that inhibit stomach acid—as well as incompatible combining of foods at a given meal.

Gentle walking before a meal, if possible, can help release anxiety from the system and encourage appetite.

Relaxing the belly with some deep cleansing breaths should be prelude to all meal situations. This helps shift the bodymind's full attention to the matter at hand. Eating while distracted or anxious is a set-up for digestive distress. Set your concerns aside for the personal ceremony of nourishing your aliveness with the food before you.

Digestive bitters taken before eating and digestive enzymes taken with the meal can each improve digestive efficiency.

Helping to disperse intestinal gas is one of the roles of the classic carminative herbs—included in foods as seasoning, nibbled at the table, enjoyed as tea. Carminative herbs are generally contraindicated in cases of gastric reflux because they may further relax the esophageal sphincter and exacerbate the condition.

- Herbal carminative teas: **Peppermint, fennel, lemon balm, ginger, lavender flowers, caraway or dill seeds**.

     To prepare, steep 1-2 teaspoons of one of the herbs in 1 cup boiled water for 10-15 minutes. With lavender, use ¼-½ teaspoon per cup.

- **Cardamom seed** [*Elettaria cardamomum*]: Carminative.

     To prepare tea, combine ½ teaspoon dry seed with 1 cup boiled water. Steep, covered, for 30 minutes. Enjoy half a cup at a time.

- Nibble on **fennel, anise** or *Nigella sativa* [aka black seed, black cumin] seeds: Carminative.

- Ingest **bitter herbs as aperitif**—as tincture, decoction or nibbling—15-20 minutes before eating to stimulate digestive secretions. Classic bitter herbs include: dandelion root, gentian root, burdock root, ginger root, angelica root, catnip, orange peel, wormwood, mugwort. Oregon grape root and yellow/broad-leafed dock root may also be used. *Caution*: Some plants with bitter principles may stimulate the uterus, as well as digestion and the bowels and are thus avoided during pregnancy. Consult with your midwife or natural practitioner if pregnant.

- Ingest high-quality **digestive enzymes** at beginning of each meal. This can also be exceptionally helpful in cases of gastric reflux.

- Food-grade **activated charcoal** can be taken at first signs of distress. Activated charcoal literally traps gas and chemicals so they can be eliminated. Avoid concurrent ingestion with medications; take at least two hours apart.

- *Carbo vegetabilis* homeopathic: Indicated in bloating that occurs even after eating mild foods, with slow and weak digestion. *Note*: Homeopathic remedies are taken at least 15 minutes away from either food or drink.

- **Kudzu root starch**: Relief par excellence! Starch extracted from the root of *Pueraria montana var. lobata* is demulcent and profoundly soothing, helping to clear gas from the digestive system and calm an upset stomach.

  To prepare: Add 1 heaping tablespoon kudzu to 1 cup cool water. Cook over medium heat, stirring constantly. When it turns from milky to translucent, cool slightly and serve. Flavor in the mug with a bit of umeboshi plum paste for salty/sour taste and additional benefit—or a pinch of ginger root or cinnamon powder. Eat calmly, sip by sip.

- See the appendix ***Food Combining Strategies*** to work that approach.

Red, Itchy Eyes

Inflammation of the eye [conjunctiva] is generically termed conjunctivitis; however, it may arise from several different causes. Typically, conjunctivitis is the term used in common reference when the cause is bacterial or viral. Either form is easily transmitted between people. This can be especially problematic when a person is immune-compromised. Stringent personal hygiene is called for to lessen susceptibility and avoid contagion. If contracted, pharmaceutical methods may be required to fully and promptly resolve so that suffering does not drag on. The most common types are noted below.

Bacterial conjunctivitis: Usually affects both eyes. Symptoms may include sense of heat and discomfort; a gritty feeling; sticky discharge, particularly in the morning, sometimes gluing the lids together.

Viral conjunctivitis: Symptoms may include reddened eyeballs; watery discharge; swollen eyelids; glassy looking sclera [white of the eye]; distorted vision; general symptoms similar to common cold, including swollen lymph nodes.

Itchy, red eyes and lids may sometimes be an allergic reaction: to an environmental irritant, to drugs, to foods. Reactive conjunctivitis usually involves intense itching and possible stringy discharge. It is often related to seasonal pollen, dust mites, smoke, chlorine, chemical fumes.

- **Compress** closed eyes with organic plant material: chamomile or calendula flowers, eyebright or red raspberry leaves, black or green tea. Either use tea bags that have been wetted with warm water, allowed to cool, and squeezed to remove excess fluid—or follow instructions below. To prevent cross-contamination, do not re-use teabags; likewise, only fresh cloth or organic cotton balls should be used for each application.

  To prepare loose tea for compress, combine 1-2 heaping teaspoons of flowers or leaves with 1 cup boiled water. Steep for 10 minutes, then strain well through double-folded gauze or cheesecloth. Cover tea and allow it to cool until safe to apply to skin. Moisten small piece of clean cloth [sterile, if possible] or organic cotton balls with some of the tea; squeeze gently to remove excess liquid. Apply moistened cloth to closed eyes, settle back and relax.

- **Organic aloe juice or gel** can also be used as soothing compress.

- **Raw, grated, peeled organic potato** or **cucumber slices**: Apply directly to closed eyes as soothing poultice. Grate just before application. Discard material after use.

- The readily available **homeopathic brand Similasan** offers **eyedrops** that can be quite effective at providing symptom relief. Even if one has to resort to prescription antimicrobial eyedrops to resolve the situation, these gentle products can offer as-needed comfort. Similasan products are safe, sterile and free of harmful preservatives. There are numerous formulations to choose from: Dry Eye Relief, Irritated Eye Relief, Stye Eye Relief, Allergy Eye Relief, and more. Some Similasan products are also offered in children's versions.

- **Eyewash**: Can be purchased commercially or prepared at home. Some commercial brands combine alcohol-water extracts of plants such as eyebright, Oregon grape or goldenseal, water, and boric acid. To use, combine 3 drops or more of extract with saline solution in a sterile eyecup and use as an eyewash up to several times a day. Take care not to contaminate the bottle or dropper. The eyecup should be boiled in water for 10 minutes before each use; tea should be made fresh daily.

   To prepare an herbal eyewash: *Make a simple herbal tea to use as the basis of a saline solution; boil the water to be used for a full 10 minutes. Best to use distilled or filtered water. Prepare tea as usual. Be sure to strain finished brew well through **unbleached** coffee filter, cheesecloth or gauze. Impeccable cleanliness is essential for this. Bring 1 cup of the thoroughly strained tea to a boil, then dissolve 1 teaspoon non-iodized salt into this tea. Allow liquid to cool before using.*

   To prepare a simple boric acid eyewash: *Boil a pint of distilled water for 10 minutes. Mix 1/8 teaspoon boric acid into 1 cup of this sterilized water. Add 1 teaspoon non-iodized salt as well to create a saline solution. Allow liquid to cool. Strain well through gauze or unbleached coffee filter or cheesecloth. Avoid using if there is any damaged skin or open wounds around eye area.*

- The flavonoid **quercitin** and/or the enzyme **bromelain**, both potent anti-inflammatory substances, may provide benefit in supplemental form. They work synergistically and are best utilized for allergic response when taken in combination —and are found thus in readily available formulas. Quercitin stabilizes the membranes of the cells that release histamine; bromelain assists in the breakdown of proteins, and enhances absorption of nutrients, including quercitin.

- **Other internal antimicrobial or immune-supporting remedies**: Colloidal silver or silver hydrosol, propolis resin, usnea lichen, astragalus root, Echinacea, garlic…

- **Calming, relaxing plant medicines**: Options include oatstraw, tulsi basil, kava, skullcap, passionflower, magnolia bark, and many more nervine plants. See chapter on *Plants to Support the Nervous System* to help select the herbs best suited for a given individual and constellation of indications.

- **Optimize nutrition**, beta-carotene, especially: Dark leafy greens, carrots, sweet potatoes, fresh turmeric, etc. Avoid simple sugars and carbohydrates. Foods rich in zinc and Vitamin C support immunity.

Dry, Reddened Skin Around Eyes

Apply oils by dabbing onto dry skin, no closer to eyeball than along top of cheekbone or onto boney ridge along side of eyes.

- **Sea buckthorn oil** [*Hippophae rhamnoides*]: Antioxidant, anti-inflammatory, emollient/demulcent, wound healing. Take internally for dry eyes. Externally, apply to dry, damaged skin. Indicated for injuries including sun- or radiation-induced damage.

- **Rosehip seed oil** [*Rosa mosqueta, Rosa canina*]: Antioxidant, nutrient rich, wound healing, tissue regenerating. Apply to red, irritated, dry or damaged skin.

- **Vitamin E oil**: Antioxidant, stabilizes cell membranes. Helps promote proper wound healing. Pierce gelcap and squeeze out oil or purchase pure oil in glass dropper bottle. Apply to dry, irritated or damaged skin.

- **Poultice**. The widely common weeds chickweed [*Stellaria media*] and plantain [*Plantago* spp.] both make soothing, cooling poultices. Apply directly to skin as needed, each time with fresh plant material.

  > ***To prepare an herbal eye-area poultice***, *mash the leaves and stem of fresh chickweed and/or the leaves of plantain with a very tiny bit of cool or room-temperature water in a mortar and pestle—using just enough water to help the leaves grind well. Lay face up on the earth or on a surface protected with a towel or other cloth. With eyes closed, apply a generous amount of the green poultice to the irritated area, cover with a clean folded cloth to hold in place, and relax. Rest there until the poultice material becomes warm to the touch. Re-apply throughout the day as desired with fresh plant material.*

Pruritis / Itchy Skin

*Pruritis is severe itching that is often a consequence of disease process, causing discomfort and fueling agitation. Topical treatments may offer temporary respite but internal support of the liver and nervous system may provide more lasting relief. Screening for iron deficiency may also be relevant. Be sure to see **Plants to Support the Nervous System** and the chapters on supporting **Liver Health** as well.*

- Monitor water intake to maintain **sufficient hydration**. See previous section discussing **Hydration** and see appendix: ***Water, Hydration and Electrolytes***.

- Ensure **sufficient beneficial oils** in the daily diet: Fish, flaxseed oil, extra virgin olive oil, extra virgin coconut oil, organic avocado, etc.

- Ensure **adequate dietary supply of skin-supporting nutrients** such as beta-carotene: Dark leafy greens, yellow and orange vegetables, seaweed, etc. The B vitamin complex is also supportive to skin and nerve tissue: Nutritional yeast powder sprinkled onto foods, whole grains, supplementation, etc. Vitamin E: Nuts and seeds, whole grains, supplementation, etc.

- **Herbal formulation**: Combine equal parts tinctures of gotu kola [*Centella asiatica*] + skullcap [*Scutellaria laterifolia*] + Oregon grape root [*Mahonia* spp.] + Vervain [*Verbena* spp.]. Can add an equal part of yellow dock [*Rumex crispus*] if bowels are sluggish. Cooling, clearing, calming. The blend expresses affinity for skin, nerves, liver. Start with ingesting one dropperful of the combination in a little water 3+ times per day—increase dose and/or frequency as needed.

- **Burdock root** [*Arctium* spp.] and **dandelion root** [*Taraxacum officinale*] decoction. Cooling, clearing, detoxifying. Together, these plants have affinity for liver, kidneys, lymphatic tissue, skin, digestion.

  > ***To prepare decoction,*** *combine 1/8 cup of each root [¼ cup total] in pot with 1 quart water. Bring to a boil, then reduce heat to simmer. Simmer for 20-45 minutes, then let stand. Start with ¼ to ½ cup of brew as a serving, up to three times per day. Can increase to 1 cup brew per serving, as desired.*
  >
  > *Can decoct a greater volume, if preferred, using the same proportions: ¼ cup total roots to each 1 quart of water. Refrigerate unused portion. Make only what can be consumed within 2-3 days.*

- **Milk thistle seed extract** [*Silybum marianum*]: Superlative liver support. Cooling, detoxifying, liver protective and regenerative, cholagogue, antioxidant; being studied for anticancer activity. Try 1-2 droppersful of tincture or 1 capsule of extract 3 times per day. *Please note* that *Silybum* has been previously suspected of influencing the metabolism of some drugs, thus potentially impacting their clinical effectiveness. Human studies have since reported conflicting results, and the latest edition of the standard reference *Botanical Safety Handbook* [2013] concludes that there are no known drug interactions.

- **Activated quercitin**: Flavonoid compound that helps quiet the internal fires of inflammation and oxidation. Typical dose is 500 mg per day.

- Support liver function with appropriate **food choices** and preparation techniques. Avoid anything fried or hydrogenated. See ***Food Considerations for Liver Health*** for more details and suggestions.

- Cooling, soothing **salves or creams** liberally applied as needed. Look for products that contain some of the following: plantain, calendula, comfrey, chickweed, mallow, Oregon grape leaf or root, peppermint, vitamin E oil, etc.

- **Aloe vera gel or juice**, applied topically, can also be cooling and soothing. Harvest from household plant or look for commercial products that are preservative-free, sourced from organically cultivated plants.

- Add **peppermint essential oil** [*Mentha piperita*] to lotion, salve, or jojoba oil to calm and cool skin. Menthol is antipruritic. For those sensitive to menthol, **essential oil of Roman chamomile** [*Anthemis nobilis*] may be used instead. Chamomile is both calming and anti-inflammatory.

- Strongly brewed **cold peppermint tea** as compress or in cool bath.

- Clinical aromatherapist Shirley Price reports combining the following to ease itchy skin: **essential oils** of sandalwood [*Santalum album*], lavender [*Lavandula angustifolia*], and peppermint mixed into lotion and applied.

- **Neem oil** [*Azadirachta indica*]: extracted from leaf and seed. Astringent, antibacterial, antifungal, insecticidal, anthelmintic. Neem is an Ayurvedic remedy for many internal and external applications. The oil is traditionally applied to the skin to treat stiff joints, wounds and ulcerations [including in the mouth], boils, ringworm, eczema, urticaria, scabies, lice, leprosy, sprains, etc. Neem has a pronounced aroma.

- Avoid sudden changes in **water temperature** while bathing.

- **Limit use of soap and water**. Glycerine- or oatmeal-based soap may work best if using soap at all.

- Commercially available **colloidal oatmeal** [or **finely ground organic oats** stuffed into a small muslin sack] can be used in the bath to soothe itchy skin.

- **Baking soda** or **sulfur powder** added to bathwater to help calm inflamed, reactive skin issues. *Caution*: Do not use sulfur powder if allergic to sulfur or sulfa drugs.

Boils

*Boils are acute, tender, inflamed nodules appearing on the skin caused by infection by the **Staphylococcus aureus** bacteria. Also called **furuncles**, boils can occur anywhere on the body, but most frequently arise on the neck, breasts, face, and buttocks. They are usually associated with an infected hair follicle or oil gland. They start as tender, red tissue, soon swelling into a lump. The initial inflamed nodule ripens into a pustule and will eventually come to a head and rupture, releasing pus. Until this drainage happens, the boil can be quite painful. It is best to allow the pustule to ripen and break open naturally or to seek professional lancing of the boil; avoid pricking or squeezing to prevent spreading infection. It is useful to quicken the ripening process with time-tested topical applications. **Carbuncle** is the name for a cluster of boils. If boils or carbuncles persist longer than two weeks, are unbearably painful, or are accompanied by fever, seek medical advice. See **Drug-Resistant Bacterial Infections** for additional considerations.*

General herbal strategy involves: Bolstering immunity and detoxification via dietary and herbal support; drawing the boil to a head; addressing and preventing infection; relaxing the bodymind so as to relieve pain and facilitate rest.

- **Avoid sugary foods**. Infections thrive when simple sugars are circulating in the system. Sucrose consumption has been shown to inhibit phagocytosis. Eating 100 gm of sugar [about the amount in two cans of soda] has been shown to suppress immune function for up to five hours after ingestion.[14]

- **To bolster immunity,** emphasize cabbage-family vegetables, onion/garlic/shallots as digestion will allow—and limit fruits and fruit juices for the run of the infection.

- **Probiotic supplementation** or **naturally cultured foods** such as yogurt, miso or kraut also bolster immunity, improving the health of the gut ecology.

- **Zinc-rich foods or supplementation** to boost immunity and wound healing. See section on **Loss of Taste/Smell** for food sources.

- **Vitamin C**, from foods or supplementation, also supports immunity and wound healing. Rosehips are an excellent source.

- **Dandelion** [*Taraxacum officinale*]: Cooling, detoxifying. Bitter tonic, mild laxative, chologogue. Root prepared as decoction, drunk 1-2 times per day.

- **Pau d'arco tea** [*Tabebuia impetiginosa*] as warm compress. Antifungal/anti-yeast, plus antibacterial, antiviral, astringent, anti-inflammatory. Also traditionally used as anticancer herb. Use topically as needed—or drink as tea for systemic support.

  To use: Dilute tincture in warm water or prepare as light decoction, simmering 2-3 teaspoons of shredded bark in 2 cups of water for about 15 minutes and dividing this brew into two to three doses during the day.

- **Poultices to speed maturation of a boil**, i.e. to draw boil to a head. **Fresh poultices**: Honey, raw cabbage, plantain leaf, burdock leaf, cleavers, tofu, raw grated potato. Various **powders**, to be used separately or in combinations: Betonite clay, baking soda, epsom salts, ginger, cornmeal, flaxseed meal, buckwheat powder, activated charcoal. Powdered root of Oregon grape [*Mahonia* spp.] or myrrh resin powder can be blended into any poultice for additional antiseptic benefit. Dispense of spent materials mindfully. Always wash hands thoroughly after tending to boils.

  To make a poultice of fresh leaves: Grind, blend [with a tiny bit of liquid] or chew fresh leaves to make a mash. Apply directly to skin. If desired, cover with clean cotton gauze, then cover all with a dry towel to hold poultice in place. Remove when plant material becomes warm. Repeat application with fresh plant material several times in one session. Poultice several times each day, if possible.

  To make a poultice of powders: Mix desired powders together with a bit of water to make a thick paste. Apply amply, cover with plastic and bandage. Example: 1 part ginger root powder to 1 part cornmeal or flaxseed meal or clay. Proceed as above. Alternately, powders may be added to honey as a base. See following entry.

- **Honey**, an ancient remedy and potent antimicrobial and wound-healing agent, can serve to promote healing when applied directly as a dressing. Honey can help to mature boils and draw heat. Broadly antimicrobial—Anti-bacterial, including drug-resistant bacteria; anti-viral; anti-fungal; immune stimulant; anti-inflammatory. Deodorizing. Can be applied to dry or moist wounds, from burns to ulcerations. All raw wildflower honeys have activity; Manuka honey from New Zealand [from nectar and pollen sourced from *Leptospermum scoparium*] is particularly active against drug-resistant strains of bacteria.

- **Internal strategies to boost immunity** and deliver *Staph*-specific antimicrobial benefit: Astragalus root, echinacea, usnea lichen, berberine-containing plants [roots of Oregon grape, coptis, goldenseal], propolis resin, isatis, red alder [*Alnus rubra*]. Deep immune support: Reishi mushroom, ashwagandha root, astragalus root, eleuthero root, rhodiola. *Please note*: Use propolis with caution if prone to allergy or hypersensitivity to bee stings, bee products, or tree resins.

- **Red alder** [*Alnus rubra*]: bark. Alterative, antibacterial, mild laxative, cholagogue. Indicated for boils, carbuncles, *Staph* infections. Formats: Tea, tincture.

    To prepare tea: Add 1 teaspoon red alder bark for each cup of water used. Bring to a boil and simmer 10-15 minutes. Remove from heat and steep another 30 minutes. Drink in half-cup doses up to 3 times per day. If the bowels become unformed, reduce intake.

- **Cleavers** [*Gallium* spp.]: fresh plant. Cooling, alterative, lymphatic drainer, diuretic. Traditionally indicated for boils, skin eruptions, venomous bites—as well as nodular swellings. Formats: 1-2 ounces of freshly juiced flowering plant may be taken internally up to several times a day. Tincture or succus of fresh plant. Topically, compress of fresh juice or poultice of macerated fresh plant.

- **Corydalis rhizome**[*Corydalis* spp.]: Acrid, bitter, warm. Analgesic, sedating, muscle relaxing, anti-inflammatory, invigorates circulation. For internal use. Contains both berberine—an anti-*Staph* alkaloid—plus constituents that have pain-relieving properties. Traditionally used in Chinese botanical medicine for pain from a variety of causes throughout the body: Chest, epigastric, gynecological, abdominal [including from the presence of masses], pain in the extremities, traumatic pain. *Caution*: Contraindicated in pregnancy and used with caution in certain deficiency states. Use with caution if taking sedative or hypnotic drugs. Consult with your practitioner to determine if this is appropriate to your situation. Available as sliced dried root, whole root powder, tincture, tea pills.

    *To use: Sliced **dried root** may be prepared as decoction and drunk as tea: 1 teaspoon root to about 10 ounces water; simmer for 15 minutes, then let steep another half hour. Four ounces of tea is typically taken up to 3 times per day. **Powdered root** may be made into capsules, directly mixed with warm water, or added to base such as small amount of applesauce. Typical dose is 1-2 grams of powder several times per day, up to 10 grams per day. Additionally, the traditional patent medicine **Great Corydalis Tea Pills** is available [Yan Hu Suo Zhi Tong Wan], which combines Corydalis with Angelica dahuricae. **Tincture**: Typical dose is 2-3 droppersful up to 5 times per day. A range of dosing is possible. Please note that a 400:1 extract is available to practitioners for treating cancer-related pain in their clients.*

- **Neem oil** [*Azadirachta indica*]: Extracted from leaf and seed. Astringent, antibacterial, antifungal, insecticidal, anthelmintic. Neem is an Ayurvedic remedy for many internal and external applications. The oil is traditionally applied to the skin to treat stiff joints, wounds and ulcerations [including in the mouth], boils, ringworm, eczema, urticaria, scabies, lice, leprosy, sprains, etc. Please note that neem has a pronounced aroma that may be unpleasant to some.

- **Gently bandage** boil to avoid scratching during sleep.

- **Calming teas** or **sedative plant preparations** can be of great help in relaxing around the discomfort and easing sleep. See the chapter *Plants to Support the Nervous System* and the Repertoire section on **Melancholy/Anxiety** for suggestions.

- **Homeopathic remedies**: *Belladonna* [for early stage with redness, heat and throbbing pain]; *Silicea* [for slow-ripening boil]; *Baptisia tinctoria* [septic conditions of the blood; foul-smelling ulcerations; acute fever]. Homeopathic remedies are taken 15 minutes away from either food or drink.

Drug-Resistant Bacterial Infections: MRSA, VRSA plus *C. diff.*

*Drug-resistant bacterial infections are a challenging and potentially life-threatening side-effect to the rampant over-prescribing of antibiotic pharmaceutical medicine both in human and veterinary practice. It is particularly an issue for immune-compromised individuals and those with exposure to medical settings, which are often the breeding ground for such virulent bacteria. Bacteria are remarkably adaptive survivors and demand our attention and deeper understanding. Preventing both the spread of pathogenic organisms and the evolution of resistance is the core challenge. Please see the article **Lessons from Bacteria** in the appendix for an overview of the microbial crisis we face collectively; that article addresses additional considerations in preventing resistance. I strongly recommend you consult the book* Herbal Antibiotics: Natural Alternatives for Treating Drug-Resistant Bacteria *by Stephen Buhner for additional background and suggestions. The complex chemistry of botanically sourced antimicrobial compounds holds great promise in managing resistant strains, but the effort to address them must be conducted holistically—simultaneously at the systems level of the whole individual, the community, and the global biological sphere.*

- To repeat, please review the article *Lessons from Bacteria* in the appendix for a big-picture view of cause, prevention and treatment. There are many, many **dietary and lifestyle factors** that play a role in meeting this challenge. Supporting beneficial microbial ecology of the gut and skin is a key concern—tend to underlying terrain.

- **Fortify beneficial intestinal microorganisms** through naturally cultured foods or supplementation. In addition, foods such as Jerusalem artichoke, dandelion root, chicory root, burdock root, and elecampane root are rich in a substance called inulin, sometimes called a prebiotic. Inulin, a non-digestible carbohydrate, is also found in artichoke, asparagus, leeks, onions, and garlic. Prebiotics serve as preferred foods for the beneficial bacteria, helping increase their numbers.

- **Myrrh** [*Commiphora myrrha*]: Antimicrobial, astringent, anti-inflammatory, analgesic, antiseptic, wound healing. Myrrh is an ancient healing remedy, an oleo-gum-resin tree exudate. That is, wound the tree, and wound-healing medicine is secreted. The tincture is used internally to enhance immune activity. Myrrh essential oil has shown activity against *Staphylococcus aureus* and other Gram-positive bacteria. Myrrh gum powder may be sprinkled into weepy wounds. Internal use of myrrh is contraindicated in pregnancy.

- **Honey**: Natural substance with numerous anti-infective and wound-healing benefits. Broadly antimicrobial—antibacterial, including drug-resistant bacteria; antiviral; antifungal; immune stimulant; anti-inflammatory. Promotes healing of wounds and ulcerations. Draws heat. Can be applied both to dry [including burns] or moist wounds. All raw wildflower honeys show effectiveness; Manuka and jellybush honey from New Zealand and Australia [sourced from the nectar and pollen of *Leptospermum* spp.] seem to be particularly active against drug-resistant strains of bacteria, without degrading the gut microbiota.[15]

- **Activated charcoal poultice**: Drawing, disinfecting, and deodorizing. Silver hydrosol may be used instead of water to thicken, lending its antimicrobial benefits.

- **Internal allies**: Propolis resin and usnea lichen—both broadly antimicrobial—and the adaptogens: Astragalus, ashwagandha, echinacea, eleuthero, reishi, rhodiola, etc. See chapter on ***Adaptogenic and Tonic Plant Allies*** for discussion of individual plants.

- **Garlic cloves** and **ginger rhizome** have been shown to be effective against multi-drug resistant clinical pathogens.

- Plants rich in **essential oils**, as well as the distilled essential oils in concentrated forms, have a key role to play in overwhelming resistant strains with antimicrobial chemical complexity. For example: Oregano, thyme, peppermint, eucalyptus, thyme, clove, cinnamon, tea tree, citrus extracts…all may be considered as potential allies.

- **Medical *Cannabis***: Calming, pain relieving, sedative, anti-nausea, mood elevation, more. *Cannabis sativa* and *C. indica* are legally available for approved medical use in some jurisdictions. Researchers in Italy and Britain have found *Cannabis* extracts to be systemically effective against multiple strains of drug-resistant bacteria.[16] Please see the Appendix article ***Lessons from Bacteria*** for more details. Consult with your healthcare provider if you think medical *Cannabis* is indicated for your situation.

- ***Clostridium difficile* [*C. diff.*] infection**: A healthcare-associated bacterial infection. Some 14,000 deaths in the United States are caused by this infection each year, according to the Center for Disease Control [CDC] in 2013.[17] All told, some 75,000 patients dealing with infections picked up in health care facilities die in U.S. hospitals each year, according to a survey published in March 2014 in *The New England Journal of Medicine*. Pneumonia and surgical-site infection were the most common infection types, and *C. difficile* was the most common pathogen. Symptoms include: watery diarrhea, fever, loss of appetite, nausea, abdominal pain. Older adults and others with immune-compromised circumstances are most at risk, particularly following courses of prescribed antibiotic medicines and exposure to medical settings. According to the CDC, *C. diff.* spores can be found on bed linens, bed rails, bathroom fixtures, medical equipment, etc. It can be passed from person to person, including from medical personnel to patients. Consult the webpage www.CDC.gov for more information. **Suggested approach**: Clean your own hands after all medical visits, using hot water and soap and/or essential oil based antimicrobial sprays. For temporary symptom relief, explore suggestions in this section and seek medical help if *C. diff.* is suspected. Consider supplementing with ***Saccharomyces boulardii***, a non-pathogenic yeast that has been prescribed for at least 30 years both to prevent and to treat diarrheal diseases caused by bacteria. Additional studies have been recommended by researchers looking into its specific efficacy with *C. diff.*[18] In my experience, *Saccharomyces boulardii* has a profoundly useful role to play, especially in combination with other probiotic strains. It may be taken concurrently with antibiotic medications. Consult with a holistic medical practitioner for guidance.

- **Keep fingernails short and clean**. All in household should practice scrupulous personal hygiene to avoid spreading resistant bacteria back and forth. *Staph* can easily be spread by touch, and can hide beneath the nails.

- **Sulfur soap** may have a role to play. Antibacterial, antifungal. *Caution*: Do not use if allergic to sulfur or sulfa drugs.

- **Shower rather than bathe**. Use washcloths and towels only once before laundering.

Neuropathy / Pain or Numbness in Hands or Feet

Peripheral neuropathy is the medical term used to describe the sensations of numbness or pain felt in hands and feet as a result of nerve damage. Such nerve damage may result from injury [including surgery], metabolic disorders such as diabetes, infections, and exposures to toxins such as radiation therapy, pesticides and chemotherapeutic agents.

The sensations can range from tingling or burning to a sense of numbness akin to wearing a stocking or glove—or beyond.

The experience of neuropathy may lessen in time, especially if underlying causes can be resolved. Supporting the body through the experience of discomfort can go a long way toward relieving its intensity. A few preventative strategies are also listed below.

- **Hand massage** and **foot massage**, self-administered or provided by caregiver, increases local circulation. Done regularly—at least daily or even twice a day, if possible—can greatly improve sensory awareness in extremities.

- If caused by chemotherapy agent, mitigate by **holding frozen object** during infusion period. Ask oncology nurses to alert you when this is appropriate.

- **Topricin Foot Gel**: A unique combination of homeopathic remedies—including those made from snake venom—to promote proper feeling and sensation to peripheral nerve endings in the feet and hands. It is rubbed in as needed or as often as desired.

- A few drops of essential oils such as **helichrysum** [*Helichrysum angustifolium*] or **rosemary** [*Rosmarinus officinalis*] added to lotion or oil can increase the effectiveness of massage. Also may be mixed with bit of liquid soap added to hand- or footbaths. Anti-inflammatory, antimicrobial, promote proper wound healing.

- **St. Johnswort infused oil** [*Hypericum perforatum*] applied topically is specific for nerve damage or inflammation; it also promotes proper wound healing. **Tincture** or **extract** [or ***Hypericum*** as homeopathic prep] can also be taken internally: Restorative to nerve tissue. Calming, anti-inflammatory, antibacterial, antiviral, astringent, wound healing. *Cautions*: Please see entry in ***Plants to Support the Nervous System***.

- **Lipoic acid**: This powerful fat-soluble and water-soluble antioxidant h as been shown to reduce pain and numbness in peripheral nerves—from multiple causes— through a variety of mechanisms. It has an important role to play in a holistic approach to metabolic syndromes, neurological/brain health, and integrative cancer therapies, among other circumstances. Therapeutic doses of the alpha-lipoic acid form [ALA] range from 50 to 400 mg. per day, usually taken in divided doses to maintain its presence in the tissues. Doses used in research have ranged from 150 to 600 mg. per day. R-lipoic acid is thought to be up to 10 times as bioavailable as ALA. *Please note*: As an antioxidant, use of lipoic acid is controversial during radiation therapy and some types of chemotherapy. Consult with your health practitioner in these circumstances.

- **B Vitamins** are key to nerve health: B_{12} and folic acid, particularly, may each have important roles to play. See **Building the Blood** for more information.

- **L-glutamine**: An amino acid existing naturally in the body, L-glutamine is a building block for proteins, produced in the muscles and distributed where needed by the blood. It is a factor in many metabolic processes including wound repair. L-glutamine can be supplemented if needed—during situations of nutritional deficiency, metabolic stress, muscle wasting [cancer, HIV/AIDS, etc.], tissue injury [surgery, radiation, etc.] particularly if the digestive/intestinal membranes have been compromised. Shown to improve gut health, immune function, and enhance wound healing. Whey protein and cabbage juice are rich sources of L-glutamine. Isolated glutamine powders are also available and are easily added to smoothies. Other food sources include miso, legumes, beef, chicken, fish, and dairy products.

- **Prickly ash** [*Zanthoxylum clava-herculis*]: bark. Pungent circulatory stimulant, anti-inflammatory. Indicated also for nerve pain. *Caution*: Contraindicated in pregnancy.

Shingles [*Herpes Zoster*]

Shingles is an acute inflammation of the dorsal root ganglia caused by infection with the herpes virus Varicella-zoster, which also causes chickenpox. Shingles usually occurs in adults, causing characteristic skin lesions and severe neuralgic pain along the inflamed nerve trunk.

Herpes zoster generally occurs in those older than age 60, and in those of any age dealing with various immune challenges, including cancer and human immunodeficiency virus [HIV]. Psychological and physiological stress tends to be associated with onset of shingles.

Herpes zoster begins with fever and a general sense of unwellness. This is typically followed within two to four days by itching, burning, tingling, or deep pain—usually on the trunk of the body and occasionally on the arms, legs, or face. Headache and chills can also be part of the picture.

Up to two weeks after initial symptoms, red nodular lesions—composed of fluid-filled blisters—erupt on the painful areas, eventually forming scabs about 10 days after first appearing. Pain may persist beyond healing of the lesions.

- **Rest**, particularly at first signs of imbalance.

- **Acupuncture treatments** may reduce pain and help the body recover more quickly. Receiving treatment at onset of unwellness would be ideal.

- **Avoid scratching** the lesions—to prevent scarring and secondary infections. Wear light cotton gloves to help encourage restraint.

- **Maximize nutrition**, particularly dark leafy greens, berries, and yellow/orange foods. Magnesium, bioflavonoids, beta-carotene, vitamin C, selenium and zinc all benefit healing. See previous section on **Herpes Eruptions** for additional suggestions.

- **Avoid nerve stimulants**, such as coffee, tea, all caffeine-containing beverages.

- **Increase B-complex vitamin consumption**, essential for nerve health. Foods that are rich in B vitamins: Nutritional yeast, eggs, fish, sea vegetables, whole grains, dark leafy greens... B-complex supplements which dissolve under the tongue seem to be more readily absorbed by the body than capsules or tablets.

- **Supplemental zinc** may also be called for, to boost immunity and promote healing. A typical dose in such a situation might be 90 mg. per day for a limited period; consult with a holistic medical practitioner for guidance. Food-based supplements are generally well tolerated. **Zinc ointments** can also be applied topically.

- **L-glutamine**: An amino acid existing naturally in the body, L-glutamine is a building block for proteins, produced in the muscles and distributed where needed by the blood. It is a factor in many metabolic processes including wound repair. L-glutamine can be supplemented if needed—during situations of nutritional deficiency, metabolic stress, muscle wasting [cancer, HIV/AIDS, etc.], tissue injury [surgery, radiation, etc.] particularly if the digestive/intestinal membranes have been compromised. Shown to improve gut health, immune function, and enhance wound healing. Whey protein and cabbage juice are rich sources of L-glutamine. Isolated glutamine powders are also available and are easily added to smoothies. Other food sources include miso, legumes, beef, chicken, fish, and dairy products.

- **Calamine lotion** or other commercial topical anti-pruretics can help calm the urge to scratch lesions. Alternatively, food-grade **bentonite clay** can be mixed into a thin paste and applied.

  To make a simple calamine lotion, *start with these proportions—In small bowl, mix 1 tablespoon betonite clay with 1 tablespoon baking soda. Gradually mix in witch hazel or water until desired consistency is reached. For the given proportions, can add up to 15 drops of essential oils for added healing benefits—antibacterial, antiviral, antifungal, anti-inflammatory: peppermint, tea tree, lavender, or Melissa. Please note: If witch hazel is used as the liquid, larger quantities may be made for use over time, as it will lend a preserving benefit; the water-based version should be made fresh daily. Also, see entry on St. Johnswort below.*

- **St. Johnswort oil** [*Hypericum perforatum*] applied topically is specific for nerve trauma or inflammation; it also promotes proper wound healing. **St. Johnswort tincture, extract,** or **homeopathic remedy** can also be taken internally. Calming, antiviral, anti-inflammatory, antibacterial, antiviral, astringent, wound-healing. *Cautions*: Please see entry in ***Plants to Support the Nervous System***.

  To prepare Hypericum-Calamine lotion, *substitute infused oil of St. Johnswort flower buds for the witch hazel or water in the basic calamine recipe above.*

- **Vitamin E oil** applied topically—alone or in combination with any of the other options—to speed skin healing and prevent scarring.

- **Kava** [*Piper methysticum*]: Preparations from root. Nervine plant useful to ease inflammation, infection, pain; also, anxiolytic, sedative, muscle relaxing—all useful benefits when dealing with neuralgia. Internally, water/coconut milk extractions or low-alcohol tinctures are best. In general, choose *either* kava preparations *or* pharmaceutical analogs—not both at once. *Cautions*: Please see entry in ***Plants to Support the Nervous System***.

- Apply **topical antiviral ointment or medicated oil** as early as possible in disease process. Antiviral essential oils specific to *Herpes zoster* include: Lemon balm [*Melissa officinalis*], peppermint [*Mentha* x *piperita*], geranium [*Pelargonium graveolens*], ravensara [*Ravensara aromatica*], and thyme [*Thymus vulgaris*].

- **Dragon's blood** aka Sangre de drago [*Croton lechleri*]: Wound healing, antiviral, antifungal, antiseptic, styptic. Can be used both topically and internally to promote healing of lesions.

- Naturopathic physician Michael Murray reports that a **combination enzyme preparation**—trypsin, chymotrypsin, and papain—has been found to be as effective as acyclovir, a standard antiviral medication.[19]

- **Proteolytic enzymes**—such as papain from papayas and bromelain from pineapples—may be of benefit when taken during the day, on an empty stomach. *Caution*: Pancreatin and other proteolytic enzymes have been reported to impair folic acid absorption. Stargrove, *et al* recommend that healthcare practitioners prescribing proteolytic enzymes suggest concurrent folic acid intake to counteract any decrease in folate absorption.[20]

- **Cool, wet compresses** may reduce pain. Try making a strong tea, either from chamomile flowers, peppermint leaves, lavender flowers, or yarrow herb. Or combine herbs, such as 3 parts peppermint with 1 part yarrow. Use this strained, cooled, concentrated infusion as the liquid for the compress and apply several times a day.

- **Sedative, anti-inflammatory,** and **antiviral herbs** and **mushrooms** all have a role to play in managing the experience. Shiitake, lemon balm, vervain, skullcap, passionflower, *Echinacea angustifolia*, turmeric. See entry on *Corydalis* in **Deep Pain** section, which follows. **Adaptogenic plants** that help to harmonize bodymind also can be of benefit: Consider reishi, ashwagandha, licorice, astragalus, eleuthero.

- **Capsaicin cream** [the active ingredient in chili peppers] applied topically. Capsaicin has been found to block pain messaging in the nerves and provide temporary relief. A cream composed of 0.075% capsaicin has shown the greatest effect.

- *Belladonna* **homeopathic remedy**. Indicated for neuralgic pain that comes and goes suddenly; heat, redness, throbbing and burning. *Note*: Homeopathic remedies are taken at least 15 minutes away from either food or drink.

- Traditional Chinese Medicine **herbal cupping therapy** has been found to offer significant benefit in reducing pain in post-herpetic neuralgia—superior in clinical observation to western treatment approaches.[21] Consult with a licensed acupuncturist who practices this technique for more information.

Deep Pain

Obviously, this is a case where pharmaceutical science can offer great relief of suffering. Lessening the experience of pain can allow the body to rest and the vital energy to focus on healing. In addition, or alternately, natural medicine approaches can also help make pain less vivid. Consult with a knowledgeable practitioner before combining prescribed drugs and pain-relieving plant medicine—combinations may result in unpredictable consequences.

- Please see *Engaging with Pain* in the Appendix for some psychospiritual strategies.

- **Fear and anxiety** can increase the sensation of pain. In addition to psychospiritual strategies mentioned elsewhere, plants that help to calm and ground bodymind can be of great benefit. See the chapters *Plants to Support the Nervous System* and *Adaptogenic and Tonic Plant Allies* to discover which plant allies resonate for you.

- Enlist a sensitive, experienced **massage therapist and/or energy worker** as part of your support team. Skillful treatments can ease the heaviness of persistent pain and help liberate the life force.

- **Acupuncture** can be one of the most blessed helps in directly addressing pain sensation. Surgeries have even been conducted under the influence of acupuncture as the sole anesthetic. Look for state-licensed practitioners [LAc].

- **Corydalis rhizome**[*Corydalis* spp.]: Acrid, bitter, warm. Analgesic, sedating, muscle relaxing, anti-inflammatory, invigorates circulation. For internal use. Contains both berberine—an anti-*Staph* alkaloid—plus constituents that have pain-relieving properties. Traditionally used in Chinese botanical medicine for pain from a variety of causes throughout the body: Chest, epigastric, gynecological, abdominal [including pain arising from the presence of masses], pain in the extremities, traumatic pain. Available as sliced dried root, whole root powder, tincture, tea pills. *Cautions*: Contraindicated in pregnancy and used with caution in certain deficiency states. Use with caution if taking sedative or hypnotic drugs. Consult with your practitioner.

  > ***To use***: *Sliced* **dried root** *may be prepared as decoction and drunk as tea: 1 teaspoon root to about 10 ounces water; simmer for 15 minutes, then let steep another half hour. Four ounces of tea is typically taken up to 3 times per day.* **Powdered root** *may be made into capsules, directly mixed with warm water, or added to base such as small amount of applesauce. Typical dose is 1-2 grams of powder several times per day, up to 10 grams per day. Additionally, the traditional patent medicine* **Great Corydalis Tea Pills** *is available [Yan Hu Suo Zhi Tong Wan], which combines Corydalis with Angelica dahuricae.* **Tincture**: *Typical dose is 2-3 droppersful up to 5 times per day. A range of dosing is possible. Please note that a 400:1 extract is available to practitioners for treating cancer-related pain in their clients.*

- **Medical *Cannabis***: Calming, pain relieving, sedative, anti-nausea, promotes mood elevation, more. This well-known plant can be of great benefit to ease a wide range of discomforts. Fortunately, *Cannabis* use is being decriminalized in numerous states, especially for those with medical need, though at the time of this writing it is still scheduled as a controlled substance by the U.S. federal government. Avoid the unhealthy complications of direct inhalation of burning herb—utilize via extracts, butter, foods, or vaporization. Whole books have been written on the history and use of *Cannabis* as a medicinal herb. In particular, recent results of studies using non-psychoactive CBD-rich strains [cannabidiol] are opening up exciting additional possibilities for therapeutic use, including direct antitumoral effects and as anticancer adjunct to conventional chemical therapies. Within the medical marijuana world, plant strains with varying levels of the cannabinoids THC [strongly psychoactive] and CBD are available—consult with a knowledgeable physician/practitioner to determine what might best suit your personality and situation.

- **Other plants used for pain relief** such as Jamaica dogwood [*Piscidia piscipula*] and Indian/Ghost Pipe [*Monotropa uniflora*] should generally be used under the guidance of a practitioner.

- **Turmeric rhizome, boswellia resin, willow bark**: all anti-inflammatory and analgesic. *Caution*: *Boswellia serrata* is recommended to be used cautiously in pregnancy, under the guidance of a holistic practitioner.

- **Rosemary** [*Rosmarinus officinalis*]: leaf. Anti-inflammatory, muscle relaxing, circulatory stimulant, rejuvenative. Strong water infusion or essential oil diluted into a bit of liquid soap may be added to baths to both relax and revive aching, tense or tired muscles. The essential oil may also be added to massage oil or lotion. *Cautions*: Avoid using at night as its circulatory stimulating properties may delay sleep. See ***Plants to Support the Nervous System*** for considerations during pregnancy.

- **Sound healing** has a significant role to play in holistic pain management. There is a wealth of recorded musical material and **guided meditation** available to help soothe the psyche, relax the body, and help the mind open into a spacious, meditative state, beyond identification with the pain. See the chapter ***Recommended Listening***.

Urinary Tract Infections

Infection can result when normal, local defenses in the urinary tract break down and allow bacteria to invade the bladder mucosa and multiply. Pharmaceutical antibiotics are usually prescribed as a remedy, but pathogens can develop resistance. Additionally, lowered general immunity, disruption of gut microflora [often as a consequence of using antibiotics or other drugs, including non-steroidal anti-inflammatories], age, and activity issues can all play a role in recurrence.

Those with in-dwelling catheters, incomplete bladder emptying, improper or insufficient hygiene, or who are bedridden or wheelchair dependent are particularly susceptible. Diets that emphasize sugars and other simple carbohydrates also predispose.

For these reasons and more, both acute and chronic infection may present.

- **Fortify beneficial intestinal microorganisms** through naturally cultured foods or supplementation. In addition, foods such as Jerusalem artichoke, dandelion root, chicory root, burdock root, and elecampane root are rich in a substance called inulin, sometimes called a prebiotic. Inulin, a non-digestible carbohydrate, is also found in artichoke, asparagus, leeks, onions, and garlic. Prebiotics serve as preferred foods for the beneficial bacteria, helping increase their numbers.

- **Avoid [or greatly limit] substances that degrade intestinal flora**: Alcohol, tobacco smoke, fluoride, chlorinated water, non-steroidal anti-inflammatory drugs [aspirin, ibuprofen, naproxen], steroid drugs, grilled foods, oral contraceptives, antibiotics in the food supply, indiscriminate or inappropriate use of antibiotic meds, antibacterial soaps [active ingredient Triclosan], and a wide array of manufactured chemicals.

- **D-Mannose**: A simple sugar that occurs in some plants, including cranberries. It prevents deleterious organisms such as bacteria from sticking to the lining of the urinary tract. D-Mannose can be used in place of cranberry juice for this purpose. Its pleasant taste helps ensure consistent use. At the low doses at which it is used, D-Mannose does not impact blood sugar regulation. Available in capsules or loose powder.

- **Corn silk** [*Zea mays*]: preparations from fresh silk. Soothing, cooling, mildly antiseptic. Found to prevent bacterial adhesion. Useful in combination with more assertive urinary tract plant medicines, such as **uva ursi** [*Arctostaphylos uva-ursi*], **agrimony** [*Agrimonia eupatorium*] or **couchgrass** [*Agropyron repens*]. Often added to such combinations, **marshmallow** [*Althea officinalis*] or **common mallow** [*Malva neglecta*] leaves and root are soothing, demulcent, cooling diuretics.

- **Yarrow** [*Achillea millefolium*]: leaves and flowers. Bitter/pungent, cooling, drying. Urinary antiseptic. Antibacterial, antispasmodic, anti-inflammatory; astringent, styptic, vulnerary [wound healing]. Circulatory support: Peripheral vasodilator, tones vasculature. Diuretic, diaphoretic, febrifuge. Bitter digestive tonic. Prepare as simple tea or use tincture added to warm water. *Caution*: Those with serious allergies to aster family plants should handle and use with caution.

- **Kava** [*Piper methysticum*]: root. Resinous, warming. Mucous membrane analgesic, among other applications. Used for inflammation, infection, pain, and irritability, particularly in urogenital tissue. Also, anxiolytic, sedative, muscle relaxing. Preparations made from root include powder in capsules, low-alcohol tinctures, powder blended with equal parts water and coconut milk, plus a bit of lecithin. *Cautions*: Please see entry in **Plants to Support the Nervous System**.

- **Avoid sugary foods.** Infections thrive when simple sugars are circulating in the system. Sucrose consumption has been shown to inhibit phagocytosis. Eating 100 gm of sugar [about the amount in two cans of soda] has been shown to suppress immune function for up to five hours after ingestion.[22]

- See section on **Yeast Infections/Thrush** for additional considerations.

Incontinence

The loss of bladder or anal control can evoke emotions ranging from embarrassment to trauma. Urinary incontinence [or bowel incontinence, as applicable] can arise through numerous causes: Natural aging and hormonal shifts; a consequence of stress; structural issues; side-effects from drugs; after-effects of surgery; cancers; obstruction; local inflammation or infection. Be sure to alert your practitioner should persistent incontinence occur; consult with your pharmacist if you are taking medications to support your heart, blood pressure, sedatives, muscle relaxants, or other drugs.

- **Monitor beverage consumption**: Drink water in smaller amounts throughout the day. Avoid caffeinated beverages and alcohol; both are diuretic and bladder stimulating. Avoid carbonated beverages, artificial sweeteners, corn syrup. Citrus, spicy or tomato-rich foods can also aggravate the bladder.

- Provide **water-proof layer on mattress** under normal sheet. Be certain to smooth this underlayer well, so that sleeping surface is uniformly smooth and even—key to maintaining skin health.

- **Position and re-position a portable commode** close to bed or favorite chair, so that there are few steps between urge and relief.

- **Discuss the possible role certain substances may play** in either urinary or bowel incontinence with your healthcare advisers: Prescribed medications, tube-feeding formulas or quantity, alcohol or caffeine consumption, food additives such as sugar substitutes, or sensitivity to dairy products or gluten.

- **Mullein** [*Verbascum thapsus*]: root. Though most people familiar with herbs may be aware of mullein leaf and flowers as support for lung health, the root is indicated here. Antispasmodic, anti-inflammatory, sedative. Indicated for urinary frequency, bladder spasms, benign prostate inflammation, and facial nerve pain. Formats: Light decoction or tincture.

  > *To prepare mullein root tea: Add 4 teaspoons of chopped dried root to 1 quart cold water. Bring to a boil, then lower heat and simmer for about 10 minutes. Remove from heat and let sit for an hour. Strain and enjoy. Usual dose: 1 cup, twice per day. Refrigerate unused portion.*

- **Kava** [*Piper methysticum*]: root. Resinous, warming. Especially indicated for nocturnal or nerve- or inflammation-related incontinence. Relaxing nervine, hypnotic, antispasmodic, locally anesthetic, analgesic, antifungal [*not* against Candida], diuretic. Demonstrated neuroprotective activity. Indications: Neuralgia; irritable bladder; urogenital inflammation, infection, pain; interstitial cystitis. Formats: Cold infusion [especially water/coconut milk extraction], decoction [slow simmer about 20 minutes], raw or freeze-dried root in capsules, low-alcohol/water tincture. *Cautions*: See entry in **Plants to Support the Nervous System**.

- **St. Johnswort** [*Hypericum perforatum*]: fresh flowering tops and leaves. Bitter/sour, cooling. Especially indicated in nerve- and inflammation-related incontinence. Useful with children manifesting fear- or anxiety-associated bedwetting; nightmares. Nerve tissue restorative with affinity for skin and urinary tract. Anxiolytic, sedative, anti-inflammatory, astringent, anti-microbial, vulnerary. Formats: Tincture [fresh preferred by most], extract in capsules. Properly fresh-dried herb may yield a pleasant tea but don't count on it for therapeutic value. *Cautions*: Please see entry in **Plants to Support the Nervous System**.

- **Horsetail** [*Equistum arvense*]: Salty/bitter/sweet, cool. The green vegetative shoot of this ancient plant is a mineralizing tonic, rich in silica—nourishing connective tissue throughout the body, including that within bone, lungs, kidneys, urinary tract. Antioxidant, anti-inflammatory. Diuretic, astringent, wound healing. Formats: Decoction or commercial products made from water extracts.

  > *To make a decoction: Simmer ¼-½ cup horsetail in 1 quart water for 20 minutes.*

- **Kegel exercises**: Pelvic floor muscle training that can benefit uterus, bladder, intestines, and rectum. To find the right muscles, imagine stopping urine mid-stream. To practice, empty your bladder and either sit comfortably or lay on your back. Tighten these muscles and hold the contraction for 5 seconds; then relax for 5 seconds. Repeat 4-5 times in a row. Breathe freely throughout. Focus on using only the pelvic floor muscles—not the abdomen, thighs, or buttocks. Work up to contracting for 10 seconds, relaxing for 10 seconds. Aim to do a kegel series three times each day.

- **Constipation** can be a factor in both urinary and bowel incontinence. See the previous section on **Constipation** for suggestions to keep the bowels emptying regularly, without creating dependency. Bulking laxatives may be especially indicated with bowel incontinence, to help give more form to the stools.

- **Biofeedback**: Studies have shown benefit for urinary incontinence. Biofeedback training may help the subject learn to control and strengthen the pelvic floor muscles. Seek a local professional who has had success working with clients in this situation.

- Additionally, certain **yoga** postures and **acupuncture** have both shown benefit for some individuals dealing with incontinence. Consult with a respected local yoga teacher and/or licensed acupuncturist for recommendations.

Radiation Burns

*A common side effect of repeated radiation therapy is an acute skin reaction that can range from a mild rash to severe skin ulceration—from dry, itching, sometimes peeling skin to moist, open wounds. As with any burn, it's best to allow the heat to dissipate—oil-based topical remedies are usually reserved for use after the acute phase has calmed—or after the full course of treatments is completed. Use other approaches between individual sessions. With radiation to the head and neck, damage to the inner mouth and throat can occur as well. See the section **Mouth Sores / Raw Mouth** for additional suggestions.*

- **Ensure sufficient hydration**. Water is essential for all healing.

- **Support systemic immunity** to prevent infection. See section on **Boils** for numerous herbal and dietary strategies.

- **Aloe vera**: Emollient, anti-inflammatory, antibacterial, wound healing. Choose an organic, preservative-free product. Drink juice internally and apply leaf gel or juice externally as needed.

- **Honey**: Great first-line treatment for burns. Draws heat; can help prevent blistering. Provides numerous anti-infective and wound-healing benefits. Broadly antimicrobial—Anti-bacterial, including drug-resistant bacteria; antiviral; anti-fungal; immune stimulant; anti-inflammatory. Promotes healing of wounds and ulcerations. Can be applied both to dry [including burns] or moist wounds.

- **Cool compresses of herbal infusions**: Cooling, soothing, astringent. Soothing plantain or mallow leaves; astringent herbs such as yarrow, green or black tea, blackberry or raspberry leaves, lady's mantle, avens, and so on.

- **Rosehips**: Rich in vitamin C and flavonoids; cooling and helps promote wound healing. Prepare as tea or simple jam.

  > *To make rosehip jam*: *Loosely fill a small jar with rosehips that have had the seeds removed. Sort through them to make sure no hard seeds remain in the batch. Cover with organic pomegranate juice or apple juice. Take a chopstick or butter knife and poke through the hips, making sure they are completely surrounded with juice. Cover with lid and refrigerate. Within some hours the dried hips will have swelled with the juice, their pectin creating a jam-like consistency. When they are soft and jammy, they are ready to be eaten by the spoonful or added to foods such as yogurt. As you take from the jar, add more juice if you like.*

- **Vitamin C-rich foods or supplementation** can speed wound healing. In addition to the usual sources, the Ayurvedic tonic **amla** fruit [*Emblica officinalis*] is one of the richest sources of vitamin C and strongly antioxidant and anti-inflammatory. Amla is used alone and is also an ingredient in the classic **Triphala** tonic as well as **Chyawanprash**, a thick jam typically made of more than 40 nutritive herbs.

- **Calendula** [*Calendula officinalis*]: Wound healing, anti-inflammatory, antimicrobial. Succus or infusion used as compress on fresh burns. Apply salve or infused oil topically as needed once heat is gone. Tea may be used orally as a swish.

- **Sea buckthorn oil** [*Hippophae rhamnoides*]: Healing fixed oil. Antioxidant, anti-inflammatory, emollient/demulcent, wound healing. Apply to dry, damaged skin. Indicated for injuries including sun- or radiation-induced damage.

- **Rosehip seed oil** [*Rosa mosqueta, Rosa canina*]: Healing fixed oil. Antioxidant, nutrient rich, wound healing, tissue regenerating. Apply to red, irritated, dry or damaged skin.

- **Vitamin E oil**: Antioxidant, stabilizes cell membranes. Helps promote proper wound healing. Pierce gelcap and squeeze out oil or purchase pure oil in glass dropper bottle. Apply directly to dry, irritated or damaged skin. May also be taken internally to support healing.

- **St. Johnswort infused oil** [*Hypericum perforatum*] applied topically is specific for burns, nerve damage, inflammation; it also promotes proper wound healing. The infused oil can be used alone, combined with other oils, or serve as base for the essential oils mentioned below. For dry, healing stage of burns. *Caution*: St. Johnswort may increase photosensitivity in susceptible individuals.

- **Lavender** [*Lavandula angustifolia, L.* spp.]: Antimicrobial, wound healing, soothing. A specific for burns. Cool tea made from flowers may be used as compress or sprayed onto skin. Lavender hydrosol [a quality byproduct of essential oil distillation] can be sprayed onto tender tissue to cool and soothe. The essential oil may be applied undiluted, though those with sensitive skin should use it diluted.

- A few drops of **helichrysum essential oil** [*Helichrysum angustifolium*] added to a small bit of lotion or oil can amplify the benefits of the base. Antibacterial, antiviral, anti-inflammatory, wound healing, analgesic. A specific for burns and to prevent scarring. Consider adding a few drops to rosehip seed oil, sea buckthorn oil, calendula oil, or honey. Helichrysum is also known as Everlasting or Immortelle. **Niaoli essential oil** [*Melaleuca viridiflora*] can be used in the same way.

- **Propolis** in honey, cream or salve applied directly several times per day. Propolis, the name given to tree resins collected by honeybees and incorporated into their hives, is a wonderful antiseptic and wound-healing substance that has an anesthetizing and anti-inflammatory effect on the tissue it contacts. *Please note*: Use with caution if prone to allergy or hypersensitivity to bee stings, bee products, or tree resins.

- **Internal prevention strategies**. Certain plants have demonstrated radio-protective benefits: American and Asian ginsengs, tulsi/holy basil, ashawagandha, amla, astragalus, eleuthero, codonopsis, reishi, and rhodiola, among others.

- **L-glutamine** consumption has been shown to lessen mouth sores in those undergoing chemotherapy and radiation—and promote general wound healing. Glutamine, an amino acid, is a component of whey protein powder and can also be supplemented on its own. Cabbage juice is also a rich source of glutamine. Cabbage juice alone or L-glutamine powder mixed with saline solution may be swished in the mouth several times a day. Please see the section **Lack of Appetite / Weight Loss** for more information on L-glutamine.

- **Hyaluronic acid** [HA], aka hyaluronan. HA is a ubiquitous natural substance found throughout the body, especially concentrated in the eyes, joints, and skin. When applied topically, it has been clinically demonstrated to improve wound healing in the treatment of second-degree burns.[23,24] Can be both ingested or used topically, as indicated.[25]

- **Sodium alginate from brown seaweed** has been long recommended [by governments as well as medical sources] as adjunct support to mediate all types of radiation exposure. Alginates help bind with heavy metals and other toxins in bodily tissues and escort them from the body. Our collective experience with large populations dealing with nuclear radiation in Japan, Chernobyl and elsewhere has led to interesting insight on the benefits of eating seaweed, particularly brown kelps, following such exposures. The natural iodine in seaweed helps protect the thyroid from radioactive forms, as well. Typical recommendation: Eat or take seaweed supplements or alginate-rich products for a week before and after exposures via diagnostic imaging or other procedures. Average dose range is about 4-14 grams [1-4 teaspoons] of dried seaweed powder per day or up to 2-3 ounces of whole seaweed per week. Concentrated alginate products are also available; follow label instructions. See the **Resource** chapter for list of quality sources of seaweed and the book *Seaweed* by former radiation oncology nurse Valerie Cooksley in the **Recommended Reading** chapter. *Please note*: Consult with a practitioner as to whether appropriate *during* radiation therapy.

Lymphedema / Edema

Lymphedema refers to the swelling of subcutaneous tissues resulting from an accumulation of excessive interstitial lymph fluid. This fluid accumulation can be caused by obstruction of lymph vessels or their destruction via surgery, radiation, or malignant disease. Infection can also cause lymphedema, sometimes accompanied by chills, fever, redness, tenderness, swelling. Lymphedema as a consequence of infection is generally treated with internal use of antibiotic drugs, particularly those active against Streptococcal strains. Edema, per se, can be caused by cardiovascular and renal factors.

*See the article **The Lymphatic Network** in the Appendix for a basic overview.*

- **Ensure adequate hydration**. In the presence of such swelling, it is natural to believe that restricting water intake will help. In actuality, sufficient water in the system is essential to promote normal blood flow and lymph drainage.

- **Dietary support**: Limit or avoid salt [increases fluid retention]. Fiber-rich diet [vegetables, legumes, nuts, seeds, etc.] promotes bowel regularity. Celery is an excellent food as it provides ample fiber, natural sodium [an essential electrolyte], and acts as a diuretic to promote urine flow.

- See the **cleansing vegetable broth** in the chapter *A Few Recipes for Gentle Foods*.

- **Aduki beans** have long been prized in Japan and China as tonic to the kidneys. May be especially helpful for edema in the lower body. They are delicious cooked with seaweed, which also can be helpful in lessening water retention.

- **Dandelion leaf and root** [*Taraxacum officinale*]: Excellent general plant support for proper kidney and liver function. Ergo, gentle, classic detoxification support. Leaf used as fresh food, tea, and in capsules of freshly freeze-dried material; root used as fresh food, decoction, liquid extract, dried root in capsules.

- **Proteolytic enzymes** are recommended therapeutically in the naturopathic community to lessen lymphedema. Proteolytic enzymes—such as papain or bromelain from papaya and pineapples; trypsin and chymotripsin made within our bodies, etc.—are proteases that help digest protein from foods. Taken between meals, on an empty stomach, they may help reduce systemic inflammation and pain, particularly in concert with lymphatic drainage massage. Take no sooner than three days after surgery—Avoid before surgery, as these enzymes can potentially interfere with proper blood clotting. *Caution*: Do not use if taking medications that reduce blood clotting.

- **Homeopathic remedies**: *Lymphomyosot* by Heel, *Nat Mur*. *Note*: Homeopathic remedies are taken at least 15 minutes away from either food or drink.

- **B Vitamin complex**: Has been shown to help reduce water retention, in addition to supporting proper nerve health as well as the body under stress in general.

- **Traditional botanical lymphatic drainers**: Certain plant medicines are known to help promote movement of lymph fluid. They tend to also possess diuretic activity—

    o **Cleavers** [*Gallium* spp.]: above-ground parts. Diuretic, astringent, anti-inflammatory. *Formats*: Tincture or juice of fresh plant, succus.

    o **Chickweed** [*Stellaria media*]: above-ground parts. Diuretic, anti-inflammatory, wound healing. Gentle, nutritive medicine—and thus useful to include regularly as adjunct to other approaches in long-term management of lymphedema. Best eaten as salad green, freshly juiced, or preserved/utilized as succus or fresh plant tincture. Grows almost year 'round in temperate regions; favors disturbed soil.

    o **Burdock** [*Arctium* spp.]: root. Mild alterative, diuretic. Gently motivates lymphatic, kidney, and liver function. Indicated in chronic lymphatic swelling and chronic skin manifestations with inflammation, among other things. *Formats*: Decoction, tincture, food, capsules.

    o **Prickly ash** [*Zanthoxylum clava-herculis*]: bark. Pungent circulatory stimulant, anti-inflammatory. Indicated also for nerve pain. *Formats*: Decoction, tincture. Generally used in combination with other plants. *Caution*: Contraindicated in pregnancy.

    o **Poke** [*Phytolacca* spp.]: root. Anti-inflammatory, anti-edematous. A potent, potentially toxic botanical that is used in drop doses in formulations. You may find poke root, in small amounts, in commercial products formulated with other herbs to promote proper lymphatic drainage. Use alone only under the guidance of a knowledgeable herbalist or natural medicine practitioner. *Cautions*: Not appropriate for self-treatment. Contraindicated during pregnancy and lactation.

    o **Red root** [*Ceanothus americanus*]: root bark. Leaves aka New Jersey tea. Astringent. You may find red root in commercial products formulated with other herbs to promote proper lymphatic drainage. Use alone under the guidance of a knowledgeable herbalist or natural medicine practitioner.

- In clinical practice, lymphatic drainers are often combined with plant compounds that **support vascular integrity and circulation** such as horsechestnut [*Aesculus hippocastanum*] and the bioflavonoid rutin.

- **Cleansing fresh vegetable juice**: Fresh cleavers and chickweed [diuretic, lymphatic drainers mentioned above] may be juiced along with fresh parsley [diuretic], celery [diuretic], some carrots, and a bit of ginger [anti-inflammatory, circulatory stimulant]. Drink in small batches; thoroughly mix with saliva before swallowing.

- **Regular therapeutic massage** from professional therapist trained in specific lymphatic drainage techniques. Ask the therapist to show you **self-massage techniques** you can do regularly at home.

- **Skillful acupuncture treatments** can help the body optimize its fluid dynamics. Always seek out a licensed acupuncturist trained in traditional holistic ways of working, not a medical practitioner only superficially trained in using acupuncture for pain relief. Traditional acupuncture [and Chinese botanical medicine] is part of a comprehensive framework of medical understanding, complete unto itself.

- **Exercise**. Unlike the circulatory system with its reliably beating heart, the lymphatic system has no pump to ensure circulation of its fluid. Lymph flow relies on alternating muscular contraction and relaxation to motivate movement. Gradually undertake an exercise program, usually including some combination of stretching and flexibility, strength training, and aerobic exercise. For personal guidance, work with a physical therapist, occupational therapist, or other professional who specializes in lymphedema management.

- **Yoga, t'ai chi chuan, or qi gong** to improve circulation and flow of vital energy.

- **Dry brushing**. Using a dry, natural bristle body brush, brush skin gently in repeated strokes. Always direct movement *toward* the heart. As circulation increases in an area, the skin will lightly pink-up in color. Move progressively from one area to another: Arms, abdomen, buttocks, legs. Shower or bathe afterward to rinse off dead skin that's been loosened.

- **For edema in general**, additional kidney support may be indicated. For this purpose, it is recommended to begin with gentle, nutritive plants such as dandelion leaf/root and stinging nettle leaf. This level of support may be sufficient. Seasoned herbal practitioners know that the more assertive juniper berries [*Juniperus communis*] or stinging nettle *seed* [*Urtica dioica*] may have a role to play in stimulating kidney function in some situations. Consult with a naturopathic physician or well-trained herbalist to determine appropriate plants and dosing strategy for your situation.

- Use **compression garments or wrappings**, if and as instructed by your healthcare advisers.

- **Rosemary** [*Rosmarinus officinalis*]: leaf. Anti-inflammatory, muscle relaxing, circulatory stimulant, rejuvenative. Strong water infusion or essential oil diluted into a bit of liquid soap may be added to baths to both relax and revive aching, tense or tired muscles—and improve blood and lymph flow. A few drops of the essential oil [eo] may also be added to massage oil or lotion. *Caution*: Avoid using at night as its circulatory stimulating properties may delay sleep. Use of the essential oil is contraindicated in pregnancy; use eo cautiously with history of seizure disorders.

- Some women have found benefit using a **poultice of fresh cabbage leaves** to ease lymphatic stagnation. Crush leaves, apply, and wrap in place. Repeat as needed.

- **Lymphology Association of North America [LANA]**—Check out their website [www.clt-lana.org] to network with certified lymphadema therapists and for an assortment of useful internet links.

Thoughts on Medi-Ports—and Other Surgeries

Medi-ports are semi-permanent central venous catheters generally installed under the skin of the upper chest wall. They provide medical staff with an easy-to-access portal to the bloodstream that eliminates the need for repeated puncturing of veins for blood draws or administration of nutrients, chemotherapy agents, saline fluid, blood products, etc. For those undergoing protracted treatment, medi-ports can be a remarkable blessing.

However, the installation process is a surgical procedure and may have consequences, both physical and emotional. Both the energy sheath surrounding the body and the bodily tissue itself are penetrated and wounded in the process. This can take quite a long time to heal, particularly if the person is immune-compromised at the time of surgery. Additionally, the ports are often left in place for many years.

The body will naturally attempt to protect the vulnerable area, and postural adaptations may occur, almost imperceptibly at times. The shoulder may roll forward, as if protecting a damaged wing. Energy and movement can become restricted, even subtly, on the side of the body where the port resides. If habitual, over time these adaptations can result in connective tissue/muscular holdings and skeletal malfunctioning that can cause pain, achiness, or impaired range of motion.

In addition, emotional material related to the body, the illness, the surgery, or essential vulnerability may become constellated in the tissue that is engaged in protecting the self. When trigger points are activated, the person who is sensitive to their experience will likely feel emotion arise. Allowing this to be released into awareness can be an important aspect of healing at a deeper level.

Physical therapy by a well-trained, sensitive practitioner can help to both prevent the musculoskeletal adaptations from becoming fixed in the first place or help remediate established dynamics that have become challenging.

It seems to me that Physical Therapy or other bodywork should be routinely prescribed as adjunct to all surgery to help the body to adapt to the changes without distorting function. These concerns, of course, are obviously amplified in the case of major surgeries that involve removal of significant quantity of tissue, such as mastectomies, other amputations, organ removal, etc. Seek out the complementary support you deserve.

Hair Growth Strategies

Hair loss can occur as a side effect of pharmaceutical drug use, as a result of nutritional deficiencies, as a sign of low thyroid function or gluten sensitivity, or as a consequence of hormonal changes associated with aging.

A wide array of drugs can cause hair loss: Non-steroidal anti-inflammatory drugs [NSAIDs], certain antibiotics, anticoagulants, select antidepressants, anti-seizure meds, cardiovascular drugs, chemotherapy agents, lipid-lowering drugs, endocrine drugs, and more. If taking drugs in any of these classes, learn if hair loss is an expected side-effect.

Some of the other possible causes are briefly described below.

Assuming underlying causes are understood and being addressed, there are also a number of topical strategies to directly soothe the scalp, stimulate circulation, and promote hair growth.

- **Ayurvedic hair oil tonic**: Such as *Hair Plus Oil* from Tattva's Herbs, formulated with amla, bacopa, bringaraja [*Eclipta alba*], gotu kola and other rejuvenating herbs, and scented with pure jasmine essential oil. [Or any of these plant oils used alone can offer benefit.] Soothing, cooling to scalp and promotes hair growth. Apply with gentle finger massage at night. Wrap head or simply place small towel over bed pillow to absorb any excess oil. Shampoo out in morning, if desired. The formula's cooling nature helps balance inner heat rising through the scalp, particularly in the days following chemotherapy infusion.

- **Essential oils** such as rosemary or lavender can be added lightly into any fixed oils used for scalp massage. These two plant essential oils stimulate follicles and scalp circulation. Water-based infusions can be used as hair rinse when appropriate. *Caution*: Avoid rosemary essential oil in pregnancy or with history of seizures.

- **Jojoba oil** [*Simmondsia chinensis*], technically a liquid wax, is calming and soothing to all skin, and particularly helpful with dry or itchy scalp. Can be used alone or combined with follicle-stimulating essential oils such as rosemary or lavender. If stimulating essential oils are added, do not apply before bed; otherwise, jojoba has no scent and can be used at any time of day.

- **Infused oil of burdock seeds** [*Arctium* spp.] helps support normal sebaceous gland secretions—can be used alone or added to a jojoba-based formula. Both root and seed oil are used as a topical treatment for scalp health.

- **Infused oil of yarrow flowers and leaf** [*Achillea millefolium*]: massaged into scalp to improve local circulation and strengthen hair growth.

- Apply **gentle, loving touch to the scalp**. Do not forsake this newly vulnerable exposed skin. Stimulate gently with your fingertips; appreciate the beauty of your noggin'. Once hair begins to re-grow, be gentle with the new sprouts.

- **Let the scalp b-r-e-a-t-h-e** as often as possible, though you may often be wearing a scarf or hat to manage your body temperature. Choose natural fabrics such as cotton, silk, or soft merino wool for headgear as much as possible.

- **Read labels of all bodycare products carefully**, particularly products marketed to promote hair growth. Synthetic fragrances and commonly used preservatives such as parabens are known endocrine disruptors and carcinogens.

- **Potentially beneficial ingredients** that can appear on shampoo labels: jojoba oil, selenium, avocado oil, aloe vera, vitamin A and various carotenes, etc.

- **Kidney/Adrenal support**. As individually appropriate, tonics from the Asian and Ayurvedic herbal *materia medica* are used to bolster kidney/adrenal vitality, which is seen to be associated with hair growth and health. Such plants include: He shou wu [*Polygonum multiflorum*], eclipta [*Eclipta alba*]–often combined with amla for this, aduki beans, seaweeds, and others. Stinging nettles, a nutritious tonic food with affinity for kidneys/adrenals used in Western herbal tradition, is wonderful as an infusion, a steamed fresh vegetable, or powdered dry leaves added to a smoothie.

- **Ensure sufficient protein in your daily diet**. A steady supply of protein, and the full range of amino acids that compose it, is essential for maintenance of all body tissue, including skin, hair and nails. Sufficient consumption of quality proteins—such as from fish, eggs, whey protein isolate, lean meats—is necessary for the extensive repair and replacement of cellular building blocks which occurs constantly. This is particularly essential during periods of illness, during and following treatments such as chemotherapy and radiation, during recovery and recuperation, and following surgery, injuries, burns, blood loss, etc. Daily smoothies are often a key method of supplementing protein during such periods, particularly if appetite or taste is altered. See *Power Smoothie Recipe*.

- **Low thyroid function can manifest as hair loss**. Discuss this possibility with your health practitioner. Meanwhile, increasing consumption of mineral- and iodine-rich sea vegetables—ideally harvested from uncontaminated waters—may be of benefit even if blood thyroid hormone tests register as normal. Additionally, those taking the drug Synthroid [Levothyroxine] to boost thyroid function may experience hair loss in the initial stages of therapy. See *Resources* for high-quality sources of seaweed.

- **Nutritional deficiencies**—of zinc, vitamin A, essential fatty acids, and iron—might be contributing to hair loss, particularly in women. This can be due either to insufficient intake of foods rich in these nutrients or inadequate digestion and assimilation. Improving endogenous digestive enzyme secretion via intake of herbal bitters before eating or supplementing with high quality digestive enzymes may be an important initial strategy. Supplementation of one or more of these individual nutrients may also be indicated. Consult with your healthcare practitioner to assess whether—and which—nutrient deficiencies might be playing a role.

- Barring other obvious causes, hair loss **may also be a sign of gluten intolerance or sensitivity**, whether or not gastrointestinal symptoms are also present. Explore this with a holistic health care practitioner.

Helpful Items to Have on Hand

- Abundance of fresh cloths and towels for sponge baths, etc.

- Basin or bucket for potential vomiting.

- Bed pan or commode.

- Extra clean bed linens and up-and-about clothes.

- Extra pillows; backrest for sitting up in bed.

- Walker/stool/small chair to help with various bedside and bathroom postures, as necessary.

- Nursing gloves for suppository insertion, etc.

- Comfortable, cozy, non-binding cotton clothing that can be easily laundered. Fabric scissors and safety pins for *ad hoc* alterations of clothing to make dressing more comfortable and less traumatic.

- Bendable straws. Bent stainless steel straws are now an alternative to plastic.

- Leak-proof water bottle.

- Lip balm that is made from natural plant-based ingredients.

- Healing herbal salve.

- Glass eyewash cup.

- Body thermometer, non-breakable.

- Arrowroot powder for body dusting: Pure, unscented, non-irritating.

- Notebook or pad for caregiver or ill person to chart remedies administered, bowel movements, dreams, insights, etc.

- Small monitor that can be strapped around wrist for checking blood pressure and heart rate. Inexpensive, yet can be invaluable when questions arise. Easy to self-administer and can provide helpful information any time of night or day. Available at most pharmacies.

Citations for *The Helping Repertoire* are located in *Reference* section at back of book.

Questions to Ask Practitioners

You deserve to make decisions from a place of informed consent. When presented with a course of medical action by a practitioner, be sure to pause, breathe deeply and insist on understanding the context and implications of what is being recommended to you.

Answers to the following questions will help you to participate in your healthcare more fully empowered and will help you to know what to expect from proposed strategies. Your physician may certainly offer the information requested here on their own, as part of explaining the logic of their thinking. Having these questions with you during a consultation will help ensure that when you leave the office, you leave with all you wished to know in the present moment. Ideally, give this list to a companion so that they can also support this process.

Remember that even when you choose to use technological medicine to assist in diagnosing a problem or assessing its progress, you are not obligated to then also choose a technological or pharmaceutical response to what is learned. You are always free to choose the course of therapy or therapies that best makes sense to your way of understanding your health, your body, and your psyche. Pause, consider, seek alternative opinions. Ultimately, the choices are yours alone. This is your body and your life.

When a test is recommended:

- What is the reason for it? What are we looking for? What are we trying to rule out?

- What, specifically, will this test or procedure tell us? How accurate or reliable do the results tend to be? Can other circumstances lead to false-positive results?

- What are possible side effects or consequences in submitting my body to this test? What have you seen with other patients? What is described in the medical literature?

- If the test detects a problem, what will happen next? What will your recommendation likely be?

- If the test does not detect a problem, what might your recommendation be?

- Is this test essential to truly understand my health status at a deeper level or is it primarily necessary for you to feel that your professional liability has been exhausted? Please be frank with me about this.

- What are my other options in this moment, from your point of view?

When a treatment plan is proposed:

- What is the problem you perceive? How urgent is it that we begin treatment, from your point of view?

- Please describe the treatment you are suggesting: How is it administered or accomplished? How likely is it to resolve the problem or improve my condition?

- How and at what point do you evaluate if this has been successful?

- Are there potential consequences to ending this treatment prematurely if my body cannot handle it?

- If the treatment does not succeed, what are the next steps you might propose?

- Are there risks or side effects to the treatment? Are they typically temporary or long-term? Are there ways we can minimize them?

- What are my alternatives [including doing nothing at this time and maintaining mindful vigilance] from your point of view?

- Be sure to ask similar questions about any alternatives that are suggested.

I hope that this line of reasoning and questioning helps you remain calm and present in your interactions with your allopathic healthcare practitioners, who may perceive your situation from a different frame of reference than you do. They are trained to apply a certain medical logic that may or may not align with the path you choose to walk.

Remember that unless faced with life-threatening emergency, one rarely needs to make an important decision while in the medical office. It is certainly appropriate to give any proposed intervention some thought, and to seek a second opinion if you feel the first recommendation seems too life altering. It is within your power to slow the momentum of the allopathic healthcare system so that you are more able to navigate your options in a way that resonates with your own research and timing. Certainly, there are situations that call for more immediate action but I have found it important to distinguish between the urgency of the physician to cover their liability concerns and the actual medical urgency to one's own well being. You deserve clarity in this regard.

These are not the only questions that might be asked, only a guide to help empower you in your discussions and decision-making process.

I encourage you to assume the best and be focused and intentional in preparing for medical appointments. In my own interactions with the medical world, I like to make a blessing before seeing a health practitioner of any type that I will meet them from a grateful heartspace and that they will be guided in their interactions with me from a place of insight, authenticity, wisdom, compassion, respect...and for the highest good of all.

Questions first inspired by the teachings of Penny Simkin, internationally known childbirth educator.

Waiting for Test Results:
Dealing with Anticipatory Anxiety

Waiting for test results consigns us to a sort of mental and emotional limbo. Or, at least, that is a very common response to the state of not-knowing such waiting shifts us into. This sort of limbo often stimulates the stress response in our glandular systems, adding anxiety-promoting hormones into the mix. Some people choose to imagine the worst, figuring that they won't be disappointed should the outcome they fear the most turn out to be true. The power of our imagining thusly only adds to our anxious state of mind.

Spiritual teachers of all traditions remind us that not-knowing is actually the very circumstance that is our essential predicament as human beings: A predicament *and* an opportunity. Not-knowing is not just a glitch in some normal stream of certainty—it's a basic truth that we like to think is the exception.

When we step back to look at the big picture, we see that to believe that we definitively *know* this or that, in absolute terms, is merely a reassuring illusion. What we call "facts" or the objects of intellectual understanding are as relative and transitory as any other mental constructs. We are as we are as we are.

Not-knowing is actually the very condition we are advised to become comfortable with, our essential relationship with our lives—our direct exposure to aliveness—rather than dependency on superimposed definitions and labels and descriptions of our life in any given moment. To find rest, relaxation and poise in not-knowing is fine practice for living fully…and for the peaceful allowing of this life *as it is* as it endlessly transforms into death and renewal. The state of unlimited, undefined, limitless potential is both the ground from which conditions for life originate and the ground to which such conditions dissolve. This is a seemingly infinite cycle, the one dynamic we *can* know. Somehow, for each of us, apprehending this truth while spirit still animates the physical body opens our awareness to the infinite rhythm of change and possibility. Resting in not-knowing is freedom. As Krishnamurti named it, this provides "freedom from the known."

The following selection is a recorded moment from my own health journey— first posted August 17, 2010 on CaringBridge.

Housesitting at a friend's place on the water, I was awaiting the results of yet another biopsy. Skin beneath a curious dark stripe on a thumbnail had been harvested more than a week ago. What would the pathologist report of that tissue sample? Was I at the cusp of another trip through Cancerland?

I had been doing my best just to rest easy in not-knowing. This marking had showed up well before the lymphoma diagnosis and my oncologist had recommended waiting to explore it until my alchemical regime was finished. Now, six months later and in remission from lymphoma, seemed the time to rule out melanoma as an explanation.

That is how I have been framing it. The doorway being framed is a passage from dealing with cancer in the present tense to healing from cancer. This nail pigmentation has been a lingering question mark for many months now. Given an "all clear" message from the universe, it's then undistracted focus on recovery and renewal.

When I didn't receive the expected physician's phone call yesterday—despite my two calls to make sure the clinic had my current number—I let a small group of family and friends know by email, then took another walk. What to do? The evening was sublime.

This morning, I again felt the anticipation arise in my body. Would I hear today? What would I hear? Out of a lovely morning's reading and meditation, I remembered a favorite mantra: "Don't postpone joy!" Regardless of the impending phone call, I was fully alive and blissed out, listening to the water's heartbeat rhythms as wake from a passing boat reached the shore below me. I did not need to keep anxious vigil for the diagnosis, as if holding my breath. I chose to live my day in joy and contentment. I felt healthy and animated. I headed out for a long walk in the gloriously clear sunshine.

My vision was relaxed and open, scanning for agates as I walked the beach. Here and there a shell or stone would catch my eye and I would stoop to look closer or to touch. One such time a seal's head surfaced in the water not far beyond. It seemed completely at ease in its element, gazing steadily at me. At length, it disappeared underwater. I stood looking out at the waters of the Sound, the reflected sunlight dancing and pulsing. I stood looking for quite some time, thinking the seal might surface again in my sight. Eventually, silent laughter welled up from my belly to my chest: Yes, *this* is the sort of vigil I am more than willing to give my life energy to!

This journey I've been on has had many of these moments, of living with a heightened sense of not-knowing. Abiding in the mystery is one thing; knowing that defining information is coming one's way is another. In either case, it seems pure folly to delay pleasure or peace. This moment remains like every other, vibrant with possibility.

I bent toward the beach and picked up a well-worn stone that fit perfectly in my hand; I felt its warmth and smooth contours. It gave pleasure to rub it with my fingers. How much this journey has worn my own edges, softening me. Certainly, there is beauty in the glistening stones that still have sharp angles and roughness, but the smoothed, worn-down stones were the ones that caught my attention. Their edges had been sanded by time and turbulence and, because of all they had been through, their form could now offer me this warm comfort. It was another reminder to direct compassion and kindness toward my self, to breathe through yet another dangling question, and to exhale gratitude for the many, many gifts of this life journey—this beautiful day of aliveness, first of all.

———

Some Considerations During Waiting Periods

Certain questions seem worthy of asking ourselves at such moments of not-knowing, or of considering whether to agree to specific diagnostics in the first place: What is it that *I* actually need to know? What information is for the physician's benefit, in terms of fulfilling liability concerns? What information is for the benefit of friends, family, and employers—to present them with labels and prognoses, to soothe their own discomfort with not-knowing? Circling back to the core question: What is it that I, myself alone, truly need and desire to know?

Make a list of questions you have for the doctor *before* the test is conducted:

- What will this test reveal? What are its limitations—how definitive do you hope the results to be? What are my alternative options for getting this sort of information about my condition?

- What are the potential side effects of this test method and where can I learn more?

- How can I best prepare for this test? Fasting, hydration, avoiding supplements, etc.

- How long will it be before results are known?

- How will I learn the results?

    o Will the physician call? Will an appointment be scheduled? Will results be posted on my online medical chart?

    o Should I call for the results? If so, whom should I contact, at what phone number, and during what hours?

Assert your connection with physical aliveness:

Be present for your life as it is in this moment. Celebrate the opportunity to experience this flavor of what it means to be in a human body.

As appropriate for your circumstance, remember the beauty of pleasurable physical movement such as walking or yoga, gentle dance, prayer, toning/chanting, meditation, humor, and loving companionship in keeping oneself oriented toward joy and gratefulness in aliveness.

To fully live life is to trust life absolutely.

That whatever arises into experience is natural perfection,
arising out of divine order and intelligence ~
though small mind might imagine alternate preferences.

To trust life absolutely is to rest in not-knowing,
in the unborn wholeness,
and to allow this natural perfection its flow.

To resist, to constrict, to contract is to precipitate out of our own fulfillment,
to believe again in separation and substantive 'self,'
to fall into the trance of 'loss' and 'other.'

"Watch and Wait"

When being assessed for a known or suspected medical condition—or a mysterious symptom that has arisen—physicians typically present a logic tree of medical options as they see them in that moment: this or that further diagnostic step; this or that intervention; and, thirdly, the choice to attentively "watch and wait."

Sometimes, as a medical client, we are upset to know we must live with mystery. For some personality types, this is the absolute worst circumstance—to not have a name for what is going on with them, let alone to not have a clear medical solution. To be told that a reasonable option is to "watch and wait" can feel like a sentence of prolonged emotional torture.

At the other end of the spectrum, some people rejoice in not knowing—in the fact that whatever is going on with their health, it is not a clearly definable medical circumstance. The truth may be as equally benign as worrisome. Whatever is happening, it is not a disease entity that can be nailed down given the remarkable diagnostic tools of the present moment. Not to say it is either/or—it simply is not available to be perceived and classified. For these personalities, living in the mystery offers rich possibility.

For those who are comfortable living with uncertainty—or, if not comfortable, at least open to the possibility that this is even a state available to contemporary humans—being told or choosing to simply "watch and wait" becomes a powerful opportunity.

When a diagnosis is not fixed, it seems to me that we have choices. On the one hand, we can allow the fears that can arise from "not knowing" to overwhelm us and depress our life force. We can *presume* the worst, though in fact we simply do not comprehend all that is going on. We can live as if we actually have been given an assured sentence—toward death or disability—for the near future. In our worry, we can constrain our lives and limit our capacity to feel alive. We have, in effect, sentenced ourselves to an immediate shrinking of our aliveness.

Alternately, when a diagnosis is not fixed, despite felt symptoms, it also may be far easier to find the space within where "All is well." This may seem an impossibility to some, or may seem an attempt at self-hypnosis. But for anyone practiced in looking within—through meditation, prayer, mindful movement, or other methods—this is a profound possibility. And many books have been written, including many by enlightened physicians, that explain some of the known physiological consequences that can flow from such an orientation.

On a continuum ranging from collapsing the spirit in full resignation that "all is lost" to the open, peaceful space of "all is well" exist a host of emotions and ways of being. What I am saying is not to negate the truth of anyone's state, emotion, perceptions. For most of us, any given period of our lives will evidence a flow of changing states and understandings. My point is to pose the question, once again: How shall we live in this moment?

Yes. In this moment, I am alive: I am living and breathing. How shall I live? What is available to be experienced? Here? Now?

From my own personal experience dancing with cancer, I can testify that "Watch and Wait" can become transformed into "Live and Flourish." It is a matter of orientation. I feel confident in asserting that our time on this earth has never been guaranteed—either in its duration or its quality. This, right now, is the life that we have. Shall I cease experiencing the joy and delight in being in this body—this day, this moment—because of the possibility that I will not live as long or as pain-free as I had imagined?

And while this process of investigation may begin for some as a mental exercise, with dedication to meeting our lives with gratitude, self-compassion and curiosity, it may soon open into a heightened aliveness that is quite embodied—A freshness, a tenderness, a willingness to stay open and vibrant in the presence of mystery.

———————

For more on this theme, please see the following section *Living with Chronic Disease* as well as Stephen Levine's remarkable body of work for masterful guidance from a compassionate meditation teacher who has long worked with those facing serious illness, death and dying. See the ***Recommended Reading*** chapter for details on his books.

Gear for the Chemo Lounge

While specific for taking to the chemotherapy infusion clinic, this list has some overlap with the Hospital To-Go Bag, which is detailed in the following section. Asterisks [*] indicate items that are also useful in the to-go bag.

☐ A small, cozy **blanket**. These may be offered but it is prudent to have one's own.

☐ **Clothing to keep you warm and comfortable**: Hat, scarf [easy warm-up item that is also infusion port-friendly], shawl/fleece vest/sweater, etc. While some chemo agents heat up the body, many cause a sensation of chill. Wear clothing that easily opens to give access to either your inner elbow or medi-port area.

☐ ***Cellular phone**. If you have one, many items such as contact phone numbers and calendar may be readily available to you. Also, you can load it with music or guided meditations. See note below.

☐ ***Digital music player**. Earphones. Sometimes group infusion pods can host chatty patients. In such cases, if you need respite, having earbuds dangling from your ears—with or without actually listening to your device—can be a clear signal to others that you seek solitude.

☐ ***Earplugs**. Again, these are a way to turn down the volume on the conversations and the hum of activity going on around you. Experiment also with staying connected to the conversations one overhears in the pod; these can be informative and sometimes almost oracular…or lead to unexpectedly beautiful connections with others.

☐ **Electrolyte beverage**. Coconut water provides efficient hydration without the artificial dyes and flavorings of standard-issue sports drinks.

☐ ***Water bottle**. The clinic may offer water in plastic bottles—which, paradoxically, may leach cancer-promoting toxins. Filtered water may be available to refill your own glass or stainless steel [preferably] bottle. Ask at the clinic.

☐ Likewise, your own **stainless steel or porcelain travel mug for hot beverages**. Some clinics may offer paper hot cups; some may provide polystyrene foam cups, which have been shown to leach carcinogenic substances into hot beverages!

☐ **Healthy snacks or lunch foods**. You may want some light food on hand to sustain you through your session. Salty foods such as seaweeds may be especially welcome. Be mindful of unhealthful clinic offerings loaded with sugars or hydrogenated oils.

☐ Stash of **ginger tea in bags**, preferably organic. Welcome aid in preventing nausea.

☐ **Sunglasses** [if feeling sensitive to fluorescent lighting]; **sleep mask**, if desired.

☐ ***Reading material**. Some clinics provide a selection of books and magazines, but of course it's nice to be independent and have your own.

☐ ***Journal or notebook, pens**. Some may wish to bring sketchpad and drawing pencils. You may be surprised by what inspiration comes.

☐ ***Treatment journal** for recording dated details of infusion strategies, dosages, infusion rates, other info learned each session. This should be the same notebook you bring to visits with your doctor, so that all information is in one place. If you are not up for making such notes, ask a companion to take responsibility for this.

☐ **Your calendar** to facilitate scheduling decisions.

☐ ***List of friends/contacts with phone numbers**.

☐ ***List of drugs or supplements** you are currently taking. Note any known interactions or adverse reactions you have experienced in the past.

☐ ***Names, addresses and phone numbers of your referring physician, primary care doctor, and other practitioners** who are part of your healing team. You never know when you'll have to fill out *another* form.

☐ ***Small supply of any pharmaceutical drugs or supplements** you will need to take during your clinic visit. Consult with oncology staff before using.

☐ ***Copy of your Medical Power of Attorney**. This may already be scanned into the system computer, but just in case….

☐ ***Small personal-sized hand sanitizer with natural essential oils** to use upon leaving the clinic for the day. Be mindful of introducing any scents into the shared space of the chemo lounge itself as some folks will be highly sensitized to aromas and may easily become nauseous. The clinic, in fact, may insist that all patients and companions arrive "scent free."

Pack a To-Go Bag
for Unexpected Hospital Stays

It's before dawn and you get a phone call from your oncologist urging you to get to the hospital as soon as possible—your most recent bloodwork has shown you need an immediate transfusion. What should you grab on the way out the door? Or, in any circumstance where you are uncertain where a visit to the clinic will lead, having a small duffle bag or daypack packed with essentials and ready to take with you is the way to go, ensuring you'll have what you need no matter where the day takes you.

☐ Copy of your **Medical Power of Attorney**. It may already be scanned into the healthcare system's computer, but just in case….

☐ Copy of your **current supplement and medication list**. Notes on any allergies or previous adverse reactions to pharmaceuticals, etc.

☐ Copy of **names and phone numbers of relevant practitioners**.

☐ Copy of **phone list of friends and support network**.

☐ **Cellular phone**. If you have one, many items such as contact phone numbers and calendar may be readily available to you. Ask about hospital rules before using.

☐ **Treatment journal**: Notes from physician appointments, other therapies.

☐ **Sleepwear**, including sleeping cap if used to keep head warm. Much more cozy than hospital standard issue!

☐ **Socks, slippers**. Forgetting these, at the hospital, you may be able to request a pair of socks that have little rubber dots on the feet to prevent slipping…

☐ Toothbrush, toothpaste, other such **articles for oral hygiene**.

☐ Small travel bottle with preferred **non-scented body lotion**: To soothe dry hands and feet, if needed.

☐ **Journal or notebook, pens**.

☐ Personal clip-on **reading light**. One that can also be adjusted to stand on its own can also serve as a nightlight, if needed.

☐ **Eye mask** for sleep!!! Almost an essential in light-saturated hospital spaces.

☐ **Ear plugs**. Ditto above.

☐ Healthful, low-sugar/high-protein energy bars or other **non-perishable snacks**. Read labels carefully to find choices that will work with your condition.

☐ A **handful of teabags** of your preferred herbal teas, tucked into a small ziplock baggie to protect from moisture.

☐ **Small supply of prescribed drugs or any nutritional supplements** you take daily.

☐ Calming, inspiring **book**. See *Recommended Reading* chapter for suggestions.

☐ Remember to grab your small **personal digital music device** loaded with soothing and uplifting music, music that makes you feel good, guided visualizations or audio teachings that help promote inner peace. No shoulds here; whatever helps you stay relaxed and in your center. Include earphones and recharging cord.

☐ **Stainless-steel water bottle** and **travel mug**. Although medical settings may offer water in plastic bottles or polystyrene cups, I greatly prefer to have my own supply with me…Carrying your own beverage container, when emptied, then provides you with independence and a non-toxic vessel for securing water from other sources.

Organizational Strategies
During Treatment and Homestay

Having things you need where you need them when you need them becomes a priority with home healthcare. Organization helps everyone involved feel more relaxed and comfortable, perhaps except for those who are challenged to be so. The goal of this section is to help simplify the organizing process.

Bedside —

- Water bottle.

- Thermometer, non-breakable.

- Blood pressure/pulse wrist cuff monitor [very useful].

- Small personal reading light—table lamp, booklight, lightweight headlamp, etc.

- Tissues.

- Small tape or digital recorder for voice messages to friends and family, journaling.

- Relevant phone numbers. Telephone within easy reach—speaker phone, if possible.

- Small, personal digital music device loaded with music [soothing, uplifting, energizing, etc.], guided meditations, spiritual teachings—whatever the individual finds helpful, pleasurable, companionable.

- Light reading material or inspirational book to help calm the mind if restless, to read until sleep comes.

- Sleep mask [or light-blocking window shades]: Essential for deepening sleep. Blocks ambient light that filters into sleeping space from surroundings. Darkness instigates the brain's production/secretion of the pineal hormone melatonin, which helps promote sleep and proper biorhythms, among many other health benefits.

- Sleeping cap to keep a bare noggin warm, as needed, through the night. Soft cotton is ideal as it allows the scalp to breathe.

- Small notebook/pen to easily record dreams or thoughts without fully waking or getting up out of bed. Booklight or headlamp-style flashlight allows note-making with minimal light disturbance.

Bathroom —

- Accurate scale for keeping track of weight gain or loss.

- Unscented, natural baby wipes: Soothing to a tender or irritated tush. Some chemo agents lend a burning quality to stools. Choose product wisely from natural-product source, free of unhealthful ingredients such as synthetic fragrances.

- Ditto aloe vera gel or calendula/zinc-based baby diaper ointment—apply after thorough wiping. Soothing, protective, promotes healing.

- Liquid natural soap with tea tree or thyme or other naturally antimicrobial essential oils—for handwashing. Essential to protect the immune compromised.

Elsewhere —

- Natural essential-oil-based antimicrobial handspray for visitors' use, staged at entryways.

- Pocket-size of same for car or purse. Use after clinic visits, shopping trips, all encounters with the outer world.

- Avoid personal sanitizers that contain chemicals such as the widely used *triclosan* and its chemical cousin *triclocarban* which have been associated with health concerns such as endocrine disruption, the proliferation of antibiotic-resistant bacterial strains, and the contamination of aquatic ecosystems.

Organizing your life —

- **File box or file sachel with folders for essential health-related documents**: Upcoming test instructions, diagnostic test results/reports, health insurance documents, living will/health power of attorney, random medical bills, prescription drug information [pharmacy instructions, receipts, etc.], hospital/clinic information, research/networking/contact information, financial support information, etc. Choose something small that could be easily transported—part of to-go plan—if necessary.

- Envelope/box/whatever for **storing practitioner business cards** as collected.

- Many health-support organizations provide **journals for keeping track of background medical details** [ask nursing staff for recommendations]: Your health history, dates of procedures and diagnoses, names and phone numbers of physicians involved, your personal emergency contact information, medical insurance name and identification numbers, critical medication or food allergies, current pharmaceuticals [prescribing physician, dosing information], name and phone number of pharmacy, current nutritional supplements [name and dosing information]. Keeping this sort of journal can simply life considerably when repetitively filling out intake forms, applications for financial assistance, and so on. **Once you have filled out some extensive intake form that includes much of this information, photocopy it and carry it with you to all medical appointments for quick reference.**

- **Desktop calendar/planner** in which all medical appointments, health-promoting sessions [Reiki, massage, acupuncture, yoga class, physical therapy, etc.] can be noted…as well as phone calls to be made on a given day, fasting that needs to happen before blood tests or procedures, etc. Use this to also note name of anyone who will be driving or accompanying you to any appointments or procedures. Write everything in pencil, as this schedule may often be changed or amended!

- **"Health Journey" notebook/journal as a tracking tool**, kept by your dining table in which you record *daily*: Foods eaten; meds and supplements taken—what and when; comments about sleep, urine color, bowel movement frequency and consistency, bodily or emotional sensations; etc. This may seem like an overly detailed task, but the chronicle it creates offers a great view over time. This sort of record keeping can prove invaluable to help you remember what you did when—and for assessing how what you take in effects your ability to sleep, to eliminate waste material, and so on.

- This notebook can also be the place to **record questions** you or your support circle wish to ask your medical team at the next visit. Take this notebook both to scheduled visits and to the hospital, should you require a stay.

- **Make a list of important contacts**—friends, family, neighbors, pharmacy and medical helpers—with phone numbers and email addresses. This is not only so everything can be found in one place; this list can be duplicated for your purse, hospital to-go bag, "Health Journey" notebook, multiple telephone sites at home, distribution to your regular helpers.

- Create yourself or have a friend **organize addresses on your email software** so that multiple friends/family can easily receive a single message updating test results or scheduled procedures. Think: how can I most easily communicate with the least expenditure of energy?

- Alternately, or in addition, create or have a friend **create a webpage on one of the free online health-notification systems such as CaringBridge**. With these, you can easily post messages and photos—and easily stay connected and receive support from loved ones and community. Highly recommended. See the chapter *Networking and Medical Fundraising* later in this book.

Organizing drugs and nutritional supplements —

- Have a special place for these, so that their physical location helps you remember to take what you need—when you need.

- Create, or have a friend help you create, some chart that lists your daily protocol in a helpful manner.

- If a drug labels list the name of the substance in tiny type, print it larger yourself with a marker. Obviously, do not cover essential information.

- For the supplements, write the number of capsules per dose right on the front of the label or on the cap so that you don't need to refer to your protocol after a while. Be sure to note AM, PM or AM/PM, etc.

- Alternately, small packages can be made up in advance of those supplements that are taken together at a given time. A cupcake tin makes a handy sorting tray. Compartmentalized pill-storage boxes and tiny baggies are available: Be sure to indicate when the contents are to be taken [eg. Monday AM; Monday PM; Monday lunch, etc.] Do not make up more than a week's supply of such packages, though, in case you wish to change your protocol—Once supplements are removed from their labeled bottles, they can be impossible to identify. ***Pharmaceutical drugs should always*** *be kept in their original containers, however.*

- Try to have backstock of what you are taking so that you don't run out. Sometimes, with nutritional supplements, you may be able to save money by buying multiple units as well. These can be stored in a box or bin close to the open containers so you or a helper can easily replenish and keep track of your supply. Make a list noting which supplements you get from which source, to help yourself or your helpers to keep things straight and to facilitate repurchasing as needed.

- Partially refill emptied drug and supplement bottles with the ***exact same*** items to create a small stash of such essential items that you might need should you be hospitalized or need to travel unexpectedly. Place these in a stuff sack or other organizer and keep them stowed in your to-go bag, just in case.

Random aids —

- **Soothing essential oils as tolerated**: Calming lavender at bedside or added into sheets or towels when laundering, etc. Aromatherapy candles to be lit to calm the stomach while eating, freshen bathroom or bedroom, etc. *Avoid all synthetic fragrances as they may likely contain carcinogenic compounds.*

- **Images of the divine**, any images that evoke a sense of peace or affirmation of health and healing. These can be placed around your space: At your bedside, on a personal altar, at your dining table, in the bathroom, where daily drugs and supplements are staged. For example, near my own collection of such bottles, I placed a photo of turkey tail fungus, a beloved medicinal mushroom ally, and a favorite image of the *shri yantra*, an ancient sacred mandala describing the relationship of essence and form. On my personal bedroom altar are images of compassionate divinity from various traditions, favorite stones, and meditation tools such as my singing bowl.

- Do your best to **harmonize and calm your bodymind whenever you feel anxious or distressed**, especially before or after sessions involving the medical system. Use whatever tools work for you: Prayer, meditation, singing sacred songs [or whatever type inspire peace or joy], toning, playing a singing bowl, reciting the rosary or reciting chants with a mala, biofeedback [hand-held types that promote cardiac coherence are easy to have with you wherever you may be], listening to soothing music, Reiki, yoga/t'ai chi/Qi gong, walking, rattling, drumming, being in a green space, and so on. All efforts toward clearing, calming and harmonizing the bodymind support cellular order and immune system functioning.

- **Establish a regular rhythm within your day**, to the best of your ability to do so. Rhythm promotes health and healing, and creates a sort of container for your activities. Rhythm helps create some sense of predictability in a life that has become more unpredictable. Try to schedule appointments and visits within the structure of the rhythm you find works best for you. This rhythm is built around morning practices, bowel movements, regular meals and snacks, exercise of some nature, rest, and sleep. Be sure to build time for quiet and relaxation into every day, *especially* if your day includes trips or appointments when it can be most challenging to maintain your health-promoting routines.

- **Sufficient hydration** is essential to good health at any time, and particularly for those going through chemotherapy and/or radiation therapies. Carry a stainless steel water bottle with you on all outings. At home, stage your daily intake of water in a way to easily keep track of your consumption. In the morning, while boiling water for tea, I would fill two half-gallon glass canning jars with fresh water and sit them in the counter. That way, whenever I passed through the kitchen there was a visual reminder to drink more water. Likewise, when sitting down with a visitor or to watch a video or listen to music, bring a large glass of water with you so it's in front of your face, so to speak. Sufficient water each day keeps the body's systems of detoxification and elimination working as smoothly as possible, and helps protect delicate tissues such as those of the kidneys. Adequate water consumption can help limit chemo-induced headaches and skin eruption issues.

- As you are able, **embrace the chemotherapeutic agents as healing elixirs, radiation as the enlivening light of life**….not demonizing or resisting these treatments…welcoming, accepting, surrendering to their potency with gratitude. Then, equally turn attention toward supporting the body's healthy tissues with clean, vibrant food and water—and complementary nutritional supplements as appropriate.

- If this resonates for you, **visualize all therapeutic efforts as dissolving disordered cells into primordial substance**…envisioning that the body will eliminate what is no longer needed and recycle basic building blocks into new and healthy cells. Intend that disorder will be eliminated, with only harmonious, cooperative, properly organized cells arising…Disorder resolved, for the good of the whole, the good of the system, the good of the body maintaining its physical life and existence.

Prayer and Visualization

Voluminous research has shown that the power of prayer and visualization—both directed and non-directed to specific outcomes, originating both locally and non-locally—can be profound healing tools.

In addition, including sacred healing sound both as preface and container for our intentional efforts offers another layer of benefit, as so many religious traditions demonstrate in their worship formats. The use of sound based on ancient healing principles to create the ambient space for meditation, prayer and visualization allows us to sink more deeply into brain states that support harmony of mind, body and spirit. These sacred sounds, particularly if recorded, may then be repeated at other times throughout the day to generate healing space.

The extensive research presented by notables such as Larry Dossey MD, Bernie Siegel MD, Deepak Chopra MD, Jeanne Achterberg, Joan Borysenko PhD, and many others documents the specific ways all this is understood to occur. A selection of relevant books is included in the **_Recommended Reading_** chapter; suggested recordings can be found in **_Recommended Listening_**.

Whatever you might choose to practice in this regard, keep it simple and personally meaningful.

Most of us need no research to convince us that our environment and inner attitude greatly influences the nature of our experience. When we are sick or exhausted or discouraged, finding an inner space where we are relaxed and can focus calmly on praying for something specific, or surrendering to the greater flow and purpose, or simply resting in wordless thoughts or wordless images of _being_ love, _being_ gratefulness, _being_ deeply well can re-align and refresh our beings—physiologically, emotionally, spiritually…

Do not take my word for it and do not waste too much time intellectually seeking out the clinical provings of this ancient wisdom—they are increasingly abundant. Right now, in this moment, put down this book, ensure that you are in a comfortable posture, take some deep cleansing breaths, soften the belly and relax the body and mind. With each fresh breath, settle into timeless space, the space within which all occurs. As thoughts come and go, return attention to the breath. Allow a gentle, sweet recognition of aliveness to permeate every cell. Open to the soft, inner smile that can become our default setting, given practice.

No matter what the outer circumstances or physical experience, this infinite inner space awaits as refuge, as temple. From this formless space, what might arise?

Living with Chronic Disease

Untold millions of people around the world deal each day with the physical limitations and emotional challenge of chronic disease and unwellness. A variation on this theme is living very delicately on a hair-trigger line between health and distress. Such often seems to be part of the burden and cost of inhabiting a human lifetime. Yet, it is also clear that the attitude we bring to our life in general is an important factor in how chronic disease, the shadow of disease recurrence, or high sensitivity impacts daily living.

How do we inhabit our days with joy and peace when we know that at any moment our equilibrium may be upset or that pain or disease process might flare? These are the questions of being alive in a human body—and material addressed by religions and varied spiritual practices. We each live with these questions, though some more consciously than others.

During a lifetime, each person has the opportunity to deeply explore the nature of anxiety and suffering—whether during an acute episode or if living with more chronic challenges. And, truly, it *is* an opportunity—that's not just some palliative language. From my own experience and from my interactions with others I have seen the truth of this. Somehow, the deeper we open to experience our emotions and our physical sensations—allowing them to be as they are without crystallizing them, identifying with them, or constricting or rejecting them—the more easily they move, shift and potentially transform.

I very, very highly recommend the work of Stephen and Ondrea Levine in exploring this topic for yourself or with a loved one. Their early books *Who Dies?* and *Healing into Life and Death,* and the more recent *A Year to Live: How to Live this Year as If It Were Your Last* are exceptional. Long-time meditation teachers, they have spent a lifetime working with the severely ill and dying. Their work first opened my own heart and being to explore the distinction between *my* pain and *the* pain, and to soften around sensations and concepts within both body and mind—thus lessening personal identification with an essentially energetic experience.

In such a process of investigation, what may at first seem fixed and rigid may ultimately be known as fluid and dynamic. Within this awareness, great healing may unfold. The nature of this healing is both utterly individual and beyond the personal. The gateway is meeting our experience with curiosity, openness and acceptance.

It is important to note that what I am calling acceptance is not resignation. These are two very different dynamics.

With resignation, there may be passivity and, potentially, a victim mentality can arise. With resignation, there may be a collapse of lifeforce, a constriction in the flow of the very energies that sustain and support health and aliveness. Resignation implies that there is a fixed state from which our physiology can never recover.

Acceptance, on the other hand, is non-resistance. It is an allowing of what *is* simply to be, even if that is impending death. With acceptance, we remain open to life, to all that life brings. With this sort of acceptance, our physical, emotional and energy bodies are free to be fully alive in each moment. We are here, now, and what shall this moment be?

Soft-bellied acceptance allows that life is constantly flowing and transforming as it moves through all form, including our selves—That our existence is a precious gift and, until our last breath, it is not yet over. Acceptance is not about hope, *per se*, but about living each moment fulfilled in its beauty and recognizing the grace that is presenting.

Take the time to investigate the difference between resignation and acceptance within yourself. Acceptance is a keynote in living comfortably with whatever presents on our journeys—whether the path suddenly turns steeply uphill and rocky or whether it smoothes and levels. Either way, we can find our strength and our footing by accepting what has shown up and knowing that, eventually, this too will change. For the moment, though, this is the way through—one moment, one step at a time.

Additional Support

Nutritional considerations: As an active way to say Yes! to Life, view each meal as direct communion with the life force. Choose foods that are colorful, vibrant and whole —which deeply nourish and renew the physical dimension and help harmonize the neurological/hormonal dynamics that support adaptability. This essentially means avoiding processed foods—all foods laden with salt, sugars, sugar substitutes, artificial colors and preservatives. Choose organically cultivated, chemical-free foods, particularly oils, seeds, nuts, eggs, meat and dairy products. Strictly avoid hydrogenated or partially hydrogenated oils. Whatever its origins, bless your food with heartfelt appreciation.

Activity considerations: Activity can be challenging in some health circumstances, yet to whatever degree movement is possible it should be part of each day. Whether aided by a therapist, a friend, a walker, or whatever it takes, the body needs to be moved in order to signal to itself that it remains alive and in need of renewal each day. To keep bones strong and muscles from atrophy, find some level of movement and exercise that works for you—walking, yoga, Qi gong, t'ai chi chuan, aerobic activities—guided by your health advisers. Movement benefits proper metabolism including digestion, assimilation, detoxification, elimination, and renewal. If you share the activity with a friend or loved one, so much the better. For a highly motivational discussion of life as movement, see the chapter on "Movement and Exercise" in *Radical Healing* by Rudolph Ballentine MD.

Attitudinal considerations: To stay connected with wise companionship and inspiration, take advantage of the wealth of books, audio/visual teachings, sound healing, and practices from all traditions that are currently offered. Surely there is a voice, a teacher, a language of healing to suit every individual. Find what resonates for you and use these materials and tools to help you meet the circumstances of your life in a way that enables you to be more fully alive. Please see the sections on ***Recommended Reading*** and ***Recommended Listening*** for lists of annotated books, music and other resources.

Repairing the Garment:
Surgery & Beyond

"Within this fathom-long body is found all of the teachings,
is found suffering, the cause of suffering, and the end of suffering."
— **Shakyamuni, the Buddha**

One of the most challenging aspects to preparing for surgery, I believe, is the coming to terms with the full implications of inhabiting a fragile human body—a body whose tissues and functionality can fail and may require such drastic intervention. A body that is constantly changing and ultimately will cease to function entirely. Prior to a diagnosis that may include a recommendation for surgery, we may be able to lull ourselves into a state of mind that precludes the awareness of the ultimate preciousness of a human life and the fragile tether by which a particular embodiment hangs. But a need for surgery can certainly wake us up. All of life is in flux—emerging into form and dissolving into formlessness. This is happening even as we observe forms that appear to be solid and unchanging. Transformation and reconfiguration is occurring everywhere, before our very eyes—the work is about cultivating our vision to perceive such energy in motion.

Preparing for surgery and dealing with its aftermath can be perceived as a wonderful opportunity to reconfigure our lives and come into greater harmony with the life force that animates our physical vehicles. We are, in large part, able to determine the breadth and depth of our healing based on our willingness to investigate and allow.

And so, with the prospect of subjecting our flesh to the scalpel or the laser, we are presented with an opportunity to perceive more clearly the nature of a lifetime. We get to explore gratitude for the elegant system design of the human body, which is inherently so remarkable in its capacity to sustain wellness. We get to explore our attitudes and behaviors regarding daily maintenance of our physical bodies. We get to explore our relatedness with all phenomenal existence. We get to explore what it is that explores such things.

In this way, consenting to surgery of any type can be life-altering, no matter the degree of urgency or invasiveness. We hope, of course, never to come to the place where surgery is necessitated at all. And yet, facing the temporary nature of our physical vehicles and investigating our relationship with our personalities and our mental concepts about our lives helps prepare us for the inevitable relinquishing of the material body—absolute surrender to what is—the ultimate release of the "I" into all-pervading suchness, within which arisal and dissolution pulse. Such surrender can open us to the healing that is possible.

General Preparation for surgery —

The approach here is influenced by many factors, including the invasiveness of the procedure. The degree of support undertaken should be customized to the individual, their constitution, current health situation, fitness level, pharmaceutical regimen if any, nutritional status, lifestyle, and so forth.

An overlighting intention is to refine harmony of vibration within the being and within their immediate field. In addition, a goal is to maximize energy reserves so to minimize the trauma associated with the intervention and to speed recovery. We look to plant allies, dietary choices, spiritual practices, sound healing, and the breath to provide a deeper resonance with life force.

Please be certain to follow your physician's guidance as to categories of natural products from which to abstain prior to surgery. *A naturopath or herbalist can help interpret which nutrients and plants fall into those categories. For instance, garlic, ginkgo, turmeric, and the ginsengs theoretically might increase the risk of bleeding and are usually discontinued for seven days before surgery. For the same reason, vitamin E at doses exceeding 200 IU per day and fish oils are generally discontinued two weeks prior to surgery. There are diverse opinions about the timing and even the rationale for such cessation, but the above represents a conservative approach.*

In addition, it is generally considered prudent to avoid some nerve-influencing herbs such as kava, St. Johnswort, and valerian for about five days prior to receiving anesthesia or analgesics, based on speculative concerns about their concomitant use with these drugs. Explore other methods to promote calm as discussed below.

Please use the material that follows as a guide to further research and to enable a collaborative discussion with your physician. This presentation outlines general principles and practices—only you, in concert with a trained practitioner/healthcare adviser can decide what is appropriate to your situation.

- **Adaptogenic herbal tonics**: Traditionally esteemed plants to support optimum harmony of body systems and optimum resiliency potential. Moderate the impact of stressors on the bodymind. Depending on constitutional considerations and lead-time, look to eleuthero, codonopsis, ashwagandha, American ginseng, *Panax ginseng*, he shou wu, schisandra, stinging nettles, rhodiola, chyawanprash Ayurvedic herbal jam, and so on. Confer with holistic practitioner or refer to the section on ***Adaptogenic Plant Allies*** for descriptions of individual plants and some congenial combinations.

- **Immune system tonification**: Synergistic with previous category. Consider astragalus root, reishi, maitake, shiitake, turkey tail [*Trametes/Coriolus versicolor*], cordyceps or some combination of mushroom species [both fruiting body and mycelium]. Many such medicinal organisms are also considered adaptogenic. Please see section on ***Adaptogenic and Tonic Plant Allies*** for further discussion and one suggested recipe for an immune broth. In general, these medicines may be beneficially utilized as water extractions—simmered into broths, foods, or beverages—or ingested as well-prepared extracts. Some, such as shiitake and maitake, are delicious as foods.

- **Related to the above**, consider working with a licensed acupuncturist/Chinese herbalist to focus on a customized series of treatments and herbal formula to tonify the vital force and maximize proper wound healing capacity in the 3-4 weeks preceding surgery.

- **Enhance health of beneficial intestinal bacterial**: Balance and vigor of this essential microbial terrain is related to immunity, digestive health, and overall wellness. Because pharmaceuticals typically used in support of surgery degrade intestinal microbes, it is important to both precede and follow their use with cultured foods and well-prepared probiotic supplements to offset this negative impact. It has also been shown that taking supplemental probiotics provides benefits even when taken within the same day as pharmaceutical antibiotics—separate dosing of these agents to whatever degree possible to maximize benefit.[1,2]

- **Ensure copious hydration** with water as free of chemicals as possible. Sip on water between meals throughout the day. Keep a water bottle with you for both convenience and as a visible reminder.

- **Two-plus weeks of sattvic eating**, including no alcohol or stimulants. This practice is deeply calming to both body and mind. Focus on organically cultivated vibrant fresh foods as much as possible: Freshly pressed vegetable juice, lightly steamed vegetables, soaked nuts and seeds, whole grains, high quality protein. Limit salt, stimulating condiments, fiery spices, congesting foods such as cow's milk dairy products. Avoid refined sugars.

- **Enhance nutritional status**:

  o **Supply readily assimilated vitamins and minerals to tissues**. Look to overnight infusions of stinging nettle leaf, horsetail, alfalfa, oatstraw, red raspberry/ thimbleberry leaf; sea vegetables; chlorella; freshly pressed green juices in moderation; dark leafy greens, dark orange vegetables; high quality liquid chlorophyll.

  o **Ensure adequate intake of protein** to build flesh, particularly if currently in a deficient state where weight has been lost. See the section in *The Helping Repertoire* on **Lack of Appetite/Weight Loss** for specific suggestions.

- **Vegetable juice**: Fresh organic carrots combined with congenial companions such as beet [no more than ¼ small beet per serving], celery, parsley, ginger, dandelion greens, etc.: Take in small quantities, mixed well with saliva, up to 3-4 times per week.

- **Vibrational hygiene**: Where you have a choice, apply careful discernment as to media and public impressions taken into your energy field. Avoid television, newspapers, agitating music, crowds, violence, frenzy, disturbing situations or images.

- **Be generous in time allowed for sleep and rest**. What is it that you really must "do"? Be your own most compassionate, protective guardian.

- **Enjoy appropriate degree and form of exercise for your situation**. Know your body and its limitations and proceed accordingly.

- **Secure private time for reflection, reading, journaling, spiritual endeavors**. Stay mindful of your inner process. Sleep alone when that feels most sacred. Pay attention to your dreams. Take notes. Make art. Deep healing may be upon you.

- **Clear your mind and heart of perturbing thoughts or feelings**. Allow what comes up to be fully felt. Speak what needs to be said, channeling it through your heart center. Release whatever separates you from an experience of true peace.

- **Quiet and calm the bodymind**: Meditation, calming practices, prayer, entrainment with soothing music.

- **Enhance your vital force**: Assign focus to Qi gong, t'ai chi chuan, yoga, reflexology, toning/chanting, time in nature: Invigorate the life force surging through your body, saturating and enlivening every cell.

- **Gather support in advance**. Arrange for a helper to companion you for the first day or two of recovery—or longer, depending on the severity of the procedure. Ask a friend to organize meal deliveries if this will be needed. See *Networking and Medical Fundraising* for internet-based support.

Week Before Surgery —

- Avoid all herbs and supplements that might interfere with pharmaceutical sedatives and anesthesia or with blood clotting mechanisms. Some of these include: **Vitamin E** [up to two weeks prior], **proteolytic enzymes**, **fish oils**, and **gingko**. **Garlic** is often on lists to avoid for potential anticoagulant impact. Stargrove *et al* conclude that moderate garlic consumption is generally safe prior to elective surgery and that the "general risk associated with garlic tends to be overstated in the secondary and derivative literature."[3] The nerve-influencing herbs **kava**, **St. Johnswort**, and **valerian** are generally recommended to be discontinued at least five days prior to anesthesia: The clinical bases of these prohibitions are still being explored, though surgery candidates should prudently abstain as directed unless otherwise guided by a naturopathic physician who is familiar with one's case.

- **Continue with other general preparations** noted previously.

- **Follow all instructions provided by your medical team** regarding fasting, medications, and other possible preparation.

- **Write up affirmations** that you plan to ask surgical team to read aloud both before surgery and before you are wheeled to recovery. For example—**Before**: "The surgery will [whatever specifics you wish it to accomplish]. Bleeding will be minimal. All will transpire with grace and ease." **Afterwards**: "Your [body area impacted] will readily return to normal functioning and all incisions will heal quickly and properly." Something along those lines. Place these on a card you can hand to a surgical nurse or surgeon. See Dr. Bernie Siegel's wonderful book *Peace, Love and Healing: Bodymind Communication and the Path to Self-Healing* for more on this approach.

Day of surgery —

- **Allow time to prepare yourself and find your place of balance**—allow time for meditation, prayer, deep, slow breathing. Calming practices.

- **Attune with the soothing music or chants** to which you have been entraining so as to ground, align, center and relax. Small digital music devices allow you to carry a personal musical soundtrack easily. Some people ask their surgeons to play such music in the operating room during the procedure or wear headphones themselves.

- **Generate gratitude** for all that will be done today to benefit your healing. Pray that those who assist you in this process may benefit many times over for their heart-felt efforts. Meet your physician and their assistants with an open heart and imagine them treating you like a beloved family member.

- **Observe that you are not your physical body—yet, wish it well.**

- **Apply Yarrow Special Formula** flower essence blend [Flower Essence Society] to your forehead, wrists, chest or belly to support the integrity of your energy field.

- **Request that the surgeon meditate or pray with you**, depending on your inclination, before anesthesia is administered. Attune your energy bodies, focus, and attention.

- **Hand he or she your affirmation card** and make your request that they speak these words to you as you go under the anesthesia and before you leave the surgical space.

- **Modified citrus pectin [MCP]** is recommended by some holistic practitioners as a non-toxic means to help reduce the body burden of heavy metals. MCP, taken orally, is seen as a potential alternative to conventional chelators.[4] It may have a role to play following diagnostic tests that involve radiation exposure. In addition, some naturopathic authorities recommend ingesting MCP before and after biopsies and other surgical procedures to limit possible seeding of cancerous cells into the bloodstream.[5] *Caution*: MCP, a gel-forming substance, has been shown to interfere with the absorption of some oral drugs and should therefore not be taken concurrently with such drugs.

First few days post-surgery —

- **Allow yourself to receive comfort, compassion, and care.** Allow yourself the space to rest and recuperate, no matter how minor you view the surgery.

- **Use homeopathic remedies to support healing**. *Arnica* internally for tissue trauma. *Hypericum* [St. Johnswort] for nerve damage or nerve trauma.

- Proprietary formula **Traumeel gel** [includes *Arnica* and *Hypericum*]: Apply topically for tissue trauma. **Hypericum infused oil** can be used topically for same. Avoid applying directly to open wound.

- Attend to liver support with **milk thistle seed** [*Silybum marianum*] extract, three times a day, to recover equilibrium following anesthesia and antibiotics. *Please note*: If on continuing pharmaceutical treatment, please note that *Silybum* has been previously suspected of influencing the metabolism of some drugs, thus potentially impacting their clinical effectiveness. Human studies have since reported conflicting results, and the latest edition of the standard reference *Botanical Safety Handbook* [2013] concludes that there are no known drug interactions.

- **Ginger rhizome** can ease post-surgical nausea and bloating as well as gently prevent constipation. Use as tea of fresh or dried sliced root or as carbonated brew, extract, candied/crystallized root, or capsules. See **Nausea** section of ***The Helping Repertoire***.

- Also, including **ginger rhizome** in foods and teas can benefit overall circulation as well as being anti-inflammatory.

- **Proteolytic enzymes** such as bromelain [from pineapples] and papain [from papayas]—taken *away* from food—can help reduce tissue swelling and inflammation, and assist in promoting lymph flow. Avoid or use with care within first three days post surgery if issues with blood clotting. *Caution*: Pancreatin and other proteolytic enzymes have been reported to impair folic acid absorption. Stargrove, *et al* recommend that healthcare practitioners prescribing proteolytic enzymes suggest concurrent folic acid to counteract any decrease in folate absorption.[6]

- **Emphasize wound healing nutrients** in food or supplementation: Zinc, selenium, vitamin C, vitamin E, B complex vitamins, flavonoids in colorful fruits and veggies.

- **Replenish beneficial intestinal microbiota,** likely compromised with antibiotics and other drugs associated with the surgical procedure. Probiotic supplements, naturally cultured foods such as kraut, miso, natto, yogurt, and so on. See sections on **Yeast Infections/Thrush** and **Diarrhea** in *The Helping Repertoire* for detailed suggestions. Also see *Lessons from Bacteria* in the Appendices.

- **Continue to drink plenty of water** throughout the day to support cleansing, proper healing, and normal execution of all cellular functions.

- **Emphasize simple nutrition**: Broths, soups, steamed vegetables, herbal infusions, smoothies. See the chapter on *A Few Recipes for Gentle Foods* for ideas.

- **Sufficient protein intake** to optimize wound healing mechanisms in the body: Isolated whey protein concentrate is ideal to supplement protein intake.

- **L-glutamine**: An amino acid essential to muscle metabolism and wound healing, helps improve tissue recovery from trauma. Found in whey protein, cabbage and/or can be supplemented as needed as an individual nutrient in powder or capsules.

- **Nutrient-dense smoothies**, particularly if appetite is suppressed or eating is difficult.

  *To make a basic smoothie: In a blender, combine—2 cups water; ½-1 cup fresh or frozen blueberries; 1-2 tablespoons freshly ground flax seeds [or blend of chia, flax, sprouted seeds, etc.]; 1 scoop micro-filtered whey protein-isolate powder or sugar-free eggwhite protein; probiotic powder or yogurt; 1-2 tablespoons concentrated green foods [stinging nettle powder, alfalfa, barley grass juice powder, or commercially available "superfood" blends]; L-glutamine, if desired, to help build and heal flesh; 1-2 teaspoons adaptogenic herb powders as indicated [ashwagandha, eleuthero, or other powdered nutrients as desired—see chapter **Adaptogenic and Tonic Plant Allies** for selection of these allies]; warming ginger powder or cinnamon powder or vanilla extract to taste. Blend all but the protein powder together; add the whey or eggwhite protein, then briefly pulse to mix. Drink promptly after blending, as the flax or chia seeds will thicken the drink over time. See **Power Smoothie Recipe** for additional ideas.*

- Arrange to receive an in-home **energy-balancing treatment** if possible: Reiki, therapeutic touch, healing touch, Zero Balancing, and the like. Gentle hugs and foot massage from a loved one are pretty effective as well.

- Again, consider working with **acupuncture** following surgery to speed healing, limit complications, and support recovery both from the trauma of the procedure itself as well as from the anesthesia used.

- Continue intake of **modified citrus pectin** if relevant to particular circumstances and as recommended by practitioner.

Thereafter —

- **Continue dietary strategies**, particularly: natural ferments [probiotic supplements, cultured foods]; sufficient protein; anti-inflammatory, antioxidant-rich fruits and vegetables; water…

- Continue with **smoothies** and **milk thistle seed extract**, as appropriate.

- Continue **bromelain** as needed to moderate inflammation and proper lymph drainage.

- **Gotu kola** [*Centella asiatica*] extract: To promote appropriate wound healing, gotu kola is typically recommended as 1 capsule of extract or 1-2 droppersful of tincture 2-3 times per day. In addition, gotu kola can be used topically as an oil [known as Brahmi oil in Ayurveda] to improve scar tissue formation.

- A few drops of **helichrysum essential oil** [*Helichrysum angustifolium*] can be added to a small bit of lotion or oil to allow it broader application and to amplify the benefits of the base fixed oil. Antibacterial, antiviral, anti-inflammatory, wound healing. A specific for burns and to prevent scarring. Consider adding a few drops to rosehip seed oil, sea buckthorn oil, calendula oil, vitamin E oil, or honey. Helichrysum is also known as Everlasting or Immortelle. Ditto **niaoli essential oil**.

- **Vitamin E**: 400 IU per day of mixed tocopherols is a typical recommended dose to support tissue healing. Pure, undiluted vitamin E oil can also be applied topically as appropriate to limit scarring.

- **Grapeseed extract**: Typically recommended dose is 1-2 capsules per day. Can be taken with vitamin E for synergistic antioxidant and tissue healing benefit.

- Ditto **Vitamin C**: Typically recommended dose is 500-1,000 mg, 1-4 times per day as individually indicated. Can be used in combination with Vitamin E and grapeseed extract to extend their benefits.

- **Continue to replenish beneficial intestinal bacteria**.

- **Warding off microbial imbalance**: After cessation of antibiotic course, should yeasty challenges arise despite your best efforts, consider following up with **Propolis**[7] or **Neem** [*Azadirachta indica*] extract or powder: 2 caps per day to protect against antibiotic-promoted overgrowth of *Candida albicans* and other microbial opportunists. Also, consider these as essential to replenish healthy bowel ecology: Supplemental probiotics, live-culture yogurt, kefir, miso, natto, and other personally appropriate naturally fermented foods. **D-Mannose** is a simple sugar that occurs in some plants, including cranberries. It prevents deleterious organisms such as pathogenic bacteria from sticking to the urinary tract lining. It is available in powder or capsule form. See **Urinary Tract Infections** in *The Helping Repertoire* for more.

- Continue personally preferred **adaptogenic herbal tonic** and **immune support** to speed and ease recovery.

- See **Thoughts on Medi-Ports—and Other Surgeries** for additional considerations.

Citations for this chapter are located in **Reference** section at back of book.

Chemotherapy / Radiation Considerations

While potentially life saving, these interventions can also take a toll on healthy tissue—resulting either in immediate distress or so-called "late-stage side effects" which may manifest somewhere down the road. Suppressed immunity and altered blood values typically occur with many agents of treatment. The heart, the kidneys, the liver, and the digestive tract are especially vulnerable to many of these substances—long-term integrity of these tissues can be supported with holistic complementary strategies.

This section is in no way intended to be anything other than an introduction. The intent here is to simply highlight some relevant health factors and natural substances that are most generally applicable as adjuncts to allopathic oncological treatment approaches. A given person's overall health status and particular pharmaceutical and radiological regimen should **always** be matched individually with any complementary agents.

Some practitioners warn against using natural substances—particularly antioxidants—during treatment, believing that they protect cancerous cells as well as healthy ones. Addressing that complicated issue requires an extended conversation well beyond the scope of this book. Complementary protocols adjunct to chemo and radiation are getting increasingly sophisticated as we learn more and more about the synergy and interaction between these approaches. Please see the books by herbalist Donald Yance in ***The Recommended Reading*** chapter, as well as the incomparable resource ***Herb, Nutrient, and Drug Interactions: Clinical Implications and Therapeutic Strategies*** by Stargrove *et al* that go deeply into these questions. That said, the bottom line is that concentrated nutritive substances can provide powerful support during harsh pharmaceutical and radiation treatments—used, ideally, under skilled professional guidance as to timing, substance, and dosage level. The "typical dose," when noted here, is mentioned for educational purposes only and is not prescriptive.

This is where assembling a personal healthcare **team** can be of extraordinary benefit. Combining the best practices of medical oncology, herbalism, naturopathic medicine, holistic nutritional science, acupuncture and energy medicine, bodywork, and spiritual practice seems to yield the most promising results. When we do so without fear, from a place of honoring the wisdom of each modality, we engage the highest human aspirations for healing. In this we align with the wisdom of our natural state of health and balance.

Please note: As always, one should confer with both the inner physician and outerworld practitioners in considering any of these adjunct therapies for oneself or another. Please consider that statement repeated under each of the following entries.

While some side-effects are mentioned in this chapter, please refer to ***The Helping Repertoire*** for detailed discussions of particular issues typically experienced while undergoing allopathic chemotherapy and radiation treatments.

- One needs to have certain amount of vitality, vital force, physical energy reserves to survive chemotherapy and radiation successfully. **Building life force with tonifying foods, herbs, and energy techniques before and during treatment may be of great benefit**. Consider current nutritional status and focus on resolving or improving any depletion as much as possible. If one has lost weight involuntarily, emphasis on high-quality protein may be especially important. Likewise, blood supply of some essential nutrients may be diminished and vibrant, nutrient-dense foods especially needed. Nutrition-packed smoothies can be of great value in bolstering daily requirements. Consult with trained helpers, if possible, to figure out what approach makes sense in the situation at hand.

- What are termed **adaptogenic herbs** are indicated here to help build resiliency, stamina, and mediate the consequences of stress: Ashwagandha root, codonopsis root, eleuthero root, astragalus root, stinging nettle leaves, and so on. Please see the chapter on *Adaptogenic and Tonic Plant Allies* for discussion of these plants. Typical dose: 1 teaspoon to 1 tablespoon of powdered herb added to smoothies, or otherwise included in food. These are also available in supplemental forms.

- Traditional Ayurvedic adaptogenic herbal jam called **Chyawanprash**—composed of some 40 herbs—is a delicious way to support almost every system in the body and improve immune function in particular. It helps replenish vital reserves and revitalize normal body functioning. This thick jam is a super-concentrated mix of nutrient-rich herbs in a base of vitamin C-rich amla fruit, honey, sesame oil, and clarified butter [ghee]. It is eaten by the spoonful, added to warm water, spread on crackers, and so on—a typically recommended dose is 1 teaspoon twice a day. Because of its warming nature, this tonic is used cautiously in the presence of diarrhea or peptic ulcer.

- These medical interventions may damage heart muscle. **Coenzyme Q$_{10}$**—also known as ubiquinone and present in most cells—is especially concentrated in the heart tissue. It is particularly active promoting metabolism within the mitochondria, the energy production centers of the cells. CoQ$_{10}$ or, preferably, its more bioactive **Ubiquinol** form helps protect the heart and enhances energy levels. Typical dose: 100 mg twice per day taken after a meal that includes oil or fat for best absorption.

- **Various traditional plant allies are known for their cardioprotective benefits**. **Hawthorn** [*Crataegus* spp.] has a role to play as a gentle, food-like tonic for cardiovascular tissue. The leaves, flowers and berries are used. **Rosemary** [*Rosmarinus officinalis*] leaves are used as another traditional, antioxidant-rich cardiovascular ally. **Numerous adaptogens** have demonstrated cardioprotective benefit, including the ginsengs, eleuthero, ashwagandha, amla, codonopsis, astragalus, reishi, cordyceps, rhodiola, and schisandra. Again, see the chapter *Adaptogenic and Tonic Plant Allies* for further discussion of these plants.

- **Kidney support** is another focus of attention during chemotherapy and radiation treatments. The death of cancer cells resulting from such therapy can cause a buildup of uric acid, among other challenges. Oncologists typically prescribe the drug Allopurinol to limit uric acid buildup in the bloodstream and promote excretion. It is a powerful drug and may typically be prescribed for those days in each treatment cycle when die-off is highest. Natural substances traditionally used to support renal function in this process include juiced celery, celery seeds, stinging nettle seeds, burdock roots and seeds, bladderwrack [*Fucus vesiculosis*], black cherry juice concentrate, and others.

- **Turmeric rhizome** has been extensively researched and utilized in the treatment of cancer. Activity observed: Liver-protective, cell-protective in general against DNA damage, inhibits the promotion of tumors, anti-inflammatory, fibrinolytic. Seems to have a synergistic effect when combined with the enzyme therapy of bromelain. Typical dose: 1 capsule of extract two or three times per day. Turmeric is generally *not* well-absorbed into the bloodstream, and previously touted 95% curcumin extracts—the best available for many years—usually combined black pepper and/or bromelain to enhance absorption. A novel, proprietary method known as BCM-95 is now being employed to create forms that are significantly more bioavailable and may remain in circulation for up to 8-10 hours—combining turmeric extracts, distilled turmeric essential oil, and phospholipids. These products are now available in the marketplace. Some, with access to fresh, organically grown rhizomes, may want to prepare a more traditional drink—juicing the roots and blending with organic coconut milk as a drink or to add to foods. See *Jamu* in *A Few Recipes for Gentle Foods*. *Cautions*: Previous advisories to avoid concurrent use with blood-thinning medications are being reconsidered in the most current reviews of the scientific literature. Stargrove *et al* conclude that "extrapolated warnings may be considered speculative and overstated." The *Botanical Safety Handbook* [2013] concurs and places turmeric in its safest class for use. Because of its antioxidant potency, concurrent intake with chemotherapy agents remains a realm of considerable debate; refer to Stargrove *et al* for detailed discussion per pharmaceutical agent.

- **Bromelain**, a proteolytic enzyme extracted from the green part of pineapple, is sometimes used during chemotherapy, etc. to make tumors and cancerous cells more vulnerable to the allopathic treatment. In addition, bromelain is anti-inflammatory, a digestive aid, and an anti-edema agent used to promote post-operative healing. Inflammation processes are being carefully studied in relationship to the expression of cancers and their level of invasiveness. Typical dose: 1 tablet or capsule, 2000 GDU potency, two or three times per day, taken on an empty stomach.

- **Bone marrow suppression** is a side effect of most chemotherapeutic agents. The bone marrow is the site of blood cell production—red blood cells, white blood cells, and platelets. Red blood cells circulate oxygen to the tissues, white blood cells fight infections and respond to tissue trauma, and platelets manage clotting and bruising. Bone marrow suppression can lead to anemia, rapid heart rate, shortness of breath, fatigue, dizziness, heightened susceptibility to infection, rash, bleeding [gums, nose, in urine], easy bruising, etc. Formulations such as **Marrow Plus** [Health Concerns] and **ImmuneCare I** [Natura Health Products] are based on classic botanical formulas to nourish bone marrow function; taking them during chemotherapy may improve production of essential blood factors. Consult with your holistic practitioner about appropriateness in your situation. Also, see next entry.

- **Suppressed immune function** is generally a consequence of treatments. Astragalus root [*Astragalus membranaceus*], extract of reishi mushroom [*Ganoderma lucidum*], maitake [*Grifola frondosa*], turkey tail [*Coriolus/Trametes versicolor*] or combination formulas containing assorted medicinal mushrooms can help maintain more vigilant immune function—helping to protect against opportunistic infections and supporting quicker recovery from the allopathic treatment. In addition, these allies are often employed to reduce or prevent other typical side effects of such treatments. These botanical medicines are typically used in various combinations with each other and often with adaptogens and liver-supporting herbs as well. Consult with your holistic practitioner about appropriateness in your situation.

- **Milk thistle seed extract** [*Silybum marianum*]—used as adjunct therapy to protect the liver from chemotherapy and pharmaceutical damage. Promotes more efficient liver cell regeneration and detoxification. [The therapeutic agents in milk thistle seed are best extracted in a full-spectrum standardized extract or tincture.] Typical dose of milk thistle: 1 capsule of extract [or 2 droppersful of tincture] in the morning and one before bedtime. *Caution*: Please note that *Silybum* has previously been suspected of influencing the metabolism of some drugs, thus potentially impacting their clinical effectiveness. Human studies have since reported conflicting results, and the latest edition of the standard reference *Botanical Safety Handbook* [2013] concludes that there are no known drug interactions.

- **Oral use of L-glutamine** [swish and swallow twice per day] has been shown to reduce the severity of mouth sores [mucositis] in human subjects undergoing chemotherapy.[1] See the entry **Mouth Sores / Raw Mouth** in *The Helping Repertoire* for more suggestions. Supplementation may also protect integrity of the gut lining.

- **Ingestion of probiotics before receiving abdominal radiation** has been shown to protect the intestine from damage, according to animal research. The bacterial strains used were those commonly found in yogurt and commercially available probiotic formulas.[2]

- **Slippery elm bark** [*Ulmus* spp.]—contains calcium and other nutrients. Nutritive, soothing, helps with nausea and upset stomach. Helps protect and soothe the lining of gastrointestinal tract. Used as lozenges, cold infusion or porridge. Make classic gruel with bark powder [see **Simple Nutrition** entry in section on *The Helping Repertoire*]. A pinch of ginger or fennel seed powder could be added to further calm digestion, as long as reflux is not an issue. *Please note* that elm tree populations have been ravaged by disease in the past several decades and this medicine should be used with mindfulness. Slippery elm's traditional nutritive use in severe deficiency and recuperation seems its most justifiable use in these times; the easily cultivated marshmallow root and ever-abundant kudzu root starch—see below—are excellent choices when soothing the digestive tract is the primary goal.

- **Kudzu root starch** [*Pueraria lobata*] is a true blessing for nausea, gas, and indigestion. Also, helps resolve food or alcohol poisoning. It is prepared as needed and taken away from food, supplements, and oral medications. Traditionally used as a thickener in cooking, kudzu root starch is readily available in the Japanese or macrobiotic foods section of natural food grocery stores. See preparation instructions under **Hydration** in *The Helping Repertoire*.

- **Sea veggies**, rich in iodine and other micronutrients, may help protect the thyroid from damage as a consequence of radiation exposure. In addition, research in Japan following the bombing of Hiroshima and Nagasaki—and in Russia following the Chernobyl nuclear disaster—demonstrate the ability of sodium alginate in the seaweed to bind with heavy metals and escort them from the body. Also, it is thought that the mineral complexes in foods such as sea vegetables may have a protective effect on healthy tissue during radiation therapy. Consider ingesting for several weeks prior and following radiation-based diagnostic scans or treatments. **As food**: Wakame is great for soups, cooking with grains, or prepared as a salad; nori is nice for rice rolls; chopped dulse is easy to add as a condiment to foods; whole dulse, nori, and toasted sea palm are wonderful eaten out of hand. Broth made from traditionally prepared **miso** plus seaweed combines their mutual benefits. Miso itself has been studied for its radioprotective benefits.[3] Seaweeds and extracts are also available in **encapsulated form**. Typical recommended consumption range is about 4-14 grams [1-4 teaspoons] of dried seaweed powder per day or up to 2-3 ounces of whole seaweed per week. **Concentrated alginate-rich detoxification products** are also available; follow label instructions. In the northern hemisphere, always seek seaweed foods harvested from the less polluted northern seas, especially the North Atlantic. See *Resources* for list of mindfully harvested products. Also see the book *Seaweed* by former radiation oncology nurse Valerie Cooksley in the *Recommended Reading* chapter. *Please note*: Consult with a practitioner as to whether concentrated extracts are appropriate for you *during* radiation therapy and given your overall health picture.

- **Modified citrus pectin [MCP]** is recommended by some holistic practitioners as a non-toxic means to help reduce the body burden of heavy metals. MCP, taken orally, is seen as a potential alternative to conventional chelators.[4] It may have a role to play following diagnostic tests that involve radiation exposure. In addition, some naturopathic authorities recommend ingesting MCP before and after biopsies and other surgical procedures to limit possible seeding of cancerous cells into the bloodstream.[5] *Caution*: MCP, a gel-forming substance, has been shown to interfere with the absorption of some oral drugs and should therefore not be taken concurrently with such drugs.

- **Aloe vera gel or juice for radiation burns**, taken both internally or applied externally as needed. Soothing and healing to damaged mucosa all along the gastrointestinal tract. Use organically cultivated, preservative-free preparation or fresh leaf gel. See **Radiation Burns** entry in *The Helping Repertoire* for more.

- **Epsom salt, sea salt, bentonite clay, baking soda, seaweed soaks** to detoxify from treatments. Consider doing such a soak each time following a treatment as a cleansing ceremony, if you like [and if you have no cardiovascular contraindications]. Lavender essential oil may be added in a bit of liquid soap, if desired. Light a candle, make the bath space sacred, slip carefully into your salty tub. Give thanks for the healing light energy the radiation process offered to you and now release all that is no longer needed for your greater experience of wellness.

- **Intention and visualization on wellness and vitality**. This deserves an extended conversation, which many books and teachings elaborate. Essentially, our inner experience of aliveness and well-being can stimulate our cells and tissues toward greater harmony and vibrancy—as well as inform our emotional response to whatever life presents. How we see ourselves and how we relate to our experience are key factors in how comfortably we might traverse challenging terrain. Please see the excerpt titled ***Entering the River*** at the very end of this publication—an excerpt from my forthcoming book—for more thoughts on this. Several articles in the ***Appendices*** also offer relevant support, particularly *Reflections on Environmental Influences, Engaging with Pain, Toward Preventing Cancer*, and *Breathing Practices*. Also, please see the ***Recommended Reading*** and ***Recommended Listening*** chapters for books and guided meditations by other authors that may surely help inform and inspire. Especially for those whose ability to move is compromised, the short and immediately useful book *Exercise without Movement* by Swami Rama [Himalayan Institute, 1984] is available for download online and offers simple exercises for using the power of mind to stimulate circulation and energy flow when more active movement is restricted for whatever reasons.

For additional discussion of these and other considerations, please see the following books listed in the bibliography as well as those mentioned previously in the text:

Adaptogens: Herbs for Strength, Stamina, and Stress Relief—Winston and Maimes; *The Tao of Medicine: Ginseng and Other Chinese Herbs for Inner Equilibrium and Immune Power*—Fulder; *The Encyclopedia of Nutritional Supplements*—Murray; *How to Prevent and Treat Cancer with Natural Medicine*—Murray; *The Definitive Guide to Cancer*—Alschuler and Gazella; *Medicinal Mushrooms*—Hobbs; *Milk Thistle: The Liver Herb*—Hobbs; *The Fungal Pharmacy*—Rogers; *MycoMedicinals*—Stamets; *Natural Compounds in Cancer Therapy*—Boik; *Prescription for Nutritional Healing*—Balch and Balch; *Naturopathic Oncology*—McKinney.

Botanical Safety Handbook, 2ⁿᵈ edition—Zoë Gardner and Michael McGuffin, editors [Boca Raton, FL: CRC Press, 2013]

Herb, Nutrient, and Drug Interactions: Clinical Implications and Therapeutic Strategies—Mitchell Bebel Stargrove, ND, LAc Jonathan Treasure, MNIMH, Dwight L McKee, MD [St. Louis, MO: Mosby/Elsevier, 2008]

Additional citations for this chapter are located in **Reference** section at back of book.

Convalescence

In our fast-paced, high-pressure culture, allowing time to rest and recover from serious illness, trauma, or medical treatments and procedures is not a given. Sometimes the individual's need is obvious; at other times the need may be more invisible to others. In either case, setting aside adequate time for convalescence is essential to help the bodymind heal and renew itself to the maximum degree possible.

The word *convalescence* itself is from the Latin "to become strong." Surviving an immediate threat is not the same as being fully recovered and renewed in strength.

Support and understanding from family, community and workplace is essential to allow an individual full benefit of this process. In addition, specific factors are key to support the bodymind in recovering from physical [and emotional] trauma or disruption. A few of the most important are noted below.

The need for the caregiver to restore themselves after a period of intensive tending to another is also a high priority, though their help may still be required during their loved one's convalescence. This is where a network of support continues to be ideal. Many understanding hearts and willing hands allow for the best outcomes for all concerned.

- **Resting when tired**; **getting sufficient restorative sleep**. The body needs this downtime to focus on repair and recalibration toward homeostasis. See the earlier section on **Disturbed Sleep/Insomnia** in *The Helping Repertoire* for support.

- **If there has been protracted bed rest or immobility**, the muscles will need to be toned and reinvigorated through gentle movement over time. Likely, medical physical therapy will be recommended. Ask your healthcare provider if there are any contraindications regarding massage—a wonderful way to stimulate circulation and enliven the muscles while receiving compassionate touch.

- Poor circulation can cause **dizziness** in a shift from stillness to movement. If this is the cause of any dizziness experienced [see section on **Dizziness** for fuller discussion], herbs that stimulate peripheral circulation can be of benefit. A favorite for this is **rosemary** [*Rosmarinus officinalis*], which is also uplifting to the spirit. Rosemary tea can be drunk or added to foot or full-body bath; a few drops of rosemary essential oil may be added to massage oil or body lotion. Best to avoid using rosemary at night; for some, the increased sense of circulation can delay sleep.

- **Intestinal ecology**: Many types of pharmaceutical drugs disrupt the beneficial bacteria composing the gut microbiota. To follow courses of drug treatment or anesthesia by focusing attention on restoring the health and balance of the gut ecology is wise—as up to 70% of our immunity happens in the gut and these bacteria are responsible for other life-support, including proper nutrient assimilation. Probiotic supplements and naturally cultured foods, such as miso, kraut, yogurt, kefir, etc., can provide what is needed. Also, see the appendix *Lessons from Bacteria* for a discussion of factors involved in promoting gut health in a holistic way.

- **Stimulate appetite** if it is dulled. See the sections on **Lack of Appetite/Weight Loss** and **Loss of Taste/Smell** for discussion and strategies.

- **Optimize nutrition** with foods and nutritional substances that are nutrient-dense and easy on the digestive system. See sections on **Loss of Appetite**, **Fatigue**, **Building the Blood**, **Simple Nutrition** and the chapters *Repairing the Garment: Surgery and Beyond* and *Recipes for Gentle Foods* for suggestions that will help meet your needs where you are.

- **Protein is essential** to supply the body with the full range of amino acids it needs to rebuild tissues and complete proper wound repair. Choose clean wholefood sources such as fish, eggs and tempeh as well as sugar-free versions of well-assimilated protein powders: Whey protein isolate, eggwhite protein, pea protein, etc. See basic smoothie instruction under **Simple Nutrition** as well as the *Power Smoothie Recipe*, a detailed version with calorie- and protein-counts that follows the chapter *Natural Strategies for Tube Feeding*.

- **Green food concentrates** are excellent ways to ingest significant quantities of helpful whole food-sourced nutrients when the appetite is weak. Again, see the smoothie recipes mentioned previously as well as the *Resources* chapter for some quality brands. These powders can also be added into various dressings and seed-butter based sauces.

- **Royal jelly**, discussed in **Lack of Appetite/Weight Loss**, is a concentrated honeybee product that can help maintain and build muscle, bone and flesh.

- For many, focusing on the health of the liver and gallbladder may also be indicated during convalescence. Please refer to the chapters *Food Considerations for Liver Health* and *Plant Allies for Liver Support*.

- Be sure to see the chapters on *Living with Chronic Disease* and *"Watch and Wait"* for additional considerations. Also, see the appendix *Toward Preventing Cancer* if recurrence is a concern.

- Please peruse the *Recommended Reading* chapter, particularly the books focused on *Natural Therapeutics and Wellness Support*. There is a wealth of wisdom and detailed health counsel available through these offerings.

- Most of all, **do your very best to enjoy this precious moment of life**. Here you are and here you be.

A Few Recipes for Gentle Foods

The question of what to eat during illness is beyond the scope of this book. This chapter simply aims to offer some suggestions of easy to digest, nutritious, comforting foods to help provide nutrition during times when appetite and digestion may be challenged.

Healthful food begins with the soil, the farming method, the consciousness of the farmers and stewards. Please assume here that all ingredients mentioned are ideally grown organically or sourced from organically grown plants. Choose wild-harvested over farmed fish, organically fed free-range lamb, chicken and eggs. Seaweeds hand-harvested in the northern oceans are the best available at the time of this writing.

Recipes for a number of other soothing foods can be found in *The Helping Repertoire* in the sections **Hydration**, **Simple Nutrition**, and **Lack of Appetite / Weight Loss**.

Vegetable Broth

Choose from among these: carrots, celery, zucchini, onion, potatoes,
   turnip, parsnip, leeks, Swiss chard, dandelion root, nettles, oatstraw
   infusion, raspberry or thimbleberry leaves, etc.
2 slices or so fresh organic ginger root
2 or more slices of dried astragalus root
Shiitake mushrooms, fresh or dried[‡]
Seaweed such as kombu, wakame, sea palm, if desired
Pure water

This is a no-stress formulation. Pick and choose ingredients based on availability and preference. Slice vegetables you have on hand very thinly and place into pot. Add about twice as much water as veggies. Simmer for 1-2 hours, covered. Adjust water level if necessary. Strain. Enjoy this gentle broth freely. Prepare only enough for about two days at a time. Add miso to individual bowls upon serving, if desired. Refrigerate leftovers.

[‡]Alternate/additional mushrooms include maitake, turkey tail, reishi. Maitake is a delectable edible and can be added directly to pot fresh or dried. The tough turkey tail or reishi should be chopped or ground and cooked alone in water for several hours, then strained. Use this broth as tea or base for soup.

Barley Broth

Simmer 1 cup of organic barley in 6 cups of water. Bring the water to a boil for a couple of minutes, and then remove from heat. Let it stand for 15 minutes. Strain out the barley and set it aside. The barley water can be drunk as a broth or, if desired, don't strain and eat the barley with the soup. Or, after separating broth from grain, the cooked barley can be mixed with honey and enjoyed as a strengthening 'pudding.' Adaptogenic or tonic herb powders can also be selectively added to the cooked barley as desired.

Vegetable Puree

1-2 small yellow-fleshed potatoes
1 cup vegetable broth or pure water
Choose: onions, carrots, zucchini, celery, mushrooms, nettles, etc.
Optional: bit of sea salt, herb salt, dulse flakes, or kelp powder to taste
Optional: organic sunflower seeds cooked into mix for nutrition and to add texture

Cube potatoes and coarsely chop whatever else. Simmer with liquid over low heat until tender. Allow mixture to cool somewhat. Carefully puree in blender or food processor. Add more liquid as necessary to reach a creamy consistency. Enjoy.

If desired, **powdered** herbs or other amendments may be added to the puree in small amounts upon serving, to taste. Choose one or two from among: stinging nettle leaf powder, barley grass juice powder, astragalus root powder, eleuthero root powder, codonopsis root powder, slippery elm bark powder, freshly ground flaxseed, flaxseed oil, tahini, sunflower seed butter, pumpkin seed butter, fermented miso paste, ghee, etc.

Bone Broth

Bone broths are essentially decoctions of animal bones and cartilage, in which the abundant nutrients they contain extract into the cooking water over time. They are an ancient practice for getting the most out of animal foods. Minerals, collagen, and many corollary nutrients become available as the animal parts soften or disappear into the broth with sufficient cooking.

In a large stock pot [or slow cooker], combine bones with enough cold water to cover by an inch or so. Add a tablespoon of organic apple cider vinegar to improve mineral extraction and let all sit for about an hour. Then cook over low heat until the magic happens. Any desired vegetables and herbs are generally added toward the end of cooking. Imbibed on a regular basis, these readily available nutrients particularly help to maintain and nourish the bones and essential structure of the body.

Baked Yam with Tahini

Sweet, satisfying, comforting—yet low in terms estimated dietary glycemic load. Rich in fiber; good source of vitamin C, carotenes, potassium. Tahini provides tissue-building fat, plus calcium, magnesium, iron, and other nutrients—fats and oils also make the carotenes more available. Wonderful paired with some fish or chicken to provide a full range of amino acids.

Organic yams
Extra-virgin olive oil
Organic tahini [hulled raw sesame butter]
Gomasio/sesame salt or seaweed sprinkle to taste [Gomasio recipe follows below]

Preheat oven to 350°F. Meanwhile, scrub, dry and pierce yams. Massage each yam with a little olive oil and place in baking dish. Depending on size of the yams, bake about 45 minutes or as long as it takes for a fork to pierce through easily.

On the plate, halve the yams and drizzle 1 tablespoon or more of tahini over all with perhaps a bit of olive oil as well. If the need to gain weight is an issue, be liberal with the tahini. Top this with gomasio or seaweed powder or flakes to taste.

Gomasio / Sesame Salt

Gomasio is a classic macrobiotic condiment—a nutritious way to spark appetite and satisfy the palate. It is available as a ready-to-use product, but for those wishing to create their own versions, the recipe is offered below. *Thanks to Shari Trnka for the nettle idea.*

6-7 T. sesame seeds
1 tsp. sea salt
Kelp powder or dulse flakes, to taste
Dried stinging nettle leaves, to taste

Lightly toast the sesame seeds in a dry heavy skillet—cast iron is ideal. Tend mindfully and stir often; be careful not to burn them. Remove from skillet and allow seeds to cool.

In a small bowl, combine cooled seeds and other ingredients. For best flavor and nutrition, the mix is stored in an airtight jar and ground into a crude powder just before adding to food on the plate.

Alternately, the combination can be ground all at once in a ridged ceramic bowl called a suribachi or pulverized in a small electric grinder or blender. Either way, grind or pulse only briefly; the finished blend should still have large pieces of seed. Use this ground blend whenever desired but the flavor may degrade over time; make small batches.

Cauliflower Mashed "Potatoes"

This dish can be as simple or as seasoned as desired. Let the current state of digestion be your guide. Most are surprised that this is made from cauliflower. It delivers the soothing taste and mouth feel of a comfort food, made into a healing food by using this satisfying cruciferous vegetable as the base.

5 cups cauliflower, coarsely chopped
1 cup organic coconut milk [regular or diluted "light"]
2 T. organic coconut oil
1 ½ tsp. sea salt or kelp powder
1 tsp. black pepper or nigella seed, freshly ground
1 ½ tsp. garlic powder or several baked cloves—optional
1 ½ tsp. onion powder—optional
2 T. fresh chives, chopped—optional

Steam cauliflower until very soft.

Place cooked cauliflower in blender or food processer with some of the coconut milk and blend until smooth. Proceed in batches, if necessary, until all cauliflower is pureed. Add a little of the cooking water, if needed, to obtain desired consistency.

Stir in the seasonings and coconut oil. Sample for flavor and adjust seasoning to taste.

If desired, top the cauliflower mash in the serving bowl with freshly chopped chives.

Congee

Rice porridge, or congee, is an ancient food prepared throughout Asia. They are warming and soothing, easy to digest, and considered a stabilizing influence on the stomach and digestion. They are an easy way to incorporate healing herbs into food. They are used in convalescence and any time giving ease yet also nourishing the system is desired. In India, they are called *kitcharee* or *khichri*; in English they are referred to as congee (from the Indian 'kanji' for 'boilings'); in Mandarin Chinese they are called *zhou* ('jook') or *shi fan*. The basic formula is rice plus water (between four to nine times as much water as grain) plus herbs. Obviously, the more water added, the soupier the end result. The congee can be as simple as rice, water, and a single herb such as astragalus root, codonopsis root, or fresh ginger. Or it may be more complex. Whole books are written giving recipes for therapeutic herbal additions to congee. Easy-to-digest vegetables may be added to the cooking pot as desired; chopped greens and onions are a typical addition in India. It is important to use a heavy-bottomed pot to distribute the heat evenly. A crock pot would be another option, especially for easy overnight preparation. Although rice is the most globally utilized grain for making congee, do experiment with others, particularly quinoa, a pseudo-grain that is exceptionally high in quality protein.

> 1 cup organic grain [rice is best; also try quinoa]
> 9 cups pure water
> 1 ounce herbs [whole or powder]

Fill large pot with water, grain and herbs. Cover pot. Bring to a boil, then turn down heat to lowest possible setting. Cook slowly and gently, about 6-9 hours. Congee is done when soupy, but having a thick, porridge consistency. Eat, as needed, one bowl at a time.

If desired, melted ghee or flaxseed oil may be drizzled into the individual bowl.

Congee will keep for one day or so if refrigerated. Gently reheat before eating.

Quinoa

Quinoa [pronounced "keen-wah"] is a nutritious, protein-rich, comforting food that can be used whenever a grain is desired. Tiny quinoa spheres, like buckwheat and amaranth, are seeds rather than true grains—although used in similar ways. Cooked quinoa may be dressed with olive or flax oil, ghee, or a tahini dressing; added to soups or stew-type foods; combined with vegetables hot or cold; or used as an accompaniment to egg dishes. It is extremely versatile, delicious, and light on the digestion.

Quinoa [*Chenopodium quinoa*] is in the same botanical family as beets, spinach, and lamb's quarters. The seeds are protein rich, with one cup of cooked quinoa providing 8 grams. It also contains manganese, potassium, phosphate, magnesium, zinc, calcium. Quinoa is low in terms estimated dietary glycemic load

The outer coats of many varieties contain bitter compounds called saponins—to remove these, quinoa should always be rinsed well before cooking. For more digestibility and even better taste, soak quinoa for several hours *after* rinsing first. Soaked quinoa cooks in 10-15 minutes; quinoa simply rinsed and cooked immediately takes about twice as long.

— Eggs —

Poached, boiled, scrambled, baked—eggs are a marvelous food that is easy to eat and excellent for building the body. Eggs from free-range chickens are rich in protein, vitamin A, vitamin D, vitamin B_{12}, selenium, and more. Each egg provides 6 grams of complete protein. Having boiled eggs on hand makes for easy healthful snacks and travel food. Here are a couple of recipes to help keep eggs interesting.

Mediterranean Egg Salad

Boiled eggs
Black pitted olives, chopped finely [Kalamata olives are divine]
Extra-virgin olive oil
Sea salt, herb salt, or seaweed powder
Shallot or scallion or red onion, minced [optional]
Celery stalk, minced

Mash the desired number of boiled eggs into a crumbled mass. Add minced celery and shallot/scallion/onion if wishing to include. Mix in. Add chopped olives as desired. Mix in. Flow a ribbon of olive oil over the salad and mix all together thoroughly—Adjust to taste; less olive oil is preferable in this dish than too much. Taste before adding any salty seasoning. Adjust proportions if needed. Refrigerate before serving.

Serve on toast, fresh lettuce leaf, steamed collard leaf, on top of cool quinoa, with kale salad or lightly steamed broccoli, and so on.

There are countless variations on egg salad. For one alternative, the basic recipe may be **curried** using a salt-free curry powder, omitting the olives and substituting a healthy brand of mayonnaise for the olive oil.

Curried Egg Custard

1 quart organic coconut milk
5 eggs
some sea salt, herb salt, or seaweed powder
1-3 teaspoons curry powder [or less of nutmeg or 5-spice powder]
shredded coconut
pinch of Stevia extract powder [optional as sweetener; nice if using nutmeg]

Preheat oven to 300°F and boil up some water for use at the end. Gently and briefly warm the coconut milk. Meanwhile, whisk or blend eggs and combine with seasonings. Gradually add the warm coconut milk into the eggs, whisking as you do. If you like, add in enough shredded coconut to give the mixture some tooth, so to speak.

Pour mixture into a baking dish [or individual custard cups or ramekins] greased lightly with coconut oil. Set into a larger baking pan partly filled with hot water. Bake for about 45 minutes or so [or about 30-40 minutes for custard cups or ramekins]—when done, the center should still quiver a bit in the center. Serve either warm or cold.

Shiitake Baked Egg Custard

1 T. ghee or organic butter
2 T. onion or shallot, finely chopped
2 T. fresh shiitake mushrooms, chopped
2 cups hemp or almond milk [choose brand *without* added sweetener]
2 eggs plus 2 extra yolks [set aside extra whites for use in smoothie]
pinch nutmeg or cayenne powder
½ tsp. sea salt, herb salt, or seaweed powder

Preheat oven to 300°F and boil up some water for use at the end. Melt the butter in heavy skillet over medium heat. Add shallots or onion until softened. Add shiitake and cook with attention until tender. Lower the flame and add the nut or seed milk. Heat gently for a couple of minutes until the liquid barely begins to steam. Remove from heat; set aside.

Combine eggs, seasoning and salt in a mixing bowl. Whisk or beat until blended. Gradually add the milk/mushroom blend into the eggs, whisking constantly.

Pour mixture into a baking dish [or individual custard cups or ramekins] greased lightly with coconut oil. Set into a larger baking pan partly filled with hot water. Bake for 45 minutes or so [or about 30-40 minutes for custard cups or ramekins]—when done, the center should still quiver a bit in the center. Serve either warm or cold.

Non-Dairy, Wheat-Free Quiche

Preheat oven to 300°F [325°F if using a typical flour crust]. Meanwhile gather ingredients and prepare the nut crust first so it will be at the ready. Then proceed with cooking and creating the filling. Assemble all and place in hot oven. Bake about 30-40 minutes until top is lightly browned and almost firm to the touch. Cool on wire rack; eat while warm.

Nut Pie Crust

Dairy free, gluten free. Thanks to the creative Shari Trnka for developing this crust recipe. Any of the nut options work well; Shari's favorite choice is hazelnut. If using walnuts, take care that they are very fresh as they most easily become rancid. Shari supported me profoundly by providing wonderful healthful food during the many months of chemotherapy treatment. The recipes she devised deserve a book all their own!

Easy and delicious, this high-protein crust that works for savory or sweet recipes. This browns faster than a flour crust so perhaps lower the temp 25 degrees from a recipe using a flour crust—or bake it for a shorter time at the higher temperature, keeping an eye out.

2 cups organic nuts (walnuts, hazelnuts, pecans, or almonds)
¼ cup brown rice flour
¼ tsp. high quality salt (optional)
3/8 to ½ cup water

Grind raw nuts to a coarse meal in a food processor, not too fine. Mix in brown rice flour and salt if using. Add water gradually to fully moisten.

Instead of rolling out this crust, simply pat it into a glass pie plate that has been greased with coconut oil.

Quiche Filling

4 T. ghee or extra virgin olive oil
4 cups thinly sliced onion
2 cups fresh shiitake, sliced [steamed leafy greens can replace all or half of the mushroom portion]
6 eggs, room temperature
2 cups hemp or almond milk [choose brand *without* added sweetener]
½ tsp. dried thyme
Pinch of nutmeg powder [opt.]
Sea salt, herb salt, or seaweed powder
1 T. nutritional yeast
Freshly ground black pepper [or ground *Nigella sativa* seed]

Heat a deep, heavy skillet over medium flame. When pan is hot, add ghee. When ghee has melted, add the onion and salt. Increase heat somewhat and cook about 20 minutes until the onion is soft and beginning to brown. Modify temperature to ensure that onion doesn't scorch. Remove from pan and set aside.

Add a tad more ghee to the skillet and add sliced shiitake. Cook them until soft, stirring frequently. When done, set aside.

Combine eggs and remaining ingredients in a bowl; whisk or beat well. Add onions and shiitake and mix together.

Put pie pan[s] with crust onto a baking sheet and pour in the egg mixture, careful to spoon in the veggies without splashing.

Bake about 30-40 minutes until top is lightly browned and almost firm to the touch. Cool on wire rack; eat while warm.

Seaweed Salad

1 ounce dried wakame
3 T. tamari [a wheat-free, low-sodium version is available]
3 T. rice vinegar
2 T. dark sesame oil
1 tsp. white miso paste
1 T. sesame seeds
1 T. scallions, sliced thinly [optional]

Soak the wakame in cool water for about 5 minutes. Bring a pot of water to a boil, add the soaked wakame and simmer a couple of minutes. Drain and let cool. [Save the cooking water for soup stock, if you like.] Meanwhile, gently toast the seeds in a heavy skillet just until they smell delicious, then set aside removed from pan. When the wakame is safe to handle, remove central spine and cut remaining veggie into about ½" strips. Whisk together tamari, vinegar, oil, and miso into a dressing, then add in the toasted seeds. Toss dressing with wakame in a bowl, then top with the sliced scallions if using. Chill. Keep in a jar in the refrigerator and use as side dish.

Jamu

Jamu is the name for Indonesian traditional medicine and also the name for this herbal healing beverage. The most popular ingredients used are fresh turmeric, ginger, galangal, and tamarind. At its core, Jamu is anti-inflammatory and antioxidant, with a range of other benefits contributed by the individual plants used in a particular batch. It is a powerful way to ingest these healing plants.

The traditional Balinese way to prepare Jamu is to peel and chop the fresh roots used, add to pot containing water, add any additional herbs such as cinnamon, simmer on low until desired concentration is reached—about 30 minutes. This is then strained through muslin cloth, sweetened with honey to taste, drunk hot or cold. Coconut oil can be added while brew is still warm, to improve bioavailability of turmeric's healing constituents.

One can easily experiment with various combinations, keeping turmeric as the foundation. **A simple basic recipe would be to use 2 parts fresh turmeric to 1-1½ parts fresh ginger**. For example, peel and chop about 7 inches of turmeric rhizome and about 3½ inches of ginger. [Remember that ginger is warming and stimulating, and adjust proportion accordingly. I suggest you don't drink a ginger-rich Jamu at night as this might prevent restful sleep.] Add chopped roots to a quart of **water** and simmer on low heat until it is golden and the concentration you desire. Strain and stir in 1 teaspoon of **coconut oil**. Instead of sweetening with honey, try substituting one pint of **coconut water** plus, optionally, the juice of a **lime**. Drink in moderation, a glass at a time. Store in glass jar or bottle in refrigerator.

Variations:

• When the initial decoction is complete, cool water can be added to lower the temperature; instead of straining out the root, the whole batch can be blended together.

- The turmeric and any other fresh herbs can be juiced, then blended with water, coconut water, coconut milk, or some combination thereof.

- Alternatively, a couple of inches of turmeric root may simply be juiced with celery, carrot, ginger, raw greens.

Be forewarned that vividly colored fresh turmeric will stain yellow whatever it touches—hands, cloth, utensils used [if wooden or porous]. In parts of its growing range, it is purposely applied to color the skin golden.

Cacao-Avocado Pudding

2 avocados, organic
¼-1/3 cup raw cacao powder
¼-½ tsp. organic vanilla extract
Up to ½ tsp. stevia extract pwd [OR 1/3 cup honey, if sugars are not an issue]

Blend all until smooth. Refrigerate about an hour and enjoy. Rich, soothing, sweet—and nutritious—treat. One cup [230gm] of pureed avocado yields 384 calories, 4.5gm of protein, 15.6gm fiber, 35.44gm fats [22.5gm of which are monounsaturated], plus potassium, vitamin A, vitamin C, vitamin K, phosphorus, magnesium, calcium, and other nutrients. *Thanks to Becky Cobb for the basic proportions in this delicious recipe.*

Roasted Beets

Beets [*Beta vulagaris*] are a nutritious and satisfying food, rich in potassium, sodium phosphorus, magnesium, calcium, folate, vitamin A. Their natural sweetness combined with fiber content can satisfy a craving for less nutritious sweet choices. They are an ancient food, offering fresh, chard-like greens on top as well as the dense underground part. The red pigments beets contain are called *betains* or *betalains,* now known to be particularly strong antioxidants and anticarcinogenic compounds—protecting cell membranes against the lipid oxidation that can degrade them and promoting programmed cell death [apoptosis] in some cancer cell types. Betalains are very soluble in water, thus making roasting an ideal cooking method.

Roasting beets is also an especially easy way to prepare them and have them on hand for several meals at a time. **Choose 4-6 fresh beets**, firm to the touch and all a similar size.

Preheat the oven to 400°F. Meanwhile, wash the beets well. Place them on a lightly oiled roasting pan and cover all with foil.

Bake as is for 45-90 minutes. To check for doneness, pierce with a thin-blade; there should be minimum resistance to insertion when done. Carefully remove each beet when it is ready; cooking similar sized beets helps synchronize this.

Store unused roasted whole beets in glass container in refrigerator. Peel just before eating.

Other Healthful Foods of Note

The **cabbage family**, or *Brassicaceae*, is an extensive and health-promoting group of vegetables. It is beyond the scope of this book to explore them in detail; let it be said they are a worthy and delicious class: Brussels sprouts, kale, cauliflower, broccoli and broccoli seed sprouts, cabbage, bok choy, collards, mustards, nasturtium, turnip, radish, horseradish, wasabi, and so on. Obviously, for those with challenged digestion, choices with lesser amounts of pungency will be most appropriate. Metabolites available through ingestion of these vegetables—to varying degrees according to vegetable eaten and preparation method—have been shown to have immune modulating and anticancer properties, helping to promote estrogen metabolism and liver detoxification efforts.[‡] See *Food Considerations for Liver Health* for instructions on sprouting organic broccoli seed. Aside from enjoyment as food, supplements containing concentrated forms of particular *Brassica* vegetables are being used clinically to protect hormone-sensitive tissue such as breasts and prostate from cancer process.

Edible medicinal fungi are an endlessly amazing category and deserve books of their own; several excellent ones are noted in the *Natural Therapeutics* section of the *Recommended Reading* chapter. The fruiting bodies of these mushrooms are ancient medicines and have been shown to possess a wide array of therapeutic activities. Current research is yielding exciting insights on the medicine of the underground mycelia as well. Each mushroom displays its own particular genius, its distinctive profile of health-supporting benefits and system affinities. Each in their own way, they are known to play a role in preventing cancer and bolstering proper immune function. Shiitake [*Lentinula edodes*] and maitake [*Grifola frondosa*] are particularly delicious eaten cooked as food, prepared either fresh or reconstituted from the dehydrated state. Shiitake powder can easily be cooked into soups, stews, grains or porridge; it is a nice addition to congee. Leathery and woody, respectively, turkey tail [*Trametes/Coriolus versicolor*] and reishi [*Ganoderma lucidum*] are not directly edible, but may be long-simmered to produce nutritious medicinal broth, which can be drunk as a beverage or used as a base for soups and other foods. Of course, freeze-dried powders, encapsulated and liquid forms of medicinal mushroom extracts are also available commercially. See the *Resources* chapter for suggested sources.

Salad greens or cooked vegetables may be pureed in a blender or small food processor to make them more easily eaten by those dealing with oral cavity issues or the inability to chew sufficiently. Add a very small amount of liquid of choice—olive oil, a little water or broth, etc.—to facilitate the blending. Try processing first without any fluid at all to assess how much may be needed to obtain the desired consistency.

USDA National Nutrient Database for Standard Reference.

[‡] *Herbal Constituents: Foundations of Phytochemistry*—Lisa Ganora [Louisville, CO: Herbalchem Press, 2009]

Natural Strategies for Tube Feeding
[Enteral Nutrition]

There are times when swallowing is either impossible or so difficult and painful that alternatives must be employed to provide nutrition on a daily basis for an extended period. Medical science has come up with remarkable methods for achieving this, particularly the feeding tube inserted directly into the system. This technique is doubtless responsible for extending many lives. Nonetheless, it is not a perfect method.

Typically, medical personnel recommend a protein- and nutrient-rich commercial liquid to administer through the feeding tube. This standard formula is widely available and many people will choose to use it and benefit from it. The original formula of the most widely recommended brand contains corn syrup, corn sugar [maltodextrin], corn oil, sugar [sucrose], soy protein isolate, artificial flavor, plus assorted USP-grade vitamins and minerals. For some, this will be the most expedient route and no one should be judged as to their choices in this matter. Each person and family constellation needs to work with the energy, focus and resources at their disposal and make their choices accordingly.

Some people will choose to work one-on-one with registered dietitians to compose alternative formulas. One friend recently going through radiation for oral cancer did just this. She was given the following formula using baby food: ½ cup dry rice cereal, 2 jars beef, one jar each carrots, green beans, applesauce, and chicken. To this is added 1 cup orange juice, 2¼ cups whole milk, 1¼ cup cream, one cooked egg, 1 T. corn oil, 3 T. karo syrup. All this was to be blended into a slurry and administered throughout the day.

"This sounds disgusting," my friend wrote to me, asking for alternatives. "Tube feeding doesn't have to mean 'we don't care about what we put into our bodies.'"

Where do we even *begin* to comment on the recipe she was given? Poor quality oils, highly suspect manufactured sweetener, bizarre food combining [citrus with milk, with animal protein? Beef *and* chicken?], no mention of choosing organic eggs or dairy products, and so on. More could be said, but let it suffice to suggest that this is clearly a recipe based on very limited concerns, certainly not the *quality* or *digestibility* of the calories provided.

Essentially, the goal for enteral nutrition is to provide **about 1,800 calories and 71 grams of protein per day**. Can this be met using higher quality foods? It would seem possible, perhaps only a matter of orientation.

For starters, using the same premise as the above-mentioned nutritionist, **pre-blended baby foods** can provide a welcome short cut to save effort and energy. With quality in mind, however, it seems worthy to note that these days there are numerous manufacturers of baby food that offer organic fruits and vegetables, as well as high quality chicken and turkey. Some of these brands are listed in the *Resources* chapter.

In addition, some people who have sufficient support cook and **blend their own home-cooked foods**. This is obviously a much more arduous path, but one that some will wish to undertake. This can also be a task assigned to friends or family looking for ways to help. For home preparation, either a hand-cranked baby food blender will be needed—or, more conveniently, a heavy-duty blender and/or food processor such as the VitaMix. Look for BPA-free work bowls. In addition, check out the website **www.wholesomebabyfood.momtastic.com** for recipes, tools, and storage ideas.

In your creations, be sure to remember ripe organic avocadoes [**one cup of pureed avocado yields 384 calories, 4.5gm of protein**, 15.6gm fiber, 35.44gm fats—22.5gm of which are monounsaturated], plus potassium, vitamin A, vitamin C, vitamin K, phosphorous, magnesium, calcium, and many more nutrients.[‡]

Another option is to create **a calorie- and nutrient-dense smoothie** that can be diluted as necessary and administered through the feeding tube. Some suggested ingredients toward that end are listed in the *Power Smoothie Recipe* that follows. Counts for calories and protein are included with that recipe so that appropriate combinations of ingredients may be selected.

Ask around your community network to discover **holistic nutritional counselors** who can support you or your loved one in creating liquid meals that take into consideration the quality, nutrition and synergy of the foods combined—aiming for a sustaining balance of calories, good fats, proteins, and nutrients. Of course, **always follow the basic guidelines given by your medical team** regarding daily nutrient mix required and the consistency of liquids introduced into feeding tubes—including diluting properly and straining to remove any chunks or globs from the mixtures used.

Given the range of considerations that must be taken into account, certainly health-promoting—not simply life-sustaining—liquid formulas can be created to satisfy those who are not willing to sacrifice their basic understanding of quality nutrition for the ease of commercially available products. Already, some initial attempts to fill this gap are appearing in the natural health marketplace and—both fortunately and unfortunately given the prevalence of need—more are certain to be introduced in the future.

[‡] USDA National Nutrient Database for Standard Reference.

Power Smoothie Recipe

<u>General Smoothie Base —</u>

1 cup **blueberries** [defrosted if previously frozen] — **84 calories, 3.7 gm protein**

2 cups **water**, room temperature — using other liquid could provide added calories, protein

1 heaping T. **VitaMineral Green** [or similar blend] — **1½ T. = 34 cal, 3.64 gm protein**

1 T. **Stinging nettle leaf powder** — ~ **22 calories, 2 gm protein**

1 T. **Coconut butter** or **coconut powder** — **100 calories, 1 gm protein**

1 T. **flax oil** — **120 calories**

<u>Main Protein, to be added at end —</u>

Whey Protein Isolate, Microfiltered [**1 scoop = 105 calories, 25 gm protein**]

Perhaps alternating w/ **Eggwhite Protein** [**1 scoop = 100 calories, 20 gm protein**]

<u>Possible Additions to Base —</u>

1½ T. **lecithin** granules [non-GMO] — **70 calories**

Astragalus root powder or 5:1 concentrate powder

Freshly juiced kale, celery, dandelion leaves, chickweed, turmeric and/or ginger root

Seaweed powder [source of minerals, iodine, alginates]

L-glutamine powder [protects intestinal lining and nerve cells from chemo damage] **OR Beyond Whey** [L-glutamine, creatine, whey, etc. [**1 scoop = 40 calories, 6 gm protein**]

Nutrigenomic Berry [or similar] powder for additional nutrition and anticancer benefits.

Coconut oil [1-3 tsp.], liquefy! — **each tsp. = 42 calories**

Fiber formula [e.g. sprouted Super Seed] — Source of lignans. Thickener: Avoid or add immediately before use in tube feeding. [**1 scoop Super Seed = 70 cal, 6 gm protein**]

<u>Directions</u> —

- Thoroughly buzz base ingredients—plus any additions—together in blender.

- Add whey protein isolate or eggwhite protein and pulse briefly, just enough to mix well. 'Chew' every mouthful to mix with saliva. Enjoy!

- If administering via feeding tube: Strain to remove any chunks or globs. Add additional water to achieve proper consistency. Make in smaller amounts to divide total throughout day.

- Take with proteolytic enzymes to improve nutrient utilization.

Base + whey protein isolate = 360 cal + whey pwd [105] **= 465 cal, 35.34 gm protein**

Add lecithin + coconut oil = additional 112 cal, totaling **577 cal, 35.34 gm protein**

Add Beyond Whey = additional 40 cal, 6 gm protein, totaling **617 cal, 41.34 gm protein**

Add Super Seed = additional 70 cal, 6 gm protein, totaling **687 cal, 47.34 gm protein**

Very important: If utilizing a feeding tube to deliver liquefied nutrition, **always follow the basic guidelines given by your medical team** regarding daily nutrient mix required as well as the consistency of liquids introduced into tubes—including diluting properly and straining to remove any chunks or globs from the mixtures used.

Food Considerations for Liver Health

Support of the liver is a foundational aspect of natural medicine, whether in maintaining wellness or restoring health.

From the Western perspective, the liver is an incredibly complex organ of transmutation: metabolizing hormones and other native substances and altering foreign chemicals in a way that often renders them less toxic. It is the liver's job to make sure the body absorbs everything it needs and eliminates what it doesn't. It stores nutrients and alters unneeded materials to facilitate their excretion.

In addition, we can envision the Liver (with a capital "L") and the Traditional Chinese Medicine view of its nature and sphere of influence. It is said that the most important of all the Liver functions is that it ensures the smooth flow of Qi, or vital force. It is about regulating and harmonizing the flow of energy throughout our internal universe.

Within this perspective, it is understood that the Liver is influential in the process of deliberating and making plans, in addition to playing a key role in the balance of our emotional experience. Prolonged or excessive anger as well as anxiety, irritability or depression can arise as consequences of relative disharmony within the Liver sphere.

In our current era, mainstream commercial food supply and contaminated water and environments place burdens on this crucial organ that tax its innate capacity to function at life-sustaining levels. The full implications of this are not yet widely understood in the collective awareness.

When the liver is presented with the additional load of pharmaceutical chemicals and radiation exposure, it is eminently sensible to undertake dedicated support of the liver's capacity to smoothly accomplish its many functions. Thoughtful dietary choices and helpful herbs may be of great benefit in lightening the liver's load both as preventive medicine and as adjunct support to standard chemical therapeutics.

- **Choose organically cultivated foods exclusively**, or at least as much as possible—for personal as well as planetary health. Agricultural chemicals are neither friends of the liver nor the biosphere. Especially choose organic nuts, seeds, oils, dairy products. Give preference to locally grown, organically cultivated fruits and vegetables in season. Choose meat, if eaten, from animals that have been raised compassionately and free from chemical-laden feed and pharmaceutical drugs.

- **Favor foods with a sour or bitter taste**. Lemons and lemon juice, dark leafy greens—including wild weedy green foods, naturally fermented organic vinegars [as appropriate], well-prepared cultured vegetables…

- **Avoid cooked oils**, especially anything commercially fried in what is likely to be burnt, rancid oil. Heating oil, especially at high temperature, converts substances that might inherently provide benefit into toxic substances. Ideally, think of oil as a condiment, added to foods *after* cooking. Extra-virgin olive oil, freshly pressed flaxseed oil, etc. Choose oils cold pressed from organically cultivated plant sources whenever available.

- **Forget margarine and harmful fats!** Anytime oils are processed to become 'hydrogenated' or 'partially hydrogenated' they become harmful substances, not only to the liver but to cell membranes, as well, impacting proper cellular metabolism throughout the body. Read labels of all commercial crackers, cookies, cakes, pies, breads, tortillas, nut butters, snack foods, and other prepared foods carefully—these "trans fats" are ubiquitous.

- **Moderate consumption of oil-rich nuts/seeds and their butters**. They are best raw and organically grown. Strictly avoid nuts and seeds roasted in oil and salted— chances are high that they are rancid. Soaking nuts and seeds to lightly germinate them makes their nutrients more available. Refrigerating nuts and seeds lengthens their shelf life.

- **Limit consumption of substances that could potentially over-stress or over-stimulate the liver**—including alcohol, pharmaceutical drugs, over-the-counter non-steroidal anti-inflammatory drugs [NSAIDs], and excessive use of stimulating spices such as black pepper.

- **Read labels on all products to avoid voluntary toxins**. While not technically foods, household and cosmetic chemicals found in the bathroom, the cleaning pantry, the laundry, and the garage are readily ingested through inhalation, the eyes, and the skin—and are thereby brought into the bloodstream. These chemicals can promote identifiable sensitivities in compromised individuals as well as occult internal damage in others. It is the liver that is required to process and detoxify these chemicals; the more this burden is reduced by stringent elimination of petrochemical-based products, synthetic fragrances, toxic preservatives and sudsing agents, the less effort expended by the liver and the less potential damage to its specialized cells and systems. Fortunately, an ever-expanding selection of health-friendly cleaning and bodycare products are widely available.

- Consider **adjunct liver support** following any course of prescription drugs, ingestion of diagnostic fluids, or session of anesthesia. Milk thistle seed extract [*Silybum marianum*], schisandra berry [*Schisandra chinensis*], turmeric rhizome [*Curcuma longa, C.* spp.], dandelion root [*Taraxacum officinale*] are especially worthy of consideration in this regard. ***Please note***: *Silybum* has been previously suspected of influencing the metabolism of some drugs, thus potentially impacting their clinical effectiveness. Human studies have since reported conflicting results, and the latest edition of the standard reference *Botanical Safety Handbook* [2013] concludes that there are no known drug interactions.

- **Emphasize low-fat vegetable sources of protein**, such as tempeh.

- **Drink plenty of pure water and engage in sweat-inducing activities** such as physical exercise and saunas. Both sufficient water and regular sweating improve overall circulation and support the liver in its detoxification efforts and help lighten its load. *Please note*: Strenuous physical exercise and sweating therapies should be undertaken only as appropriate for one's overall condition.

- **Promote healthy intestinal microbial ecology** by eating beneficial traditionally cultured foods such as yogurt, kefir, miso, kimchee, sauerkraut, natto, etc. Consume good quality, multi-strain probiotic supplements as needed. Detoxification also occurs in the gut, given healthy, flourishing microbiota.

- If constitutionally and situationally appropriate, **consider a period of fasting or food simplification** to give the overall digestive system a well-deserved rest. **Do not** undertake a fast if deficient in vitality or physical reserves, or burdened by a heavy toxin load—consult with a nutritional counselor as to what, **if any**, type of cleanse might be safe and appropriate.

- **Include cabbage-family vegetables** on a regular basis. These vegetables—also known as cruciferous or brassica—have been shown to support proper detoxification mechanisms in the liver, among numerous health-promoting benefits. See the chapter *A Few Recipes for Gentle Foods* for more information. Organic broccoli seeds may also be sprouted in the kitchen: Well-tended sprouts 5-6 days old may be eaten as food, juiced, added to smoothies, and so on. Even more than the vegetables themselves, broccoli sprouts have been shown to powerfully support detoxification. *Please note*: Sprouts should be avoided by those with significantly compromised immune function, as they might introduce challenging microorganisms into one's system. Consult with your healthcare practitioner to determine if this caution is applicable in your situation.

> *To sprout broccoli seed*: **Sprouting time**: about 5-7 days at temperatures between 60°-80°. **Yield**: 1 T. organic seed = 1-1½ cups sprouts
>
> *Place seeds in a canning jar and cover with cheesecloth or other porous material. Secure the cloth with a rubber band. You can also use reusable sprouting lids that attach to wide-mouthed canning jars—this eliminates the need to use fresh cheesecloth for each batch. Fill the jar full with filtered water or well water and let seeds soak overnight. [Some people use distilled water for this stage, feeling that may increase the percentage of seeds that sprout successfully.]*
>
> *In the morning, drain the jar by carefully pouring out the water through the cheesecloth or screened lid. Rinse seeds with water again and let drain. Lay the container on its side in a dark location where the air temperature remains at about 70°. Rinse twice each day with water and drain. Continue this rinse cycle until they are ready to harvest. When sprouts are 1-2 inches long you can put them in the light briefly to allow them to green up.*
>
> *Before storage, if you like, rinse the sprouts to remove the tiny seed hulls or skim them off the top of the water with a spoon. The hulls are not harmful to eat but removing them helps to minimize spoilage during storage. Sprouts are best stored in an airtight container in the refrigerator and kept for no longer than a week. Compost any that start to spoil.*

Plant Allies for Liver Support

There are numerous plants that benefit the liver in one way or another, any of which could be discussed at length, over the course of many pages. Here are brief profiles of a few reliable plants which may serve as personal allies—either used alone or in some combination—to both protect the liver and improve its functioning. Reviewing the overall pattern of a given plant's affinities and attributes is the first step in choosing a plant to work with. As with any plant medicine new to you, I recommend starting with a single plant in small quantities and tuning into its effects and benefits. Please note that using plants that influence the liver and gallbladder may naturally result in loosened stool—adjust dosing strategy accordingly.

Burdock [*Arctium* spp.]: root. Bitter, cooling. Nutritive. Affinity for kidney, lymph, liver. Tonic alterative. Deeply cleansing, diuretic; helps detoxify, clears heat. Promotes bile secretion; mildly laxative. Especially indicated in skin manifestations related to liver function. Excessive initial use may worsen symptoms in cases of severe toxicity—approach with respect and patience. Think of burdock as a body opener, an energy mover, a powerful ally in staying grounded in the presence of change, in moving forward without fear, in releasing what no longer serves. A harmonizer of blood chemistry. Rich in nutrition: iron, calcium, magnesium, phosphorus, potassium, selenium, carotenes, vitamin C, and more. Works well combined with its congenial companion dandelion root. Like dandelion root, burdock root contains significant amounts of inulin, a carbohydrate found as a food reserve in some plants. Inulin provides food preferentially to beneficial bacteria in the gut and can benefit blood sugar regulation. Inulin is soluble in hot water, therefore available in foods and in traditional decoctions, and only slightly soluble in cold water or alcohol. Gobo, as burdock root is known in Japan, makes for a wonderful dish combined with carrots, ginger, dark sesame oil and tamari. Please see additional discussion of burdock in the appendix ***What About Essiac?*** **Formats**: Decoction, tincture, food.

Dandelion [*Taraxacum officinale*]: root. Bitter, cooling. Moves stagnation. Affinity for digestion, elimination, liver/gallbladder, kidneys. Tonic, protective, detoxifying, 'opens the way'. Digestive stimulant. Promotes bile secretion; gently laxative. Stimulates pancreatic secretions and hydrochloric acid production in the stomach, thereby supporting nutrient absorption and immunity. Improves fat metabolism. Contains inulin: Used as decoction or cooked into foods to support blood sugar balance and healthy microbial ecology in the gut. Used in Traditional Chinese Medicine to support breast health. A ubiquitous wonder plant, all parts of the plant are edible and health supporting. **Formats**: Decoction, tincture, glycerite, succus, capsules, as food. ***Please note***: Due to choleretic activity, caution has been suggested for persons with gallstones.

Milk thistle [*Silybum marianum*]: mature seed. Slightly bitter, slightly cooling. Affinity for liver and gallbladder. Featured constituents: Several flavanolignans collectively known as *silymarin*; flavonoids, including quercetin. Protective, regenerative, tonic. Antioxidant, cholagogue. Helps detoxify liver cells; protects liver from damage; and promotes hepatic tissue regeneration. Indicated in damaged or diseased liver, abnormal liver function, jaundice, acute or chronic chemical exposures [environmental toxins, paints, solvents, glues, anesthesia, alcohol, many pharmaceuticals including acetaminophen], complications from diabetes such as neuropathy. Clears heat and resolves toxins. Works well alone or harmoniously in combinations. A well-studied and remarkable medicine. **Formats**: Tincture, extract in capsule, ground seed in food. The absorption of silymarin is enhanced by lecithin. ***Please note***: *Silybum* has been previously suspected of influencing the metabolism of some drugs, thus potentially impacting their clinical effectiveness. Human studies have since reported conflicting results, and the latest edition of the standard reference *Botanical Safety Handbook* [2013–Gardner *et al*] concludes that there are no known drug interactions.

Oregon grape [*Mahonia* spp.]: stem and root bark. Bitter, cooling. Antimicrobial, anti-inflammatory, laxative. Stimulates production of stomach acid, bile, and other digestive juices. Used for impaired digestion, especially of fats; sluggish liver; jaundice; urinary tract infections; thrush; eruptive skin conditions; psoriasis. Those with cool or cold constitutions should combine Oregon grape with warming herbs such as ginger or cinnamon. **Formats**: Decoction, tincture, capsules. Powdered root can be applied topically to oozing sores. Well-strained decoction can be used as compress or wash for eye-area irritations and infections. ***Please note***: Most safety concerns [e.g. use in pregnancy] reported for *Mahonia* are based on studies of the alkaloid *berberine* used in isolation and may not apply to full-spectrum preparations or extracts of Oregon grape. See *Botanical Safety Handbook* [2013].

Rosemary [*Rosmarinus officinalis*]: leaf. Resinous, pungent/bitter, warming. Stimulating nervine with affinity for digestion, liver, cardiovascular. Promotes peripheral circulation. Diaphoretic. The strongly antioxidant rosmarinic acid possesses neuroprotective, antimutagenic, radioprotective, anti-inflammatory, antibacterial and antiviral properties. A bitter tonic, rosemary stimulates bile production and secretion, sharpens the appetite, strengthens detoxification, relieves flatulence. Also antifungal, astringent, anti-inflammatory, carminative, muscle relaxing. Tones and calms digestion where psychological tension is present: dyspepsia, headache, depression. It awakens, warms and brings light to our beings. See entry in ***Plants to Support the Nervous System*** for additional indications. **Formats**: Tea, tincture, in foods, as essential oil. ***Please note***: The essential oil and concentrated extracts are generally contraindicated during pregnancy; limited use as a tea or culinary herb is not.

Schisandra [*Schisandra chinensis*]: berries. See ***Adaptogenic and Tonic Plant Allies***.

Turmeric [*Curcuma longa*]: rhizome. Acrid, bitter, warming. Affinity for liver, gall bladder, gastrointestinal, connective tissue. Strong anti-inflammatory and liver-protective properties. Potent antioxidant and antimutagenic. Antimicrobial. Stimulates the gallbladder and regulates the viscosity of bile. Very useful aid in digestive issues, including gut healing. Soothes inflamed mucosa, joints, and muscle tissue. Turmeric brilliantly normalizes inflammatory response through multiple pathways. Assimilation is an issue to achieve sufficient dosage for therapeutic benefit; traditional use combines turmeric with lipids [ghee or coconut milk], black pepper, ginger, and so on. Commercial preparations are available that are based on these understandings. Please see entry in chapter on ***Chemotherapy/Radiation Considerations*** for further discussion. **Formats**: Tincture, extract in tablets or capsule, root powder in capsules, food. ***Please note***: Previous advisories to avoid concurrent use with blood-thinning medications are being reconsidered in the most current reviews of the available literature. Stargrove *et al* conclude that "extrapolated warnings may be considered speculative and overstated." The *Botanical Safety Handbook* [2013] concurs and places turmeric in its safest class. Because of its antioxidant potency, concurrent intake with chemotherapy agents remains a realm of considerable debate; refer to Stargrove *et al* for detailed discussion per pharmaceutical agent.

Yarrow [*Achillea millefolium*]: leaf and flower. Bitter/pungent, cooling, drying. Affinity for digestive, urinary, circulatory, excretory, liver/gallbladder, reproductive systems. Antibacterial, antispasmodic, anti-inflammatory, astringent, decongesting, choleretic, cholagogue, styptic/hemostatic, wound healing. Bitter digestive tonic: Helps with gas, nausea, gastric discomfort, especially associated with fat digestion; useful for spasms in the digestive tract. Indicated in chronic diarrhea, hemorrhoids. Peripheral vasodilator, tones vasculature. Urinary antiseptic. Diuretic, diaphoretic [helps move heat to the surface], febrifuge. **Formats**: Tea, infusion, tincture, fresh-pressed juice [leaves and flowers], poultice, bath [for aches and pains; sitz bath], oil infusion. Fresh leaves may be chewed into a small plug to relieve toothache. Infused oil applied to scalp to benefit local circulation and strengthen hair growth. ***Please note***: Those with serious allergies to aster family plants should handle and use yarrow with caution.

— Cleansing Root Brew —

To a pot filled with two quarts of pure water, add a handful of chopped **dandelion** root, 1 tablespoon **burdock** root, 1 tablespoon chopped **cinnamon** bark, 1 teaspoon chopped **licorice** root, and 2 teaspoons of chopped **ginger**. Let it sit for an hour or even overnight.

Bring to a boil, then reduce heat and simmer for 45 minutes or an hour. Remove from the fire and let sit another half hour or more if you can wait. Strain and store in airtight jars in the refrigerator. Stored cool, the brew will keep for several days.

Enjoy a half-cup of the warmed brew several times throughout the day as desired. Please do not microwave your tea!

Adaptogenic and Tonic Plant Allies

"In that awkward, ambiguous moment is our own wisdom mind.
Right there in the uncertainty of everyday chaos is our own wisdom mind."
— Pema Chodron, When Things Fall Apart

Feeling anxiety arising because of a pending deadline, I uprooted my body from my writing table and headed out into the misty greenworld. The colors and textures of the mosses and lichens that greeted me immediately quickened my energy field. Bright rosettes of foxglove leaves sang like spring blooms on the woodland floor. The softly percussive dripping of rain onto sword fern filled me with a sense that all was right with the world. As I walked among cedar and maple, breathing deeply the fresh moist air, I felt washed with the green energy that both cleanses and renews. My muscles relaxed and my joints opened as feelings of calm joyfulness soon accompanied the rhythm of my stride.

Returning yet again to the presence of the sacred green, so readily my mind and body find peace and poise. It is a truth I must remember daily—in the midst of all that calls for attention—even though it is so vivid a blessing. There is so much that would distract me from this ecstatic reunion with vital essence.

At all times, and especially in times of increased stress, it will benefit us to remember the healing power of simply immersing ourselves in the realm of the plant beings. It is of benefit to make pilgrimage to their abodes—the temples within cedar circles, maple groves, stream bank nooks, meadows rippling with wild carrot. This is the first and most fundamental level of plant medicine—simply to be in sacred relationship with that which heals. To recognize and to honor. To invoke assistance. To allow the vibrational attunement to occur.

At another level, we make physical communion with our plant helpers, taking them materially into our bodies. This, too, can be made a sacred exchange and the manner in which we work amplifies the healing energy. Plants that are especially beneficial in maintaining human wellness in the presence of stressful factors have been termed "adaptogens." The dictionary definition of "to adapt" is to make or become suitable for a new use or situation. Plants termed "adaptogenic" increase the ability of an organism to cope with stress and to adapt to the circumstances of the new moment with the least disruption and expenditure of energy. Adaptogens such as *Panax ginseng* have been revered in their native traditions since ancient times. Their benefits are undisputed by the peoples who honor them, although their mechanisms of action have only been understood through the filter of western physiology within the last century.

To be considered an adaptogen, a plant must fulfill three criteria, according to the Russian researcher who coined the term: Be innocuous; increase the body's overall resistance through multiple non-specific actions; restore balance and normal function. Adaptogens generally demonstrate the following activity: Support adrenal function thereby lessening the weakening effects of stress; improve cellular energy [Qi]; support elimination of toxins; build up tissue and substance; improve oxygen utilization; and regulate biorhythms.

What follows are brief descriptions of a few notable adaptogenic and tonic plants. Adaptogens work well alone or in concert with various herbs which directly influence the nerve tissue, discussed later. Please also see the appendix article *The Impact of Stress on Memory: The Plant Allies* where many of these marvelous plants are further discussed. Additional, detailed information is available in numerous books listed in the **Bibliography**. And, as always, please consider working with a skilled practitioner to determine which plants or combinations might best suit your individual constitution and circumstances.

In whatever ways you request healing assistance from these botanical allies, bless yourself, bless the ancestors, bless the plants, bless the planet—and, within it all, breathe deeply of the precious oxygen the green ones provide.

A Selection of Adaptogenic and Tonic Herbs

Ginseng [*Panax ginseng*]: root. Sweet/bitter, warming. [The "red" steamed root is considered more warming and stimulating than the raw "white" root.] Adaptogen and tonic to replenish vital energy. Rejuvenative, demulcent, stimulant, anti-inflammatory, hypotensive, anticonvulsant, blood sugar regulating. One of the most famous and valued herbs on earth. It has been shown to be stimulating and regulatory to both the central nervous system and to the endocrine system. It is the primary Qi tonic of Chinese herbalism. Ginseng helps a person to adapt to all manner of stresses, and enhances endurance and resilience under stressful conditions. Ginseng is also used to tonify digestive and respiratory functions, and to build muscle. There are various varieties of ginseng, all of which have distinct characteristics. Indications: Debility, weakness, fatigue, poor appetite and digestion, emaciation, shortness of breath, palpitations. **Formats**: Decoction, tincture, medicated wine, food, capsules. ***Please note***: Use of red ginseng may potentiate the effects of caffeine or other stimulants in sensitive people. Avoid in false or excess heat conditions; one source lists high blood pressure, though it may be skillfully used clinically for that purpose in appropriate circumstances. Some sources contraindicate use during pregnancy, though that caution is not consistent with traditional use in Asia. Use with guidance of a practitioner conversant with botanical medicine if taking pharmaceutical drugs: ginseng with its complex chemistry and amphoteric nature has been seen to have seemingly contradictory effects on physiology depending on the individual observed. Regarding the question of concurrent use with anticoagulant drugs, Stargrove *et al* conclude that the "weight of the currently available research data suggests that the reported ginseng-warfarin interaction is not clinically significant."

American Ginseng [*Panax quinquifolius*]: root. Sweet/slightly bitter, neutral or slightly cooling. A true member of the ginseng family that grows in North America. Unlike the Asian species, American ginseng is considered to be a Yin tonic herb, especially nourishing to the lungs, skin, and stomach. It builds adaptive energy without the warming effects of Asian ginseng; it is considered the preferred ginseng for people with excessively Yang energy. Adaptogen, Qi and Yin tonic, demulcent, rejuvenative, immune enhancing, anti-tumor, antiviral, antioxidant, metabolic and endocrine enhancement. Regulates basic metabolism, benefits vital energy, improves digestion and assimilation, promotes fluid production, supplements and moistens the Lungs, clears heat. It has been shown to reduce fatigue, strengthen adrenal function, enhance reproductive performance, improve liver metabolism, and enhance immunity. **Formats**: Decoction, tincture, medicated wine, in food, capsules. ***Please note***: In terms of possible interactions, Gardner *et al* conclude that "concomitant use of warfarin and American ginseng may reduce the efficacy of warfarin and should be under the supervision of a healthcare professional." Related to the comment on Asian ginseng in previous entry, Stargrove *et al* recommend further research into possible differences between American and Asian species as to their influence on blood coagulation and any possible interactions with prescription anticoagulant agents.

Ashwagandha [*Withania somnifera*]: root. Bitter, warming, drying. Aka winter cherry. Calming adaptogen, nervine, tonic, anti-inflammatory, sedative, hypotensive, astringent, diuretic, antispasmodic, immunomodulator. Keynote: flourishing in the flesh. In Ayurveda, the root of this plant is held in the high esteem given to *Panax ginseng* in Chinese herbal medicine. The horsey aroma is unmistakable, and in India the plant is said to impart the frisky vigor of the horse. A supremely regenerative herb, Ashwagandha is especially indicated after a period of illness, exhaustion or overwork. It helps builds tissue and energizes muscles. It is one of the plants to turn to when the physical body is wasting away, including a misconnection between the psyche and physique. Other indications: adrenal exhaustion, sluggish thyroid function, chronic fatigue, anxiety, depression, impaired memory, hypertension, insomnia, peptic ulcers, impotence, fibromyalgia, arthritis, asthma, multiple sclerosis, anorexia nervosa, iron-deficient anemia, adjunct support in cancer therapies. Ashwagandha is considered one of the best nutritive plants for the mind—calming, nurturing, clarifying. It promotes a deep, restorative sleep. Considered both an adaptogen and a tonic in Ayurveda, it is considered appropriate for all ages, including young children and pregnant women. **Formats**: Traditionally, it is prepared as either a water or milk decoction [honey or raw sugar may be added] or eaten as a powder on a daily basis. Capsules and liquid extracts are also available. ***Please note***: Some sources caution against ingesting ashwagandha during pregnancy; in India it is considered appropriate for all ages, including young children and pregnant women—this discrepancy may be related to the dose, frequency or format used. Because of conflicting recommendations, use during pregnancy is suggested only with the guidance of a knowledgeable healthcare practitioner.

Astragalus [*Astragalus membranaceus*]: root. Mildly sweet, slightly warming. Adaptogen, immune-stimulant, antibacterial, antiviral, anti-inflammatory, pectoral, antipyretic, diuretic. Invigorates Qi, builds stamina, strengthens superficial resistance, promotes tissue regeneration, reduces inflammation. It is also a digestive tonic that can speed up the digestion and assimilation of food. Indications: Wasting or exhausting diseases, fatigue, colds, poor digestion and metabolism, weakness, chronically weak lungs with shortness of breath, prolapsed organs, spontaneous sweating, nephritis, tumors, adjunct to chemotherapy and radiation. Astragalus has been used for more than 2,000 years to fortify the body as a whole. In Asia, it is used to strengthen muscle and improve metabolic functions. It is the main herb in a wide assortment of tonic formulations. Astragalus has been recognized as a potent immune system tonic by modern researchers and clinicians—found to be a tonic to bone marrow. **Formats**: Decoction used as beverage and as broth in soups and grains, tincture, powdered root as food, capsules. ***Please note***: Generally, discontinue use during hot, acute conditions. Chen and Chen [2001] recommend using with caution during third trimester of pregnancy. There is a theoretical concern about combining astragalus with immune suppressant drugs. Consult with a knowledgeable practitioner in such circumstances.

Codonopsis [*Codonopsis pilosula*]: root. Sweet, neutral. Adaptogenic. This food-like Qi tonic is sometimes called "poor man's ginseng" because of its more affordable price and similar applicability. Favored over *Panax ginseng* when the latter's energy may be too stimulating or too heating. Unlike *P. ginseng*, codonopsis is more universally appropriate regardless of constitution, age, or season. It may be substituted for ginseng in many formulas. Invigorates the vital force, tonifies the immune system, supports adrenal function, nourishes fluids. Tonifies the lungs; used in China to address bronchitis. Combines well with nervines to address chronic depression or stress. **Formats**: Decoction, tincture, powder, food.

Eleuthero [*Eleutherococcus senticosus*]: root, root bark. Bitter/sweet, neutral/warming. Also known as Siberian ginseng, eleuthero is one of the most clinically studied adaptogenic herbs. Reinforces the vital force, invigorates the Spleen and Kidney, calms the nerves, stabilizes energy. Many physiological effects of eleuthero have been demonstrated, including blood-sugar regulation, liver protection, increased resistance to stress, normalization of adrenal response, enhanced immunity, increased stamina, improved oxygen utilization, and protection against radiation. See page 255 for more. **Formats**: Decoction, tincture, extract in capsules, powder as food.

Gotu kola [*Centella asiatica*]: leaf. Acrid/bitter, cold. Also known as *Hydrocotyle*, Indian Pennywort, or Brahmi, this water-loving plant grows wild in India and is an essential medicine of Ayurveda. The heart-shaped leaves are highly esteemed in India as a restorative, adaptogenic tonic particularly for the brain and nervous system. It is the herb of choice for many indications including rheumatism, ulcers, leprosy, varicosities, and to normalize the metabolism of connective tissue. Both externally and internally, it is used to speed the healing of wounds, burns, ulcers, and to minimize scarring after surgery or accident. Supplementing with vitamin C further increases the rate of collagen synthesis. In addition, it can be of benefit in situations of excessive or inappropriate collagen production, such as in scleroderma. **Formats**: The dried plant may be made into a tea or, better still, ingested freshly picked or preserved by tincturing or freeze-drying. Grow your own or look for organically cultivated herb as there is much poor-quality gotu kola in the marketplace.

He Shou Wu [*Polygonum multiflorum*]: prepared root. Also known as Fo-ti. Bitter/sweet, slightly warming. Adaptogen, blood tonic, astringent, anti-tumor, antioxidant. Builds the Blood, invigorates the Liver and Kidneys, supplements the Qi. Consistent consumption of this celebrated "longevity herb" is said to help restore youthful vitality. Indications: Low energy, infertility, premature gray hair, low back pain, aging. It is a classic Jing tonic, as well as a major Blood tonic. It is said to increase energy and to be a powerful fertility tonic when consumed regularly. He shou wu is included in many classic Asian tonics utilized to nurture the hair and teeth. **Formats**: Cured root is dark reddish brown [cooked in black bean liquid]; uncured root has a laxative effect. Used in decoction, syrup, medicated wine, tablets, tincture. Combines well with ginger, cinnamon, or licorice to harmonize its energy. ***Please note***: Avoid in weak digestion with fluid retention, congestion, or loose stools.

Holy Basil / Tulsi [*Ocimum sanctum aka O. tenuiflorum*]: leaf. Aka Tulasi. Pungent, heating. Affinity for nerve tissue, respiratory and digestive systems. Adaptogenic, nervine, neuroprotective, antioxidant, anti-inflammatory, antispasmodic, antibacterial, antiseptic, diaphoretic, febrifuge. Supports normal cortisol and blood sugar levels. Helps relieve anxiety, mental confusion, inability to focus. Demonstrates significant protection against ionizing radiation. Holy basil is one of the most sacred plants in India—devotion to this plant is thought to cultivate states of higher consciousness. In Ayurvedic medicine, Tulsi is utilized to purify and stabilize the mind, emotions and body—opening the heart and awareness, strengthening clarity and compassion. Recent research has shown that holy basil has adaptogenic properties—enhancing adrenal function and the bodymind's response to stress. It is an honored tonic for enhancing memory and modern science is explaining the mechanisms involved. Clinical studies in India have shown holy basil to prevent stress-related conditions such as peptic ulcers, colitis, asthma, and hypertension. **Formats**: The leaf tea is often drunk with honey. Powdered extract in capsules. Fresh leaf juice applied topically on wounds or fungus. In India, Tulsi tea is often used for pregnant and lactating women as well as for children.

Licorice [*Glycyrrhiza glabra*]: root. Sweet, neutral. Adaptogenic, immune enhancing, antiviral, liver-protective, detoxifying, demulcent, expectorant. Licorice root builds energy and is an excellent digestive tonic. It is widely used in natural medicine for addressing gastric ulcers, usually in a deglycyrrhizinated form [DGL] to avoid hypertension. It increases immune cell production and activity, and inhibits the replication of viruses. It helps regulate blood sugar levels. Licorice root also provides basic nutrients to the adrenal glands. Licorice helps build and strengthen muscle. Licorice is included in most Chinese herbal formulations because it is said to harmonize all the ingredients. It should be used in small quantities. **Formats**: Infusion, decoction, medicated wine, tincture, solid extract, capsules, tablets.
Please note: Licorice is basically safe, but excessive amounts may cause fluid retention, heart palpitations and may promote hypertension. Therefore, Gardner *et al* contraindicate use by those with hypertension, liver disorders, edema, severe kidney insufficiency, low serum potassium, and cardiovascular disease. Avoid during pregnancy. These cautions do *not* apply to deglycyrrhizinated [DGL] products.

Reishi [*Ganoderma lucidum*] aka Ling zhi: polypore fruiting body and mycelium. Sweet, neutral. Known as "herb of spiritual potency." Reishi is more commonly thought of as an immune system tonic, but it also nurtures the heart, soothes the spirit, and calms the mind. Its ability to deeply change our experience is profound. It is widely renowned in Asia as the "mushroom of immortality" and the "herb of good fortune." It is believed to protect the spirit and to nurture the growth of intelligence, wisdom, and spiritual insight. System affinities: Respiratory, cardiovascular, immune, liver function. Adaptogen, immune amphoteric, antioxidant, anti-inflammatory, liver protective, kidney protective, radioprotective, cardiotonic, anti-hyperlipidemia, adjunct treatment for cancer. *Ganoderma* is used to tonify the blood and vital energy. *Ganoderma* is used in formulas for insomnia, palpitations, anxiety, impaired memory, general weakness and debility, heart disease, cancer, allergies and hypertension. **Formats**: Dried mushroom decoction as tea or soup base, tincture, extract.

Rhodiola [*Rhodiola rosea*]: root. Sweet/slightly bitter, cooling, drying. Adaptogenic, immune enhancing, cardioprotective, hepatoprotective, neuroprotective, antioxidant, anti-inflammatory, astringent. It is used clinically, particularly in combination with other plants and nutrients, to assist with weight gain, improve energy and strength, and to improve mood. It has been shown to be anti-mutagenic, protect against radiation and chemical therapies, inhibit cancer metastasis, improve oxygen utilization, memory, and more. A stimulating adaptogen, rhodiola is generally best taken no later than mid-afternoon. **Formats**: Tea, tincture, standardized extract. Herbalist Donald Yance reports that most of the research on rhodiola has utilized a 1:1 fluid extract of wild Russian rhodiola.

Schisandra [*Schisandra chinensis*]: fruit. Astringent, warming. "Five tastes fruit": Possesses the five flavors sweet, sour, acrid-bitter, salty—though its dominant tastes are sour and salty, with an overall warm energy. Considered a harmonizing remedy in Eastern medicine. Tonic and restorative; adaptogenic. Anti-inflammatory. Liver protective and regenerative: congenial allies include milk thistle and turmeric. Can improve sleep when liver issues contribute to insomnia or restlessness. Enhances overall detoxification. **Formats**: Decoction, tincture, extract, or capsules. ***Please note***: Schisandra may influence the way the liver metabolizes drugs, therefore avoid concurrent use with pharmaceuticals. Avoid during pregnancy—may stimulate uterine contractions. Traditional Chinese botanical medicine cautions against use in cases of excess heat in the interior or where an exterior disorder such as rash has not been cleared. May occasionally cause heartburn in susceptible individuals.

Stinging Nettles [*Urtica dioica*]: leaf. Astringent, cooling. Mineralizing tonic, fortifying, affinity for lungs and kidney/adrenals, blood building, improves blood clotting and bone mineralization, diuretic. Vitalizing, nutritive tonic to entire organism. Useful in formulas for depression, fatigue, anemia. A fabulous way to get a dietary serving or two of leafy green vegetation, especially when the appetite is depressed or otherwise unreliable. **Formats**: Tea, infusion, fresh leaf as vegetable or juice or blanched and frozen, powdered leaf in food, capsules.

Recipes Using Adaptogenic and Tonic Plants

Immune Support Decoction

3 T. Astragalus root, cut
3 T. Codonopsis root, cut
2 T. Dandelion root, cut

1 T. Schisandra berries
1 T. Ginger root or Prickly ash bark, cut
1 T. Licorice root, cut

Add the herbs to two quarts pure water. Let them hydrate a bit for 15 minutes or even much longer if you can. Place them on the stove; bring to a boil, then turn down the heat and simmer for 1-2 hours. Take off the heat and let sit for another 30 minutes. Strain and enjoy a cup. Reserve the balance in a well-sealed jar in the refrigerator, if available. This will keep for up to three days.

Drink 1-3 cups in the course of the day. Eat some of the cooked codonopsis or dandelion root if you enjoy it. Make notes to adjust proportions of ginger and licorice as desired for the next batch.

If you are able to plan ahead, prepare the herbs by soaking them in the water overnight before cooking. Discontinue use of this blend should you find yourself dealing with a hot, acute condition such as flu or fever.

Herbal Power Fudge

These are basic proportions. Increase quantities as desired to make larger batches.

1 cup creamy almond butter or tahini
½ cup+ honey
1 T. Nettle or alfalfa leaf powder
3 T. Eleuthero or codonopsis root powder
2 T. He shou wu powder
OR 2 T. Ashwagandha root powder
2 tsp. royal jelly [opt.]
Pinch of sea salt or kelp powder [opt.]

<u>Optional additions:</u>
•coconut flakes
•freshly ground sunflower seeds
•freshly ground almonds
•hempseed hearts
•chopped dried fruit [dates, raisins, apricots…]
•chopped lycii berries
Add one or more of these additions to taste.

Mix together nut butter and honey first. Gradually work in other ingredients. Mix all together until blend is consistent. Add additional almond butter or tahini as needed to adjust consistency. Form into bite-sized balls or press into a small pan to create a fudge-like depth. Optional additions can be added into the dough to create texture or used as topping or outer layer. **Tip**: Try the first batch using nettle, codonopsis and he shou wu powders…and then experiment with various alternatives from there. The base recipe is delicious as it is, so do try it first before amending it with any optional additions.

These are a fabulous energy-boosting snack to have on hand. Using adaptogens as food and teas is the most wonderful way to take in their building and strengthening energies. Store in a well-sealed container in the refrigerator. This food is based on a recipe I first encountered in the wonderful work of Rosemary Gladstar, herbalist extraordinaire.

Schizam!

Schisandra berries, whole
Lycii berries, whole

Licorice root, chopped
Poria cocos, slices

This is a delicious, refreshing, easy-to-prepare brew.

The schisandra berries are decidedly astringent; to mellow this characteristic, soak a handful of the berries in water overnight.

In the morning, strain the berries and add to one quart fresh water in a cooking pot. Add a good handful of the lycii berries, about a tablespoon of licorice root, and a slice or two of poria. [Poria, also known as Fu ling, is a water-regulating and damp-resolving medicine used extensively in Chinese herbal medicine. It is diuretic, tonic, calming, and antibacterial. Poria is another beneficial member of the polypore mushroom clan. See books by Hobbs, Rogers, Powell, Chen and Chen, Teeguarden, or Bensky *et al* in the bibliography to research more information on this mushroom.]

Bring to a boil, then turn down the heat and simmer for 15-20 minutes. Remove from heat and let sit a bit to further steep before enjoying.

Cooking with Herbs

Traditionally, herbs are included as part of the routine cooking repertoire. For instance, astragalus root slices, codonopsis root, or slices of Poria fungus are readily added into long-simmering soups or stews and then removed before serving. Decoctions made from these plants may also be used as cooking water for rice or other grains. Ground pieces of the woody reishi mushroom can be decocted freely and the strained broth used as tea or soup base; the more bitter it becomes, the more beneficial. Delicious, immune-enhancing shiitake mushrooms are wonderful cooked into many dishes, including several in the chapter *A Few Recipes for Simple Foods*. Dried stinging nettle leaves can be added toward the end of cooking into soups, stews, etc. Think of the tonic plants as specialized food and use your imagination.

Smoothies

Selected tonic and adaptogenic herbs are shelf-stable in powdered form—having well-labeled, air-tight jars of these allies in the kitchen pantry makes them very available for incorporation into foods such as the herbal fudge on the preceding page. In addition, it is easy to add personally appropriate plant powders into smoothies. A suggested recipe can be found in *The Helping Repertoire* section on **Simple Nutrition** as well as the detailed *Power Smoothie Recipe*. Some plants to consider include: Astragalus, ashwagandha, eleuthero, codonopsis, the ginsengs, he shou wu, Licorice [small amounts], and stinging nettles. Review the sketches on these plants in the preceding pages and then choose one plant at a time to include. Some cinnamon or ginger powder added to smoothies serves to harmonize the flavors, warm the blend, and they contribute their own distinct health-supporting properties to the mix.

Plants to Support the Nervous System

The nervines—plants that have a special affinity for nerve tissue—are a particularly relevant category of herbs to explore in times when stress is a keynote of our experience. The nervine herbs are truly a gift of Gaia. They can nourish, tone, stimulate, and sedate. They can help repair and refresh. They can clarify the mental landscape.

They work well individually when selected thoughtfully, and combine synergistically in formulation. Nervines work very compatibly with adaptogenic herbs. They may offer more immediate benefit during stressful times, while the adaptogens lend their optimal support through more long-term consistent use.

The nervine plants can smooth the jagged edges of mental and physical sensation. Helping to unbind energetic impediments that may be present, they allow the vital force to flow freely, strengthening us for the work at hand.

Many of the nervines extract well in water, and so the act of preparing a tea or infusion from them can become a pleasant and anticipated part of the ritual of self-care.

Depending on the plant, they may be enjoyed as a beverage, used in the bath, massaged into the skin, or inhaled for their aromatherapy. Some plants may also lend themselves to extraction—via solvents such as alcohol/water, glycerine, or carbon dioxide [CO_2]. These are noted in the *Format* section as well.

What follows is a selection of such beneficial allies and some signature indications for their traditional use. Many of these plants deserve a chapter of their own. These descriptions will hopefully also serve to aid better understanding of herbal formulas you may come across in the marketplace or be recommended by holistic practitioners.

Please note: The term *herb* denoting plant part used indicates leaf, flower, and stem [if flexible]; *whole plant* includes root.

California poppy	*Lavender*	*Peppermint*
Catnip	*Lemon balm*	*Rosemary*
Chamomile	*Linden*	*Sage*
Damiana	*Motherwort*	*St. Johnswort*
Holy basil [Tulsi]	*Mugwort*	*Skullcap*
Hops	*Mullein*	*Valerian*
Kava	*Oats*	*Vervain*
	Passionflower	

California poppy [*Eschscholtzia californica*]: whole plant in flower

System affinities: Nervous System / Liver-Gallbladder
Tastes/Temperaments: Bitter/acrid, cooling
Actions: Sedative, anxiolytic, antispasmodic, mild analgesic.
Indications: Sedative—both for adults and children—particularly when pain, spasms or anxiety is present. Soothes the spirit. Often used in combination with other plants that direct activity toward relevant tissue.
Formats: Tincture [fresh plant preferred]
Cautions: Moves blood—avoid during pregnancy. May potentiate pharmaceutical MAO inhibitors; probably best avoided with other pharmaceuticals. *Please note*: While in the same family as opium poppy, and possessing some similar medicinal properties, California poppy contains neither morphine or codeine, is not narcotic, and is not habituating. The alkaloids it does contain, however, could create chemical confusion if your urine is being tested for opiates.

Catnip [*Nepeta cataria*]: leaves and flowers

System affinities: Nervous System / Digestive
Tastes/Temperaments: Bitter, cooling
Actions: Carminative, antispasmodic, diaphoretic, astringent, mildly sedative
Indications: Tension-related digestive upset, gas, nausea, colic; fever, cold/flu
Formats: Tea, tincture
Cautions: Some older herbals list as contraindicated during pregnancy, but current published reviews of the literature do not support this concern.

Chamomile [*Matricaria chamomilla, M. recutita, Chamomilla recituta*] aka German chamomile: flowers

System affinities: Nervous System / Digestive / Musculo-Skeletal / Skin
Tastes/Temperaments: Aromatic/slightly bitter, cooling, drying
Actions: Sedative, antispasmodic, anti-inflammatory, antimicrobial, carminative
Indications: Same as catnip plus inflamed tissue; loss of appetite, dyspepsia, colic, ulcers; insomnia; anxiety; diarrhea; aches and pains of influenza; headaches, migraine; neuralgia; tooth and gum pain; motion sickness; conjunctivitis.
Formats: Tea, glycerite, bath, essential oil [e.o.]
Cautions: Roman chamomile [*Chamaemelum nobile*] is not used during pregnancy. Those with serious allergies to aster family plants [e.g. feverfew, yarrow, Echinacea, etc.] should handle and use chamomile with caution.

Damiana [*Turnera diffusa*]: leaves

System affinities: Nervous System / Urinary / Reproductive
Tastes/Temperaments: Aromatic/slightly bitter, warming, drying
Actions: Considered restorative; mild stimulant, endocrine tonic, bitter tonic, urinary antiseptic, mild laxative

Indications: Stress or depression related to sexual activity; excessive or insufficient sexual/creative energy; tendency to experience urinary tract infections. Tonic to nerve tissue and hormonal system.
Formats: Tea, tincture, cordial

Holy basil / Tulsi [*Ocimum sanctum* aka *O. tenuiflorum*]: leaves

System affinities: Nervous System / Digestive / Respiratory
Tastes/Temperaments: Pungent, warming, drying
Actions: Adaptogenic, calming nervine, neuroprotective, cardioprotective, liver protective, immuno-modulating, antispasmodic, antioxidant, antibacterial, antiviral, antiseptic, anti-inflammatory, carminative, expectorant, diaphoretic/diuretic, febrifuge. Shown to protect against cellular damage caused by ionizing radiation, and inhibit cancer process. Normalizing effect on blood sugar metabolism.
Indications: Stress and stress-related digestive, immune, and cardiovascular issues; depression [in formulations]; tonic for memory and cognitive function [contains rosmarinic acid]; managing coughs, fevers; warding off colds, influenza. In the ancient texts detailing the art and science of Ayurveda, tulsi is one of the foundational plants used to preserve and promote health.
Formats: Tea, tincture, extracts in capsules
Also see: Chapter on *Adaptogenic and Tonic Plant Allies* and the appendix *The Impact of Stress on Memory: The Plant Allies.*

Hops [*Humulus lupulus*]: strobiles

System affinities: Nervous System / Digestive / Musculo-Skeletal / Genito-Urinary / Liver-Gallbladder
Tastes/Temperaments: Bitter, cooling
Actions: Sedative, antispasmodic, anti-inflammatory, analgesic, digestive bitter, tonic, soothing diuretic, astringent, febrifuge, antibacterial, locally antiseptic, estrogenic, antioxidant. A role in cancer inhibition is being explored.
Indications: Anxiety, excitability, restlessness, tension headaches, irritability and hot flashes in menopausal women, pain, insomnia, neuralgia, nervous stomach, mild spasms [muscular, intestinal, genitourinary], urinary incontinence, restless legs, anxiety-induced diarrhea, loss of appetite [especially when associated with anxiety], nocturnal emission in men.
Formats: Tea, tincture, freeze-dried fresh flowers in capsules. Never squirt hops tincture directly into your mouth—its astringent, resinous taste is much better diluted.
Topical applications: Used as compress or poultice for swellings, painful joints, headaches, facial nerve pain or toothache, eczema, cuts, wounds, skin ulcerations— Some tincture can be added to strobile-based preparations for additional benefit. Fine lupulin powder can be dusted on wounds. **Hop pillows**, lovely mixed with lavender, can be placed near the head to promote sleep. For these, take fresh strobiles—or dried cones sprinkled lightly just before use with witch hazel or alcohol—and loosely fill a small, double-stitched casing. Use new plant material each time.
Cautions: Some sources recommend avoiding hops in clinical depression; alternative herbs abound. Avoid with hops allergies or sensitivities [primarily reported by

agricultural or brewery workers]. Some experience dermatitis in contact with plant. Many older herbal texts caution against using during pregnancy; current botanical safety reviews do not state this contraindication. Consult with botanical medicine practitioner if combining with melatonin; may have additive or synergistic effect [Stargrove *et al*].

Kava [*Piper methysticum*]: rhizome and root
  System affinities: Nervous System / Urinary / Musculo-Skeletal
  Tastes/Temperaments: Resinous, warming
  Actions: Relaxing nervine, sedative, locally anesthetic, analgesic, anodyne, antispasmodic, antiseptic, antifungal [*not* against Candida], diuretic. Demonstrated neuroprotective activity.
  Indications: Stress/insomnia especially associated with muscular tension; headache, anxiety, restlessness; fibromyalgia; neuralgia; irritable bladder; urogenital inflammation, infection, pain; interstitial cystitis. Support for withdrawal from benzodiazepine anti-anxiety drugs under professional guidance.
  Formats: Cold infusion [especially water/coconut milk extraction], decoction [slow simmer about 20 minutes], raw or freeze-dried root in capsules, [tincture].

  Kava Coconut Drink: *Combine 1 tablespoon kava root powder with ½ cup water and ½ cup coconut milk. Let sit about 30 minutes, stirring frequently. If desired at this point, add 1 tablespoon non-GMO lecithin granules to aid emulsification; blend briefly by hand or in blender. Strain, if desired, and serve. Kavalactones have low solubility in water alone; addition of fat-rich coconut milk and/or lecithin improves extraction.*

  Cautions: Contraindicated in pregnancy, pre-existing liver disease. May potentiate the effects of other substances that act on the central nervous system, e.g. alcohol, barbiturates and other psychoactive pharmaceuticals. Dopamine antagonism has been reported. Excessive or extended consumption has been reported to cause a scaly, yellowing skin condition that resolves when kava use is discontinued.

Lavender [*Lavendula officinalis*]: flowers
  System affinities: Nervous System / Digestive / Liver-Gallbladder
  Tastes/Temperaments: Aromatic/slightly bitter, neutral, drying
  Actions: Considered restorative; calming, antiseptic, carminative, antispasmodic [gut], mild cholagogue
  Indications: Digestive disturbances related to stress; tension headaches; lifting the spirits/soothing the heart center; nervous exhaustion, insomnia, restlessness, irritability.
  Formats: Tea, tincture, essential oil, hydrosol, infused oil, bath

Lemon Balm [*Melissa officinalis*]: herb
  System affinities: Nervous System / Digestive / Cardiovascular
  Tastes/Temperaments: Aromatic/slightly bitter, neutral, drying
  Actions: Sedative, antispasmodic, anti-inflammatory, antiviral [*Herpes*], carminative, diaphoretic, hypotensive

Indications: Anxiety, headaches, anxiety-induced palpitations; colds/flu, fever, stomach upset; high blood pressure; mild depression; tendency toward stress-induced *herpes simplex* outbreaks. Spasms in digestive tract, non-ulcer dyspepsia related to stress. Tonic to heart and cardiovascular system; mild vasodilation of peripheral blood vessels.
Formats: Tea, infusion, tincture, glycerite, CO_2 extract, essential oil, bath
Caution: Consult with botanical medicine practitioner if combining with melatonin; may have additive or synergistic effect [Stargrove *et al*].

Linden [*Tilia* spp.]: flowers

   System affinities: Nervous System / Cardiovascular
   Tastes/Temperaments: Slightly sweet, cooling, drying
   Actions: Anti-inflammatory, hypotensive, sedative, expectorant, diuretic
   Indications: Mildly high blood pressure. Headaches. Tendency to retain water. Occasional difficulty relaxing enough to fall asleep. Stress and panic, palpitations [*see motherwort*]. Feverish colds and flu. Topically: In lotion for itchy skin.
   Formats: Tea, tincture

Motherwort [*Leonorus cardiaca*]: leaves and flowers

   System affinities: Nervous System / Cardiovascular / Reproductive / Liver
   Tastes/Temperaments: Bitter, neutral, drying
   Actions: Antispasmodic, bitter, emmenagogue, cardiac tonic, sedative, diuretic
   Indications: Racing heart or palpitations, especially associated with fluctuating hormone levels or experience of higher frequency vibrations than one is used to. The chest sensations are themselves causing stress. Physical or emotional tension in anticipation of menstruation or potential sleep challenges.
   Formats: Tea, tincture, nibbling fresh leaf
   Caution: Contraindicated in pregnancy except under guidance of qualified healthcare practitioner.

Mugwort [*Artemesia vulgaris*]: herb

   System affinities: Nervous System / Digestive / Reproductive
   Tastes/Temperaments: Aromatic/bitter, warming
   Actions: Aromatic bitter tonic, carminative, antimicrobial, anthelmintic, mild choleretic, emmenagogue, mild NS tonic
   Indications: Digestive stimulant, especially with flatulence or craving for fats; scanty or delayed menstrual flow, especially associated with tension; uplifting. May increase the vividness of dreamspace.
   Formats: Tea, bath
   Cautions: Contraindicated in pregnancy except under guidance of qualified healthcare practitioner. Handling fresh plant has been known to cause contact dermatitis in susceptible individuals.

Mullein [*Verbascum thapsus*]: flowers, root, leaves

> **System affinities**: NS [flrs & rts] / Lungs [lvs & flrs] / Urinary [rts]
> **Tastes/Temperaments**: Neutral
> **Actions**: Anti-inflammatory, astringent, demulcent, expectorant, diuretic; mild sedative, antispasmodic and anodyne [flrs, root]
> **Indications**: Hard dry cough with soreness or spasms. Earache [infused flower oil]. Facial nerve pain, urinary frequency, bladder spasms [root]
> **Formats**: Tea, glycerite, oil infusion [dry flrs], tincture [fresh flrs, rts], decoction [rts]
> **Caution**: Small leaf hairs may cause local irritation in mouth and throat if inhaled or swallowed—handle plant material gently and filter water-based extracts well.

Oats [*Avena sativa*]: milky seed, straw, groats

> **System affinities**: Nervous System / Nutritive / Skin
> **Tastes/Temperaments**: Sweet, neutral, moistening
> **Actions**: Considered restorative; nutritive, demulcent, vulnerary
> **Indications**: Recovering from stressful physical and/or emotional period, such as substance withdrawal or great life changes. Feels raw and depleted, with desire to be soothed. Both topically and internally to soothe itchy skin and attendant agitation.
> **Formats**: Oats as food, tincture of milky oats, tea, infusion, bath
> **Cautions**: Please note that some folks with gluten sensitivity may be bothered by internal use of this remedy, as oats in commerce are often processed on equipment used to process gluten-containing grains. To minimize the challenge with decoction or tincture: Allow the liquid to settle and then carefully decant the clear liquid off the solid layer that has settled to the bottom. Use this clear liquid.

Passionflower [*Passiflora incarnata*]: herb

> **System affinities**: Nervous System / Musculo-Skeletal
> **Tastes/Temperaments**: Slightly bitter, cooling
> **Actions**: Sedative, hypnotic, antispasmodic, anodyne
> **Indications**: Insomnia, especially with overactive mind and tense muscles—eases one into sleep, no hangover. Nerve pain—neuralgia, sciatica, shingles. Elevated blood pressure. Mild seizures, persistent tremors [work with practitioner].
> **Formats**: Tea, tincture, extract in capsules
> **Caution**: Consult with botanical medicine practitioner if combining with melatonin; may have additive or synergistic effect [Stargrove *et al*].

Peppermint [*Mentha piperita*]: leaves before bloom

> **System affinities**: Nervous System / Digestive / Liver-Gallbladder
> **Tastes/Temperaments**: Sharply pungent/aromatic, initially warming/then cooling.
> **Actions**: Stimulating nervine, carminative, gastrointestinal antispasmodic, anti-tussive, anti-inflammatory, antioxidant, antibacterial, antiviral, anti-emetic, mild astringent, diaphoretic, cholagogue [stimulates release of bile by gall bladder], choleretic [stimulates production of bile by liver], febrifuge. Peppermint possesses

compounds shown to be anti-carcinogenic and chemoprotective. Topically applied, it is antiseptic, analgesic, antipruritic, and stimulates local blood circulation.

Indications: Clears the mind, reduces pain sensitivity, relaxes the muscles. Also used for stomach upset, spastic complaints of the gastrointestinal tract, flatulence, nausea; fever; sore throat; headache, nerve pain; upper respiratory congestion; itchy skin.

Formats: Tea, tincture, infused oil, liniment, poultice, compress [tea or diluted eo], essential oil [topical], gargle, in food.

Topical: The essential oil may be inhaled directly or diffused in steam—or added to creams, lotions, oils or alcohol for topical applications.

Cautions: Peppermint may worsen symptoms of GERD/reflux as it can relax the esophageal sphincter; herbal practitioners offer mixed opinions on its use with hiatal hernia. Avoid peppermint essential oil in cardiac fibrillation, epilepsy. In pregnancy, avoid essential oil internally; essential oil should be used cautiously with children. Traditional Chinese botanical medicine texts caution that because of its dispersing nature, mint should be used with care by those who are deficient or recovering from chronic illness.

Rosemary [*Rosmarinus officinalis*]: leaves and flowers

System affinities: Nervous System / Cardiovascular / Digestive / Liver-Gallbladder

Tastes/Temperaments: Bitter/aromatic, warming, drying

Actions: Stimulating nervine, circulatory stimulant, antibacterial, astringent, carminative, diaphoretic/diuretic, antifungal, anti-inflammatory, muscle relaxing. Rejuvenative. The strongly antioxidant rosmarinic acid possesses neuroprotective, antimutagenic, radioprotective, antibacterial and antiviral properties. A bitter tonic, rosemary stimulates bile production and secretion, sharpens the appetite, strengthens detoxification, relieves flatulence.

Indications: Tones and calms digestion when psychological tension is present — dyspepsia, headache, depression. Feels dull or sluggish after eating, both mentally and physically. May feel a bit blue, a bit hollow in the heart center. Tends toward cold hands and feet and/or varicosities, hemorrhoids, fragile capillaries. Forgetful, slow thinking at times. Broadly antimicrobial: traditionally used to ward off disease. Component of the celebrated Four Thieves formula used to prevent infection in Europe during the virulent plagues of the Middle Ages [+ thyme, sage, garlic, lavender]. Widely applicable plant.

Formats: Tea, tincture, as a garden nibble, whole leaves in foods, essential oil, bath

Topical: Strong water infusion or essential oil diluted in bit of liquid soap added to baths to both relax and revive aching, tense or tired muscles. Hair rinse used to stimulate scalp and hair growth. Tea or tincture diluted into water makes an effective antiseptic and astringent gargle for sore throats, gum issues, canker sores.

Cautions: The essential oil and concentrated extracts are generally contraindicated during pregnancy; limited use as a tea or culinary herb is not.

Also see: The appendix ***The Impact of Stress on Memory: The Plant Allies.***

Sage [*Salvia officinalis*]: leaves and flowers

> **System affinities**: Nervous System / Respiratory / Digestive / Liver-Gallbladder
> **Tastes/Temperaments**: Aromatic/slightly bitter, mildly cooling/mildly warming, drying. The actual temperature of preparation used influences sage's temperament.
> **Actions**: Nervine, mildly astringent, antiseptic to mucosa, anti-inflammatory, antifungal, carminative, cholagogue, diaphoretic/diuretic, uterine stimulant. A key constituent is rosmarinic acid, a powerful antioxidant and preserver of life—anti-bacterial, antiviral [including Herpes, HIV], neuroprotective, radioprotective, more. Calms the heart and spirit.
> **Indications**: Enhancing memory and cognitive function; enhancing immunity; sweats arising from deficiency [cool or cold tea]; mouth and gum health [canker sores, gum infection, thrush]; digestive complaints [indigestion, flatulence, spasms, diarrhea, challenges with fat-rich foods]; muscle aches; headaches, vertigo; irritability, restlessness, tremors. Used to reduce nasal congestion during colds or allergy. Sage tea taken hot is diaphoretic, dilating the peripheral blood vessels, opening the pores, and stimulating sweating—used to manage fevers. It is also used to moderate hot flashes in menopausal women [taken cold] and to bring on irregular or scanty menses.
> **Topical**: Excellent mouthwash to support gum and mouth health; as a gargle, sage is specific for sore throat and laryngitis. Nasal wash for sinus infections.
> **Formats**: Tea, infusion, tincture, honey, in food, footbath, gargle, rinse, poultice, compress, douche, cream, lotion, liniment.
> **Cautions**: Prolonged therapeutic doses, alcohol extract, and essential oil are contraindicated during pregnancy; limited use as a tea or culinary herb are not. Those susceptible to esophageal reflux should use sage with caution.
> **Also see**: The appendix ***The Impact of Stress on Memory: The Plant Allies.***

St. Johnswort [*Hypericum perforatum*]: flowering tops and leaves

> **System affinities**: Nervous System / Musculo-Skeletal / Skin / Urinary
> **Tastes/Temperaments**: Bitter/sour/slightly sweet, neutral, drying
> **Actions**: Anxiolytic, sedative, astringent, anti-inflammatory, antiviral, antibacterial, wound healing. Considered restorative.
> **Indications**: Anxiety. Describes themselves as occasionally sad, blue, vulnerable; tends to manifest herpes lesions when under stress—oral or genital [*Herpes simplex*], shingles [*Herpes zoster*]. Used in combination with other nervines and adaptogens for mild-to-moderate depression—particularly when associated with periods of disruption or transition. As a vulnerary, *Hypericum* is specific for nerve trauma, crushed digits, spinal injuries, radiating nerve pain [such as sciatica, TMJ], post-herpetic pain, or puncture wounds. Irritable bladder, incontinence.
> **Formats**: Tincture, extract in capsules, freeze-dried fresh flower buds in capsules, infused oil of fresh flower buds, homeopathic preparations.
> **Topically**: Topically, speeds healing of wounds, bruises, mild burns, post-herpetic lesions. Specific for deep or puncture wounds.
> **Cautions**: Can potentially amplify photosensitization in susceptible individuals. May influence metabolism and effect of pharmaceutical antidepressants, other psychiatric drugs, and other drug substances if taken concurrently; consult with naturopathic physician or medical herbalist for more information. The reference *Herb, Nutrient,*

and Drug Interactions offers an extensive monograph on *Hypericum* exploring these questions in detail, per drug category.

Skullcap [*Scutellaria laterifolia*]: leaves and flowers

    System affinities: Nervous System / Musculo-Skeletal
    Tastes/Temperaments: Bitter, cooling, drying
    Actions: Considered restorative; sedative, bitter tonic, antispasmodic, astringent
    Indications: Renews nerve tissue. Tension, muscular twitching, mild seizures; exhaustion, depression; premenstrual tension. Widely applicable.
    Formats: Tea, infusion; strongest = tincture [fresh plant]

Valerian [*Valeriana officinalis, V. sitchensis*]: rhizome and root

    System affinities: Nervous System / Musculo-Skeletal / Digestive
    Tastes/Temperaments: Aromatic, slightly warming, drying
    Actions: Sedative, antispasmodic, hypnotic, hypotensive, carminative
    Indications: Pain associated with tension. Migraine. Grief. Insomnia, hysteria, colic, cramping, worming. Topically for cramps and other muscular tensions.
    Formats: Tea, tincture, freeze-dried in capsules
    Cautions: Consult with botanical medicine practitioner if combining with melatonin; may have additive or synergistic effect [Stargrove *et al*]. Use cautiously if combining with barbiturates, benzodiazepines, and other sedative drugs—theoretical possibility of potentiating effect of these drugs. Some individuals have noted a paradoxical, stimulating effect—including agitation and increased heart rate.

Vervain [*Verbena officinalis*]: leaves in flower or bud stage

    System affinities: Nervous System / Hepatic / Digestive
    Tastes/Temperaments: Bitter, cooling, drying
    Actions: Considered restorative; sedative, antispasmodic, hepatic, diaphoretic
    Indications: "Raw" nerves, "on edge". Feels tense and angry a lot of the time. Irritable feelings especially associated with hormonal tides. Sluggish digestion—especially noticed with fatty foods.
    Formats: Tea, tincture
    Caution: Contraindicated during pregnancy.

Botanical Safety Handbook, 2nd edition—Zoë Gardner and Michael McGuffin, editors [Boca Raton, FL: CRC Press, 2013]

Herb, Nutrient, and Drug Interactions: Clinical Implications and Therapeutic Strategies—Mitchell Bebel Stargrove, ND, LAc Jonathan Treasure, MNIMH, Dwight L McKee, MD [St. Louis, MO: Mosby/Elsevier, 2008]

Congenial Combinations of Nervine Plants

1 part Vervain

3 parts Lemon balm

Nice cooling tea to chill the edge off the tightly wound.

Steep 10 minutes.

2 parts Rosemary

1 part Oatstraw

Enlivening, brightening, soothing.

Steep 15-45 minutes.

2 parts Passionflower

1 part Lavender flowers

Sedative, muscle relaxing, uplifting, soothing.

Steep 10-15 minutes.

1 part Oatstraw

1 part Skullcap

Tension-taming tea. Mineral-rich. Lovely before bed, especially when muscle twitching is an issue.

Steep 15-20 minutes.

2 parts Motherwort

1 part Linden flowers

1 part Lavender flowers

Calms and uplifts the heart

Steep 10-15 minutes.

1 part Chamomile flowers

1 part Lavender flowers

Calming and soothing to the stomach and the mind. Comforting.

Steep 10-15 minutes.

1 part Hops strobiles

1 part Chamomile flowers **Or**

1 part Hops strobiles

1 part Lavender flowers

Used to ease anxiety, headache and soothe bodymind in preparation for sleep.

Steep 10-15 minutes.

2 parts Holy Basil/Tulsi

1 part Chamomile flowers

1 part Rose petals

Calming, uplifting. Helps in relaxing into an open heart.

Steep 10-15 minutes.

Networking and Medical Fundraising

In this globally connected age it is easier than ever to develop a network of support for yourself or your loved one. Email lists and social networking can be used to direct your extended community to other, more intimate and controlled settings where privacy can be managed to various degrees. If you are not computer or internet savvy, enlist someone who is to take charge of setting up and administering this project. Whomever you ask will likely be delighted to be able to assist in this way.

There are three basic types of sites available online to benefit those facing serious illness: health-status blogs, medical fundraising sites, and helper coordination calendars. More and more, the distinct types are merging features to provide extensive support on a single site.

Well-designed **Health status blogs**, such as **CaringBridge** [www.caringbridge.org] and **MyLifeLine** [www.mylifeline.org], allow one to post updates at any and all hours of the day or night. They are easy to use and personalize. Photos may be uploaded, and viewers have the opportunity to leave comments of their own.

CarePages [www.carepages.com] is another such blog, which also offers a full online library of helping tips relevant for various disease conditions.

These types of sites are a wonderful way to expend a minimum amount of energy to stay in touch with those you care about and with those who wish to follow your journey. In turn, receiving messages of love and support on a regular basis can become a treasured healing balm.

Sites such as CaringBridge allow one to choose variable levels of access—from just one's closest, individually invited family and friends to larger spheres that must first login extending all the way to completely open public access. Having control over who may access your personal story may feel particularly comforting to many.

These sites offer easy-to-use templates so that one can create a personal page within the site's "gated" structure with relative ease. Many of these sites are free of charge and rely on donations from participants or advertising to keep them going.

Medical fundraising sites are focused on helping raise money to pay for medical treatment and other health-related expenses. They each have unique set-ups regarding fees, and one should read their terms carefully before signing on. They provide secure methods for friends and family to offer support through donations. While the recipient learns the identity of each donor, supporters may choose to give as "Anonymous" on the public layer of the site.

These sites also allow for status updates to be posted and for the fundraising campaign to be shared using social media. Examples of medical fundraising sites include: **GoFundMe**

[gofundme.com], **YouCaring** [youcaring.com], **GiveForward** [giveforward.com], and the like.

A third type of site is also appearing, helping to create another web of physical support. For example, the sites **Take Them a Meal** [www.takethemameal.com] and **MealTrain** [www.mealtrain.com] allow for the orchestration of community meal delivery to households in need of such support. **CareCalender** [www.carecalender.org] is a planning site used to coordinate meal delivery, errands, and other volunteer helpers of all sorts.

This is just a short list of some sites that were available at the time of this writing. Their numbers are increasing every day. These sorts of projects make excellent use of the available technology to help us make our needs known with relative ease. They help us stay connected to our support networks when we can feel most isolated…and allow our friends to extend lovingkindness and helpfulness in effective, meaningful ways.

Helping a Person Approach Death

Since I first began writing this manual, a wealth of truly helpful books have been written to assist in this process and in addressing the decisions that may need to be made around the physical requirements of death. The **Recommended Reading** chapter highlights some gems. This section is offered as a basic overview to gently prompt attention to these areas while the mind can focus on such things. In this way, sometimes-difficult conversations may be initiated—and loving collaboration promoted as is appropriate and desired in each given circumstance.

This sort of review is important whether or not death is an imminent, predictable outcome of the current circumstances. Whenever we find ourselves on seriously shifting ground, it bears fruit to tend to such matters. Energy may be liberated from the bodymind that has been bound up in the knowledge that such details have not yet been arranged or that particular relationships remain without desired resolution.

- **Make closure, settle accounts, guide the spiral around**:

  - Material/financial details [legal instruments: will, living will, durable power of attorney, etc.]. See the **Resources** chapter regarding models for living wills and financial testaments.

  - Letters, calls, visits with relatives and friends. Query: Is there any energy unresolved, unaddressed between myself and another? Where do I yet feel static or lack of closure? How can I address it—through physical contact, through writing, through prayer or meditative practices?

  - Finding peace in the culmination of one's work in the world. Does something still need to be completed, transmitted or disseminated? Who can best facilitate that?

- **Grieve together**. Create a safe space for even the most naked grief and fear.

- **Arrange for hospice support**, if that has not already been part of the picture.

- **Review in detail wishes** about life-support efforts, distribution of resources and possessions, names/contact info of those to be notified of one's passing, and so on.

- **Plan for death and subsequent handling of the body** [issues such as anointing, cremation, burial, religious/spiritual/legal considerations, disposition of ashes, etc.]. How long shall body remain unbothered before being removed from deathbed? Is a viewing desired? If so, shall it be public or private?

- **Plan a post-death gathering** for friends and family to grieve, express, honor, celebrate, and release. Such a coming together can be deeply healing for all involved. The planning itself can help bring peace to the dying person.

- **Arrange spiritual counsel** or support or benediction as requested. In addition to the usual religion-affiliated clergy, non-denominational end of life chaplains may also be available in your community.

- **Weave a circle of friends and family**—either directly or through helpers—who, together, can hold space for the loved one's leave-taking. This circle may include some who actually appear on-site and others who do their focus from a distance. Enlist those who can truly allow the dying to unfold as it will, can hold the departing being in the light of love, can release their own attachments to their persisting in physical form, and can unreservedly bless them on their way.

- At some point in this journey your companion may seem unresponsive or untouched by their surroundings. As the elements of the bodymind transform through the dying process, a being may become ever more sensitive to their environment—their perception and awareness may be heightened on another level. Your steady calm and sense of groundedness will **create a sacred space, a container of stability** in which their inner process—as well as your own—may unfold: releasing and surrendering this unique being into the infinite mystery that cradles us all.

May we each know
deep blessing on the journey

Recommended Reading

The distinction drawn between these categories of recommended readings is by necessity somewhat arbitrary. For the sake of creating some ease in accessing the material they offer, they have been separated into two main sections—those which focus more on mindfulness in general and caregiving in particular, and those which discuss and detail specific therapeutic issues and approaches.

There are many more wonderful books out there and more being written everyday. The ones here represent some precious jewels, from this writer's point of view.

Caregiving & Cultivating Compassion

All Sickness is Homesickness—Dianne M. Connelly, LAc [Columbia, MD: Centre for Traditional Acupuncture, 1986]. Written by a practitioner and teacher of Traditional Chinese Medicine; reading this elegant book is a healing process in itself. It helps the engaged reader reframe notions about health, illness, and concepts around helping another to heal. I have all my serious students read this book.

Being with Dying: Cultivating Compassion and Fearlessness in the Presence of Death—Joan Halifax, PhD [Boston: Shambhala Publications, 2008]. Joan Halifax is a Zen priest and anthropologist with a background in shamanic healing. For 40-plus years she has worked with dying people and since 1994 has been training chaplains and health-care professionals in the contemplative care of the dying through Upaya Zen Center, which she founded. This book is a precious distillation of her teachings and offers skillful, practical guidance through the terrain of pain, grief, loss, acceptance, dying... Could be of great benefit to both caregivers and to those for whom they care.

Boundless Healing: Meditation Exercises to Enlighten the Mind and Heal the Body—Tulku Thondup [Boston: Shambhala Publications, 2000]. "There is a dimension of human experience where all is well, where perfection reigns, where all is peace. This book teaches us how to contact this awareness and allow it to surface in our lives."—Larry Dossey, MD. Says it so beautifully.

Caring for the Sick at Home—Tineke van Bentheim, *et al* [Edinburgh: Floris Books, 1987; Hudson, NY: Anthroposophic Press, 1987]. An empowering exploration rich with specific suggestions based on an Anthroposophical worldview.

Circles of Care: How to Set up Quality Home Care for Our Elders—Ann Cason [Boston: Shambhala Publications, 2001]. Cason shares from her more than 20 years of experience in caring for the elderly. She helps cultivate empathy in the reader through stories, examples, and exercises. Discusses nutrition, finances, environment, conflict, caregiver burnout, moods and confusion.

Death: The Final Stage of Growth—Elisabeth Kubler-Ross, MD [Englewood Cliffs, NJ: Prentice-Hall, 1975]. This key pioneer helped break the silence around dying in our western culture with her insights and observations. Everything Kubler-Ross has written is grist for the mill.

Dying to be Me: My Journey from Cancer, to Near Death, to True Healing—Anita Moorjani [Carlsbad, CA: Hay House, 2012]. I read this book while recovering from my own experience with cancer and it resonated in ways that are challenging to describe in words. A beautiful, remarkable story of awakening and healing—deeply personal yet universally instructive.

The Earth House—Jeanne DuPrau [New York: Fawcett Columbine, 1992]. The true story of two women life-partners facing the illness and dying of one while simultaneously building a simple mountain home near their Zen monastery—in the process, rethinking, deconstructing, and rebuilding their lives on many levels.

Embrace, Release, Heal: An Empowering Guide to Talking About, Thinking About, and Treating Cancer—Leigh Fortson [Boulder, CO: Sounds True, 2011] After her third cancer diagnosis in three years, the author was given few options and offered little hope for healing by her medical doctors. She was introduced to the transforming idea that our thoughts and emotions influence every cell. This book shares her inspiring story and the insights gleaned from her research.

Emmanuel's Book: A Manual for Living Comfortably in the Cosmos and ***Emmanuel's Book II: The Choice for Love***—Compiled by Pat Rodegast and Judith Stanton [New York: Bantam Books, 1987; 1989]. Perennial wisdom channeled in an extremely compassionate voice. Very accessible question-and-answer format. These books offer a wise, gentle voice counseling love and trust in the presence of fear.

Final Gifts: Understanding the Special Awareness, Needs, and Communications of the Dying—Maggie Callanan and Patricia Kelley [New York: Bantam Books, 1997]. A thoroughly useful book to read and to share with friends and family.

Final Victory: Taking Charge of the Last Stages of Life; Facing Death on Your Own Terms—Thomas A. Preston, MD [Roseville, CA: Forum, 2000]. Explores the dying process from within the modern medical paradigm, offering insight into how to negotiate the information and choices that it presents from a personal place of power.

Finding Inner Courage—Mark Nepo [San Francisco: Conari Press, 2007]. Mark Nepo is a cancer survivor and poet. This book, as well as his daybook ***The Book of Awakening: Having the Life You Want by Being Present to the Life You Have*** [Conari Press, 2000] are each wonderful companions on the way through what life presents. Nepo offers fresh perspective on whatever topic he explores and helps the reader uncover their own inner wisdom and recognition of beauty in each day.

Grist for the Mill—Ram Dass, with Stephen Levine [New York: Bantam Books, 1976]. All of Ram Dass' teachings are sweet gifts of a humble, wise companion on the path of living. In this early work, see particularly the chapter on *"Dying: An Opportunity for Awakening."*

Healing into Life and Death—Stephen Levine [New York: Doubleday, 1987]. Working with pain and grief, being present for one's life, cultivation of merciful awareness. One of the classic guides to living [and dying] mindfully.

A Healing Path: A Soul Approach to Illness—Marc Ian Barasch [New York: Penguin/ Arkana, 1993]. Helps map this sometimes seemingly impenetrable terrain. Based on his own experience and the stories of many others.

Hidden Spring: A Buddhist Woman Confronts Cancer—Sandy Boucher [Boston: Wisdom Publications, 2000]. Boucher's story of being diagnosed in 1995 with Stage III colon cancer and her deep encounter with the disease. She shares how meditation techniques and application of Buddhist principles prepared her to meet the mental and spiritual challenges of her illness.

How to Heal: A Guide for Caregivers—Jeff Kane, MD [New York: Helios Press, 2003]. Kane brings 26 years of practice to this work, offering compassion and wisdom to assist caregivers in becoming unconditionally present to the sick person rather than relating to the disease. Beautiful.

In the Light of Death: Spiritual Insight to Help You Live with Death and Bereavement—Timothy Freke [Hauppauge, NY: Barron's Educational Series, 2002]. Poetry, wisdom, beauty, stimulation, comfort.

The Journey through Cancer: Healing and Transforming the Whole Person—Jeremy Geffen, MD [New York: Three Rivers Press, 2006, revised edition]. Written by a board-certified medical oncologist who has been a pioneer of integrative oncology. Helps to explain conventional diagnoses and treatment options, relevant to a variety of cancer types—as well as outlining some of the common approaches of complementary medicine. Also, explores the psychological and spiritual terrain a person [and their family] may encounter subsequent to diagnosis.

Kitchen Table Wisdom: Stories that Heal—Rachel Naomi Remen, MD [New York: Riverhead Books, 2006]. This, and the author's ***My Grandfather's Blessing*** [2000] are treasures. Remen, a founder of Commonweal cancer retreat center, is herself a wounded healer. She shares stories from her personal journey as well as those of her patients in this wonderful offering. These narrative jewels sparkle with authenticity, compassion, insight, hope, inspiration, wisdom and power. You will laugh and you will cry…and be reminded that we are not alone on this life journey.

Leaning into Sharp Points: Practical Guidance and Nurturing Support for Caregivers—Stan Goldberg PhD [Novato, CA: New World Library, 2012] A private therapist, clinical researcher, and former university professor, Goldberg has been a hospice volunteer and caregiver for many years. Valuable guidance and compassionate advice on what to expect and how to navigate the challenges.

Lessons from the Dying—Rodney Smith [Boston: Wisdom Publications, 1998]. Smith is a former director of Hospice of Seattle and a noted teacher of meditation. His offering here is a precious jewel, luminous with compassion, insight and wisdom.

Looking After: A Son's Memoir—John Daniel [Washington, DC: Counterpoint, 1996]. Daniel's poignant memoir of caring for a mother with Alzheimer's Disease is perhaps, ultimately, Everyone's story.

The Lotus in the Fire: The Healing Power of Zen—Jim Bedard [Boston: Shambhala Publications, 1999]. Bedard, a martial artist and Zen student, was diagnosed with acute myeloid leukemia and given 10 days to live. He shares his journey into impermanence to help others find the strength and cultivate the tools to venture there skillfully themselves.

Luminous Emptiness: Understanding the Tibetan Book of the Dead—Francesca Fremantle [Boston: Shambhala Publications, 2001]. The writer is a Buddhist teacher and practitioner, a student of both Sanskrit and Tibetan. With Chogyam Trungpa, Fremantle translated the *Tibetan Book of the Dead*. This amazing work is more than a commentary on that text—it shines as a penetrating, lucid teaching on awakening.

Making Friends with Death: A Buddhist Guide to Encountering Mortality—Judith L. Lief [Boston: Shambhala Publications, 2001]. Tibetan Buddhist teacher Lief shows that as we open to a mindful relationship with death, our capacity to appreciate life, change, and others deepens. Includes practices for cultivating kindness and offers caregiver guidelines for grounding actions in awareness and compassion.

Medicine and Compassion: A Tibetan Lama's Guidance for Caregivers—Chokyi Nyima Rinpoche and David R. Shlim [Somerville, MA: Wisdom Publications, 2004]. Helpful material for all caregivers, but should be required reading for professional healthcare workers to improve the dynamics of care.

Mind Over Medicine: Scientific Proof that You Can Heal Yourself—Lissa Rankin, MD [Carlsbad, CA: Hay House, 2013]. Rankin owes—and acknowledges—a great debt to the pioneer physicians and teachers who have paved the way for this book through their own published work. She brings a very contemporary voice to her story of awakening from her medical training to the realizations and research she shares about self-healing.

Never Turn Away: The Buddhist Path Beyond Hope and Fear—Rigdzin Shikpo [Boston: Wisdom Publications, 2007]. This simple advice—*Never turn away*—is powerful instruction for meeting whatever we encounter with clarity, courage, and openheartedness. This is a beautiful book—clear, practical, and inspiring.

Not the Last Goodbye: On Life, Death, Healing and Cancer—David Servan-Schrieber MD, PhD [New York: Viking, 2011] Written as the author, a physician/professor and 19-year survivor of brain cancer, deals with disease recurrence and, ultimately, with the conscious dying process. This is an intimate meditation on the topics stated in the subtitle, completed just days before he passed.

"On Being a Support Person"—Ken Wilbur [*The Journal of Transpersonal Psychology,* 1988, Vol.20, No.2.] Accessible online.

The Pagan Book of Living and Dying: Practical Rituals, Prayers, Blessings and Meditations on Crossing Over—Starhawk [New York: HarperBooks, 1997]. All of the above, plus discussion of caregiving, grieving, distributing possessions, planning memorials, providing final instructions for one's own death. Frames death as a doorway into another stage in the cycle of life.

Peace, Love and Healing: Bodymind Communication and the Path to Self-Healing— Bernie S. Siegel, MD [New York: Harper & Row, 1989]. A warm, inspiring book by this noted surgeon, encouraging the reader to bring all of themselves to their healing path—and to fully inhabit their inner capacity to influence physiological behavior. Filled with clinical stories and medical insight, this is a book you will want to hand to medical practitioners and insist they read! His work, bridging medicine with the richness of inner healing practices, has been a blessing to many.

Return to Wholeness: Embracing Body, Mind and Spirit in the Face of Cancer—David Simon, MD [New York: John Wiley & Sons, 1999] If you are facing cancer or other life-changing illness, read this book. It is elegant, clear, compassionate and a treasury of powerful support and guidance. Simon was a co-founder and the Medical Director of the Chopra Center for Well Being who beautifully wove together the healing wisdom of both East and West.

Sacred Passage: How to Provide Fearless, Compassionate Care for the Dying— Margaret Coberly, RN [Boston: Shambhala Publications, 2002]. Chronicles the path of this psychologist and hospice nurse through her own denial of death to her immersion into this "trajectory." She offers a wonderful integration of her own Tibetan Buddhist studies with practical applications of skillful means at the bedside of the dying.

Still Here: Embracing Aging, Changing, and Dying—Ram Dass [New York: Riverhead Books, 2000]. Written by Ram Dass both before and after a stroke that would radically change his life. This is a meditation turned master class on being fully present with our lives, through all its twists and turns. Ram Dass brings his usual wit to the warm wisdom he offers for facing change with grace.

The 36-Hour Day: A Family Guide to Caring for Persons with Alzheimer's Disease, Related Dementing Illnesses, and Memory Loss Later in Life—Nancy L. Mace and Peter V. Rabins, MD [Baltimore: The Johns Hopkins University Press, fifth edition, 2011]. A remarkably comprehensive survey of the questions and challenges that arise in this situation. This is essential reading for those dealing with this circumstance.

The Ostomy Book: Living Comfortably with Colostomies, Ileostomies, and Urostomies 3rd edition—Barbara Dorr Mullen, Kerry Anne McGinn RN, ARNP [Boulder, CO: Bull Publishing, 2008]

The Tibetan Book of Living and Dying—Sogyal Rinpoche [San Francisco: Harper SanFrancisco, 1992]. Compassionate wisdom and detailed practices. The practices that this honored teacher describes for various levels of proficiency are quite remarkable in their benefits.

An Unintended Journey: A Caregiver's Guide to Dementia—Janet Yagoda Shagam [Amherst, NY: Prometheus Books, 2013]. A well-informed companion on the path. This is an overview of the many issues facing family members and caregivers when mind starts to change for a loved one—assessing change, diagnosis, legal matters, caregiving, finding support, money and food issues, family dynamics, medication, assisted living, and much more.

When Life Becomes Precious: A Guide for Loved Ones and Friends of Cancer Patients—Elise NeeDell Babcock [New York: Bantam Books, 1997]. Guidance to facilitate meaningful, intimate communication and sharing.

When Things Fall Apart: Heart Advice for Difficult Times—Pema Chodron [Boston: Shambhala Publications, 1997]. What it says. An enduring offering from this venerated, accessible, compassionate teacher.

When You're Falling, Dive: Lessons in the Art of Living—Mark Matousek [New York: Bloomsbury USA, 2008]. "How does a person survive his own life, the ceaseless surprises, uncertainties, struggles, reroutings in strange, inconvenient directions?" Matousek poses this question early in this book and then proceeds to explore it. Each chapter tells a story that can stand on its own or be read in sequence. He weaves together the wisdom of the ancients with the insights of those whose stories he tells.

Who Dies? An Investigation of Conscious Living and Conscious Dying—Stephen Levine [New York: Doubleday, 1982]. A wonderful offering from Stephen Levine exploring the gifts that awareness of death has on our living ways. Based on many years of hospice work and meditation practice.

A Year to Live: How to Live this Year as If It Were Your Last—Stephen Levine [New York: Belltower, 1997]. Another masterful guide from the author. It takes the reader through the question stated in the title with great compassion and wisdom. There is also an audio CD version of this offering.

The Zen of Living and Dying: A Practical and Spiritual Guide—Philip Kapleau [Boston: Shambhala Publications, 1998]. This wonderful book by a renowned Zen teacher gently guides the reader through the many decisions, questions, and seeming dilemmas facing both the person dying and those who love and care for them during such transition.

Natural Therapeutics and Wellness Support

Adaptogens: Herbs for Strength, Stamina, and Stress Relief—David Winston and Steven Maimes [Rochester, VT: Healing Arts Press, 2007]. David was one of my core teachers in the 1980s and he is widely honored as one of the premier herbalists of our time. David's teachings have influenced my own work immeasurably through the years. *Adaptogens* is an essential read and an accessible resource on the topic. Very highly recommended.

Adaptogens in Medical Herbalism: Elite Herbs and Natural Compounds for Mastering Stress, Aging, and Chronic Disease—Donald R. Yance, Jr., CN, RH(AGH) [Rochester, VT: Healing Arts Press, 2013]. Donnie Yance is an herbalist's herbalist and his research and teaching regarding cancer and chronic disease process is very highly regarded. This newly released and long-awaited book provides an overview of his clinical approach as well as key details of primary and secondary adaptogenic plants and their clinical applications.

Anticancer: A New Way of Life—David Servan-Schreiber, MD, PhD [New York: Viking, updated edition, 2009]. When the author was diagnosed with brain cancer, his life and perspective changed completely. This is his honest and inspiring story, interwoven with a compelling, accessible compendium of well-researched, potentially life-saving recommendations. One of those rare gems that weaves together spiritual journey with practical science—mind/body tools, clinical examples, a wealth of detailed, evidence-based material. This is an amazing, life-affirming book that should be read by all.

The Body Ecology Diet—Donna Gates with Linda Schatz [Juno Beach, FL: Healthful Communications, 1996]. A thorough and immediately useful guide for addressing chronic or recurrent fungal/yeast/*Candida albicans* overgrowth—or insight for changing the terrain holistically to prevent an acute occurrence from becoming a chronic condition. This is a compassionate and practical book that helps the reader apply the principles in manageable stages of recovery. Highly recommended.

The Book of Jook: Chinese Medical Porridges—Bob Flaws [Boulder, Co: Blue Poppy Press, 1995]. Written by a respected practitioner and teacher of Traditional Chinese Medicine, this book contains hundreds of herbal porridge recipes for both health promotion and remediation purposes.

Breast Cancer: What You Should Know (But May Not Be Told) About Prevention, Diagnosis, and Treatment—Steve Austin, ND and Cathy Hitchcock [Rocklin, CA: Prima Publishing, 1994]. The emotional journey of this married holistic-oriented couple and the research they conducted as Cathy's diagnosis and choices presented themselves. Though the research could be updated, it remains a friendly and knowledgeable guide during what is often a stressful search for solid ground.

Cancer Salves: A Botanical Approach to Treatment—Ingrid Naiman [Berkeley, CA: North Atlantic Books, 1999]. Written by an herbalist dedicated to this issue, the book provides an extensive survey of the historical and contemporary application of topical plant-based salves to address cancerous growths, as well as formulations for internal use. There is nothing else like this detailed book currently available.

Cannabis and Cancer: Vol. 1, Cannabis in Context—Jonathan Treasure MNIMH, RH (AHG) [OncoHerb Press, 2016]. This ebook by a highly-esteemed herbal practitioner and researcher sets the overall use of botanical medicines in cancer scenarios in context, as well as addressing essential questions of *Cannabis* efficacy and formats per se. Very highly recommended.

Cell-Level Healing: The Bridge from Soul to Cell—Joyce Whiteley Hawkes, PhD [New York: Atria Books, 2006]. A biophysicist and practitioner of traditional Eastern healing methods, Joyce Hawkes offers precious insight into how our thoughts and feelings impact the workings of our cells. In a poetic and visually inspiring work, she provides simple yet profound exercises for accessing our innate healing capacity. This might be one of the first books recommended upon receiving a troubling diagnosis.

The Definitive Guide to Cancer: An Integrative Approach to Prevention, Treatment, and Healing—Lise Alschuler ND and Karolyn Gazella [Berkeley, CA: Celestial Arts, 2010, 3rd edition]. A wonderful and very accessible survey of holistic cancer treatment. Offers a great foundation to help readers consider botanical and nutritional support complementary to allopathic oncology therapies. Answers scores of questions that arise, including interaction considerations.

Dr. Katz's Guide to Prostate Health: From Conventional to Holistic Therapies—Aaron E Katz, MD. [Topanga, CA: Freedom Press, 2006]. A board-certified urologist, Katz is the director of the Center for Holistic Urology, Columbia University. This overview discusses prevention of disease, medication, surgery, radiation, other allopathic treatments, as well as nutritional, hormonal and other therapies.

Encyclopedia of Nutritional Supplements—Michael Murray, ND [Rocklin, CA: Prima Publishing, 1996]. Written by a respected naturopathic physician/researcher/writer, this offers a useful overview of vitamins, minerals, essential fatty acids, accessory nutrients. Includes a reference guide to specific health conditions.

Energy Medicine—Donna Eden with David Feinstein [New York: Jeremy P Tarcher/ Putnam, 1998]. Simple, effective techniques for aligning the energy body, reducing pain, promoting vitality, cultivating healthy boundaries. Clearly illustrated, explained.

Exercise Without Movement—as taught by Swami Rama. [Honesdale, PA: Himalayan International Institute of Yoga Science and Philosophy, 1984]. A precious book of simple exercises that utilize the power of mind and breath to relax and vitalize the body without vigorous movement.

Fighting Cancer: A Nontoxic Approach to Treatment—Robert Gorter, MD, PhD and Erik Peper, PhD [Berkeley, CA: North Atlantic Books, 2011]. Must reading for anyone dealing with cancer or any immune-related illness. Accessible, empowering and holistic in approach, this wonderful book helps readers to understand and benefit from the mind/body connection. Steeped in the authors' self-experience, extensive research, and decades of clinical practice. It offers detailed strategies for making treatment decisions, relieving stress, minimizing toxic exposures, bolstering immunity, and living well with a challenging diagnosis.

Flax Oil as a True Aid Against Arthritis, Heart Infarction, Cancer and Other Diseases—Dr. Johanna Budwig [Vancouver, BC: Apple Publishing Company Ltd., 1994]. European biochemist and authority on fats and healing, Dr. Budwig offers a stimulating discussion on flax oil, the role of dietary fats in health and disease, the effects of solar energy in our human biological systems, and more.

Flower Essence Repertory: A Comprehensive Guide to North American and English Flower Essences for Emotional and Spiritual Well-Being—Patricia Kaminski and Richard Katz [Nevada City, CA: The Flower Essence Society, Earth-Spirit, Inc., 1994]. A very extensive and user-friendly guide to the healing energies of flowers. The flower essence profiles included were inspired by their teachings as well as my own experience. Find them at **www.flowersociety.org** and **www.fesflowers.com**.

The Fungal Pharmacy: The Complete Guide to Medicinal Mushrooms and Lichens of North America—Robert Rogers, RH (AHG) [Berkeley, CA: North Atlantic Books, 2011]. This is truly a wonderful contribution to the field of clinical use of medicinal fungi. Beautifully illustrated, with discussions of traditional and contemporary medicinal uses, preparations, chemical constituents, folklore, and more.

Healing Lyme Disease Naturally: History, Analysis and Treatments—Wolf D Storl. [Berkeley, CA: North Atlantic Books, 2010]. Medical anthropologist and herbalist, Storl uses his personal account of Lyme disease as the springboard for this fascinating work—a blend of science, history, and healing approaches from various cultures.

The Healing Power of Sound: Recovery from Life-Threatening Illness Using Sound, Voice, and Music—Mitchell L. Gaynor, MD [Boston: Shambala Publications, 1999]. This is a foundational, inspirational text on restoring harmony through sound healing, with many examples from Dr. Gaynor's oncology practice. Immediately usable ideas on working with the voice, music, and Tibetan singing bowls. Highly recommended for both caregivers and people dealing with unwellness.

Healing Words: The Power of Prayer and the Practice of Medicine—Larry Dossey, MD [San Francisco: Harper, 1993]. Dossey has been a pioneer in mind/body medicine. Here he shares clinical evidence linking prayer, healing and medicine. Also: ***Space, Time & Medicine*** and ***The Extraordinary Healing Power of Ordinary Things.***

The Hepatitis C Handbook—Matthew Dolan [Berkeley, CA: North Atlantic Books, 1999]. A germinal and very valuable contribution to the literature on this topic.

Herbal Antibiotics: Natural Alternatives for Treating Drug-Resistant Bacteria, 2nd edition—Stephen Harrod Buhner [North Adams, MA: Storey Publishing, 2012]. An essential overview of the difficult circumstances we face with resistant organisms and solid herbal approaches to addressing them. Buhner is the author of many fine books, including *Healing Lyme: Natural Healing of Lyme Borreliosis and Its Coinfections* [2005] and *Healing Lyme Disease Coinfections: Complementary and Holistic Treatments for Bartonella and Mycoplasma* [2013].

Herbal Medicine, Healing and Cancer—Donald R. Yance, Jr., CN, RH(AGH) [Chicago: Keats Publishing, 1999]. Excellent information on supporting the vital force as well as confounding the processes of disease. Very accessible; includes recipes. Those facing Hepatitis C and other such serious challenges will also find much here.

Herbs Against Cancer: History and Controversy—Ralph W. Moss, PhD [Brooklyn, NY: Equinox Press, 1998]. A very readable overview of botanical therapies, past and present, that continue to inspire controversy as well as adamant adherents around the world. Includes a resource list for obtaining further information or actual materials.

Herbs for Hepatitis C and the Liver—Stephen Harrod Buhner [Pownal, VT: Storey Books, 2000]. A much-needed review of natural therapies as they address serious liver disease, benefit liver function and enhance vital force in general. Includes preferred modes of preparation, dosages, contraindications, recipes, and more. The back-matter is extensive and useful as well.

The Hidden Meaning of Illness: Disease as a Symbol and a Metaphor—Bob Trowbridge, M.Div [Virginia Beach, VA: A.R.E. Press, 1996]. Trowbridge brings a gentle ministerial voice to this non-judgmental work. He offers ways of working with illness, dreams, and beliefs that offer possibilities for insight and transformation.

How to Prevent and Treat Cancer with Natural Medicine—Michael Murray, ND *et al* [New York: Riverhead Books, 2002]. A very reader-friendly resource for both looking at the multiple factors involved in cancer manifestation and addressing prevention and treatment strategies using natural substances. Discusses nutritional, herbal and emotional preparation for chemotherapy, radiation and surgery, plus natural means for addressing side-effects.

Imagery in Healing: Shamanism and Modern Medicine—Jeanne Achterberg [Boston: Shambhala/New Science Library, 1985]. One of the influential modern surveys of using the ancient practice of imagery as a contemporary healing tool. Her later book *Rituals of Healing: Using Imagery for Health and Wellness* [1994, with Barbara Dossey] is more accessible for immediate application.

Integrating Conventional and Chinese Medicine in Cancer Care: A Clinical Guide— Tai Lahans, LAc [Philadelphia, PA: Churchill Livingstone/Elsevier, 2007]. This well-regarded textbook is primarily intended for practitioners of Chinese medicine, but will prove an invaluable resource to western-trained herbalists, naturopathic physicians, and as reliable research material for any well-studied reader.

Integrative Oncology—Donald Abrams, MD and Andrew Weil, MD, eds. [New York: Oxford University Press, 2009]. Intended for both a professional and lay audience, this book features extensively referenced chapters authored by a panel of international experts on issues in integrative oncology: Nutrition, meditation, prayer, exercise and bodywork, energy medicine including acupuncture, use of antioxidants during treatment, medicinal mushroom and botanical therapies, the role of marijuana, and much more. Four chapters review well-established systems of care: Ayurveda, Traditional Chinese Medicine, Homeopathy, and Anthroposophic medicine.

The Journey through Cancer: Healing and Transforming the Whole Person—Jeremy Geffen MD [New York: Three Rivers Press, 2006, revised edition] Written by a board-certified medical oncologist who has been a pioneer of integrative oncology. Helps to explain conventional diagnoses and treatment options, relevant to a variety of cancer types—as well as outlining some of the common approaches of complementary medicine. Also, explores the psychological and spiritual terrain a person [and their family] may encounter subsequent to diagnosis.

Living Well with Pain and Illness: The Mindful Way to Free Yourself from Suffering—Vidyamala Burch [Boulder, CO: Sounds True, 2010]. Burch drew on the work of Stephen Levine and other meditation teachers to learn to live with her own traumatic pain experience. She went on to develop a mindfulness-based pain management approach called Breathworks. This book is a rich and intimate guide.

Lupus: Alternative Therapies That Work—Sharon Moore [Rochester, VT: Healing Arts Press, 2000]. Moore lived with lupus for five years before her condition was finally diagnosed. Offered pharmaceuticals to manage or suppress symptoms, she sought alternative treatments and approaches. This book is the result of that research.

Medicinal Mushrooms: An Exploration of Tradition, Healing, & Culture—Christopher Hobbs [Santa Cruz, CA: Botanica Press, second edition, 1995]. One of the most complete overviews of medicinal mushrooms currently available to the lay reader. Hobbs, a highly respected herbalist and holistic researcher/practitioner, details the health-promoting benefits of more than 100 species of edible fungi.

Meditation as Medicine: Activate the Power of Your Natural Healing Force—Dharma Singh Khalsa, MD and Cameron Stauth. [New York: Pocket Books/Simon & Schuster, 2001]. Very clear, engaging explanation of ancient techniques using breath, mantra, meditation and body postures to promote balance, calm, and renewal.

MycoMedicinals: An Informational Treatise on Mushrooms—Paul Stamets, assisted by C. Dusty Wu Yao [Olympia, WA: MycoMedia Productions, third edition, 2002]. An essential reference regarding the efficacy and potential of medicinal mushroom therapy in human health maintenance and renewal, by a world-renowned mycologist.

Natural Compounds in Cancer Therapy—John Boik [Princeton, MN: Oregon Medical Press, 2001]. A pioneering work, discussing the scientific basis for natural therapies. Very detailed and thoroughly annotated, both this and Yance's book will make discussing alternative protocols much easier with an allopathic practitioner.

Perfect Health: The Complete Mind/Body Guide—Deepak Chopra, MD [New York: Three Rivers Press, 1991, 2000 revised]. One of the pioneer guides to harnessing the power of the mind in healing: how to apply ancient Ayurvedic techniques to interface with the body at the quantum level to effect balance and change. See also ***Quantum Healing: Exploring the Frontiers of Mind/Body Medicine*** [1989].

The Path of Practice: A Woman's Book of Healing with Food, Breath, and Sound—Bri. Maya Tiwari [New York: Ballantine, 2000]. An inspiring account of healing. Tiwari was diagnosed with ovarian cancer at age 23 and given two months to live. She refused to accept this prognosis and instead radically changed her life, turning to ancient holistic methods for restoring health. A user-friendly handbook filled with nutritional guidance, recipes, meditations, breathwork, and more.

Prepare for Surgery, Heal Faster: A Guide of Mind-Body Techniques—Peggy Huddleston [Cambridge, MA: Angel River Press, 1996]. Discusses relaxation techniques, visualization, support groups, healing statements, vitamins to speed healing, preparing children for surgery, lessening the side effects of treatments.

Radical Healing: Integrating the World's Great Therapeutic Traditions to Create a New Transformative Medicine—Rudolph Ballentine MD [New York: Harmony Books, 1999]. A truly remarkable and accessible synthesis of the wisdom of major healing traditions, this book offers a dynamic mind/body approach to optimal whole being wellness. Ballentine, author of the classic ***Diet and Nutrition: A Holistic Approach*** [1978], is a passionate and skillful teacher and practitioner.

Seaweed: Nature's Secret to Balancing Your Metabolism, Fighting Disease, and Revitalizing Body & Soul—Valerie Gennari Cooksley, RN. [New York: Steward, Tabori, and Chang, 2007]. This book is a gem. Cooksley is a former radiation oncology nurse who has made a study of the health-supporting benefits of sea vegetables. The book is filled with solid information and delicious recipes.

Spontaneous Healing: How to Discover and Embrace Your Body's Natural Ability to Maintain and Heal Itself—Andrew Weil, MD [New York: Ballantine, 1995]. An important and highly readable contribution to the subject by one of the pioneer bridge builders between allopathic and holistic medicine.

Staying Well with Guided Imagery—Belleruth Naparstek [New York: Warner Books, 1994] A user-friendly primer, explaining the basics of guided visualization and how to generate images in the mind to influence emotional and physical healing. Naparstek has also created an extensive collection of **recorded guided meditations** for a wide variety of health circumstances [www.healthjourneys.com].

Stress and Natural Healing—Christopher Hobbs [Loveland, CO: Interweave Press, 1997]. A well-composed overview of a truly holistic approach to soothing the mind and body. An abundance of ready-to-use material here, with detailed sketches of the individual herbs cited in the text.

The Tao of Medicine: Ginseng and Other Chinese Herbs for Inner Equilibrium and Immune Power—Stephen Fulder [Rochester, VT: Healing Arts Press, 1980]. Republished in 1993 as *The Book of Ginseng and Other Chinese Herbs for Vitality*, Fulder's book is a fact-filled, inspiring look at the role of these harmony medicines in optimizing human wellness.

Total Wellness: Improve Your Health by Understanding the Body's Healing Systems—Joseph Pizzorno, ND [Rocklin, CA: Prima Publishing, 1996]. Anyone dealing with chronic complaints should read this book before turning to pharmaceutical remedies. Written by a founder of Bastyr University, it helps the reader ascertain which core system of the body is out of balance and offers well-explained correctives via herbs, supplements, dietary adjustments, and lifestyle modifications. Truly a treasure.

Touch Awareness in Caregiving: An Everflowing Handbook for Hospice Care Providers—Irene Smith CMP [San Francisco: Everflowing, 2015 edition]. This small, precious book is a treasure of wisdom from a gifted practitioner/teacher of mindful touch. She offers insight and clear guidance in relating through touch with medically frail individuals. Smith helped pioneer the inclusion of massage into hospice care and was an assistant to Elisabeth Kübler-Ross, MD. **www.everflowing.org**

Treating Cancer with Herbs: An Integrative Approach—Michael Tierra, LAc, ND [Twin Lakes, WI: Lotus Press, 2003]. A worthy contribution to the growing body of literature on natural approaches to cancer prevention and treatment. Much of the material is based on Traditional Chinese Medicine principles and perspectives.

Viral Immunity: A 10-Step Plan to Enhance Your Immunity Against Viral Disease Using Natural Medicines—JE Williams, OMD. [Charlottesville, VA: Hampton Roads Publishing, 2002]. Williams is a well-respected practitioner of Chinese and integrative medicine. This is an invaluable resource, an accessible yet detailed and thorough text. Williams is also the author of *Prolonging Health* [2003].

What to Eat if You Have Cancer: A Guide to Adding Nutritional Therapy to Your Treatment Plan—Maureen Keane and Daniella Chase [Chicago: Contemporary Books, 1996]. Keane is a licensed nutritionist and a cancer survivor. This presents a discussion of nutritional consequences relative to cancer therapies and provides diet plans and supplemental recommendations during chemotherapy and/or radiation.

When the Body Says No: Understanding the Stress-Disease Connection—Gabor Maté, MD [Hoboken, NJ: John Wiley & Sons, 2003]. A skillful blending of clinical insights with recent biomedical understandings of mind-body unity. Effectively illustrates the relationship between trauma, emotional stress, and disease manifestation.

Your Body's Many Cries for Water: You Are Not Sick, You Are Thirsty!—F. Batmanghelidj, MD [Falls Church, VA: Global Health Solutions, 1995]. This book should be required reading for all. Those dealing with chronic conditions of imbalance would profitably explore Batmanghelidj's material as first-level response.

Recommended Listening

*Utilizing the sound of instruments, wild nature, and one's own voice is an ancient mode of healing, practiced in various iterations around the world. It is a powerful tool from which all may benefit. Whether used to create an ambient sonic texture in a space or used in a directed way, sound is healing. For details on the substantial benefits of utilizing sound, voice and music in maximizing the innate healing response, please refer to the books on sound healing listed in the **Recommended Reading** section.*

There exists a wealth of recorded musical contributions to healing. Likely, you and the person you are caring for will already have favorites that may prove especially comforting during a time of trial. Nature sounds, chants, and familiar melodies can wash away anxiety and offer a shift in focus—particularly beneficial in transmuting agitation to a peaceful sense of uplift. Healing sound amplifies the benefits of yoga, massage, meditation, prayer, and breath practices. In addition, guided meditation tapes by skillful teachers can be wonderful—to relax, to coax sleep, to prepare for surgery, to practice forgiveness, to release attachment to the physical...

Here are a few suggestions to get you started. Each person will discover recordings they resonate with during particular emotional/spiritual states. Try to sample what you can to find the precious jewels that work for you.

Sacred Chants of Devi—Craig Pruess and Ananda. The 21-minute Ananda Devi Prayer must be experienced. Pure, sublime and spacious. Wonderful for yoga, settling into meditation, entry into sleep, overall calming, before meals, entraining music before surgery or medical procedures. Try playing this on a "repeat" function for a longer soundscape of pure heart blessing.

Bija—Todd Norian. Two extended pieces that seamlessly flow as one. Soothing, grounding, yet transporting. Perfect to accompany massage or energy work or to create a calming environment at any time.

Ultimate OM—Jonathan Goldman. Wonderfully calming, centering, harmonizing. From the liner notes: "Imagine being in a temple, surrounded by hundreds of people chanting the sacred mantra 'OM' in a continuous, fluid wave of sonic vibration." Jonathan Goldman is a skilled sound healing pioneer with many recorded offerings. This ambient piece is perfect for healing sessions, meditation, shifting into sleep. Also recommended: ***Divine Name: I Am***.

Jewels of Silence—Ashana. Beautiful healing soundspace that progresses through the chakras. Excellent for energy work, prayer, before sleep: guides the listener to a space of deep relaxation. Angelic vocal improvisation to the sounds of crystal bowls, meditative keyboard, bansoori flute, esraj, and santoor.

All is Forgiven—Ashana. A tapestry of soaring angelic vocals and the healing sounds of crystal bowls creates a sacred space. Opens with a luminous rendition of *Ave Maria*.

Heart of Compassion—Ashana. An exquisite selection of heart-opening songs from several sacred music traditions, this work creates an ocean of healing sound that allows whatever is held to arise: especially allowing grief, loss, despair to transform into acceptance, forgiveness, and hope. Lovely.

Love is Space; Embrace—Deva Premal. Classic Eastern chants rendered with a respectful contemporary flavor by a gifted vocalist from the angelic realms.

Prem—Snatam Kaur. Anything by this lovely life-long singer of sacred chants is heartfelt healing medicine. Uplifting and soothing. Other recordings include *Anand*, *Grace*, *Ras*, and collaborations with others.

From Within—Nirinjan Kaur. Truly lovely. Also recommended: *Prem Siri*. A clear, inspiring, compassionate voice singing sacred chants. The arrangements are uplifting and healing as well.

Feather Light; Dream Spiral—Hilary Stagg. Stagg's distinctive harp music to lift the spirits, open the heart, and calm the mind.

Savasana—Wah. Heart-soothing Eastern chanting to lead one into deep repose. All of Wah's recordings are uplifting to the spirit.

Shamanic Dream—Anugama. Mesmerizing and relaxing.

For God Alone—Mark Kelso. Soothing piano music emerging from the heart of practice.

Ambient 1: Music for Airports—Brian Eno. An original experiment in progressive musical relaxation that succeeds in fulfilling its intention.

Angelic Harp Music—Erik Berglund. Erik is a master at invoking calming angelic presence. As with all his recordings, his heartfelt music and ethereal voice creates space for deep healing.

Atlantis Angelis—Patrick Bernhardt. A classic of its genre.

Quietude: Gregorian Chant. What the title implies. Creates a beautiful container of sacred space.

A Sufi Song of Love—On Wings of Song / Robert Gass. A chorus of angels sings from the heart and coaxes sweet peace in the listener.

Dance of the Light; Rivers of Life—James Asher. Two spacious, uplifting, flowing musical compositions to accompany mindful activity or simply to soothe, energize and delight.

Sounds of nature, such as ocean waves, river sounds, birdsong, etc.

Wavepool—Robert Rand. An amazing, effective integration of ambient Atlantic Ocean wave soundings with deep, slow melodic sound textures. The result is deeply relaxing and creates a profound soundtrack for healing work of all kinds.

Any music that suits the mood. Be prepared for favored music to change, sometimes suddenly and unexpectedly.

Sacred Sound Instruments

These may be broadcast into the space through speakers or listened to with headphones, depending on circumstance and preference. Lying down with eyes closed while listening seems to enhance the experience of these vibrations. Make yourself comfortable and cozy.

33 Bowls—Two extended sessions of meditative playing of Tibetan bowls. The sessions have been skillfully recorded to convey the healing vibrations remarkably well. Wonderful at any time of day, but especially entering meditation or sleep.

Golden Bowls—Karma Moffett. Also, ***Golden Bowls of Compasion***. Two beautiful, effective offerings from this gifted sound healing practitioner. Her wonderful ***Way to Katmandu*** is a more stimulating recording, but needs to be mentioned as a healing classic—uplifts the spirit, motivates the body, and encourages calm focus when tasks need to be done.

Tibetan Bowl Sound Healing—Diáne Mandle. A wonderful session performed by a noted teacher of Himalayan sound healing.

Sacred Sound Healing—Kristen Rubis. Sacred sound bath flowing through seven tracks, using Tibetan singing bowls, quartz crystal bowls, bells, chimes, tingshas and gong. Rubis is a licensed massage practitioner and yoga teacher.

Sedna's Prayer: Receiving Grace through Sacred Vibration—Visudha de los Santos. Deeply transporting and healing gong journey. Choose a single track or settle in for the whole sequence, which runs a little over an hour.

Tibetan Chakra Healing: Gong Bath Immersion—Richard Rudis. Rudis is a devoted Buddhist practitioner who is a master of gong healing.

Planetary Lullaby—Judy Bernard. Judy Bernard is an acupuncturist and Acutonics® instructor. Planetary gongs, Himalayan sound instruments, hand chimes.

Other styles of sound healing include **overtone chanting** by Tibetan Buddhist monastics and the playing of the aboriginal wind instrument, **the didgeridoo.**

Guided Meditations / Teachings

Deepak Chopra MD—Well-known pioneer in mindbody healing. Creator of numerous inspiring and enlightening CDs and DVDs. *The Soul of Healing Meditations* [CD] offers guided meditations. *Return to Wholeness* [DVD] with psychologist Stephanie Simonton and neurologist David Simon offers guided meditation and visualization to focus, cell-by-cell, in awakening the immune system's natural healing response. Chopra's offerings are widely available.

Belleruth Naparstek—A respected pioneer in the field, Naparstek has produced guided meditations/visualizations for an extensive range of health conditions and concerns. Topics include: Insomnia, fatigue, trauma, depression, pain, stress, addiction, chemotherapy, radiation, surgery, bone marrow transplant, dialysis, Parkinson's disease, fibromyalgia, recovery from injury, dental anxiety, grief, accepting change, general wellness, and more. Online: www.healthjourneys.com

Leslie Temple-Thurston—A wonderful spiritual teacher with a voice that calms and helps lead one to center. She offers numerous recorded teachings and meditations, including: *The Art of Gazing* [yantra gazing meditation], *Deep Relaxation and Expansion, Meditation for Healing, Gateway to Samadhi*, and more. Wonderful at any time of day, particularly in evening before sleep. Online: www.corelight.org

A Year to Live: How to Live this Year as If It Were Your Last—Stephen Levine [Sounds True, 2005]. In this audio presentation, meditation teacher Stephen Levine guides the reader through the question stated in the title with great compassion and wisdom. There is also a book by the same title.

A few of the books recommended in ***Recommended Reading*** contain **guided visualizations** that can be read and recorded by a beloved companion's voice to guide the listener into a compassionate healing space.

A Verse from the Bhagavad Gita

This verse can be recited nine times, in multiple series of nine recitations, or repeated without counting until your inner energy has shifted. It provides a way for you to both honor your loved one and to release your own attachments to their existence in physical form. This can be a powerful method for blessing their journey, no matter what direction it takes. I have worked with it both in a sitting meditation and while walking. One way to apply its healing and clarifying energy is to recite it ceaselessly while walking clockwise on some sort of loop trail. Allow emotions to freely arise and transform in the vibration of this ancient verse.

Never the spirit was born

The spirit shall cease to be never.

Never it was it was not

End and beginning are dreams.

Lightness and darkness are changeless

Remain the infant forever.

Death has not touched it at all

Dead though the house of it seems.

Appendices

CONSCIOUS CAREGIVING

Reflections on Environmental Influences:
Practicing Vibrational Hygiene

When the cancer was still actively growing in my body and throughout the months of alchemical treatments, my being was extremely sensitive to vibrations of all sorts—far beyond the high sensitivity I had known previously. Sounds, movement, and light all impacted me at the deepest molecular level. This is always true, whether we are consciously aware of it or not.

In this rarefied health state, however, I perceived and experienced this invisible impact most acutely. This awareness prompted me to withdraw from those people, activities, and scenes that seemed the most distressingly affecting. This was not a difficult choice—it felt more like essential common sense self-care and health protection. In addition, this awareness heightened motivation for my own spiritual practices involving silent meditation, cleansing and tending my energy field and chakras, chanting, and listening to consciously created music that harmonized body, mind and spirit.

It must be emphasized that this was not simply a subjective experience, relating to a given individual's sensitivity to energetic influences. Scientific research has led to exciting insight regarding the consequences of thought, sound, and movement on water and on lipid components of cell membranes.[*] These contemporary scientific "revelations"—while inspiring and paradigm shifting—really only serve to confirm the ancient understandings transmitted through the millenia by the wise sages of Ayurveda and practiced by shamanic healers of many traditions.

Essentially, our physiological status is constantly responding to vibrational influences—both from *within* the mindflow and from the *seemingly* external environment. Thoughts, emotions, vibrations, and electromagnetic fields within the setting all influence the actual biochemistry in a remarkable fashion. These are not inconsequential or even secondary factors in health and disease but rather, I would suggest, the ground of healing and well-being at the most profound level. Happily, at this level, an individual can engage in deliberate, mindful, proactive ways. In my case, the processes going on in my bodymind during the cancer journey, and my deep attunement to this experience on multiple levels, simply opened my awareness to these influences to a profound degree.

In practical terms, this meant that I could keenly feel the reverberations of energy within my environment as they affected my cellular structures. The voices and footfalls of those around me, their volume and tone, the words spoken, the stories shared—all moved through me either to soothe and harmonize or to agitate and disrupt. The same was true of musical sounds being broadcast and images projecting off the video screen. It was utterly and thoroughly clear to me as to which vibrations were assisting in restoring my being to harmony and which were unsettling and disruptive.

As a consequence of this sensitivity, I embarked on a sort of fast, being especially mindful of daily 'vibrational hygiene.' This type of cleansing and clarifying was familiar to me given my background, as such vibrational mindfulness is preparatory in learning to work with master plant teachers, to refine one's sensitivity to their healing activities and vibrational transmissions. In a similar way, this practice was powerfully useful here—beyond useful, actually; it became a requirement of my healing matrix.

I began a news fast, not reading or listening to details of what was happening in the world—the atrocities and suffering and acts of ignorance being perpetrated every day, seemingly *ad infinitum*. Certainly, I knew what was happening—this was no denial of pain, death, and destruction. It was only that I did not need details and vivid images of how these constants were particularly manifesting in the present moment. I simply cradled humanity's pain as I worked most intimately with my own.

Likewise, I chose to read only materials that inspired, uplifted or entertained. And, benefiting from the wisdom of a wise practitioner friend in such matters, I researched my medical condition and allopathic treatment options in strict 20-minute-maximum sessions per day. This allowed me to dive into the sometimes-distressing information reported in the medical literature with a clear endpoint calling me back to surface for a refreshing breath of air. And, of course, I gave myself full permission to avoid going into these realms at all. I was already significantly engaged with such energy simply through the seemingly endless string of medical appointments.

To create an ambient nurturing soundscape, I played music created by those skilled in the use of sound to promote relaxation and healing. This was particularly beneficial before bedtime or in preparation for test procedures or while awaiting test results.

I chose to watch films that uplifted my spirit or made me laugh in a full-hearted way. I was particularly drawn to a favorite television series from my youth about the journey of a Chinese Shaolin priest exiled to the American west in the 1800s [David Carradine's *"Kung Fu"*] that inspired me as to what the human is capable of attaining.

———————

I share my story primarily because you yourself or those in your care may not be able to recognize vibrational sources of agitation in the home environment [and beyond]—or, be able to clearly articulate what is being sensed. I offer this commentary to assist you in communicating what you need in these realms—and to sensitize the caregiver, family and friends to these invisible, yet profound, impacts on the bodymind.

Each of us leaves a trail of invisible—yet felt—vibrational impact in our wake as we move through our day's activities. What shall the quality of that vibration be?

———————

[‡] Please see the work of Bruce Lipton PhD, Candace Pert PhD, Deepak Chopra MD, Bernie Siegel MD, Gabor Maté MD, David Simon MD, Masaru Emoto, Theodor Schwenk, and others on the scientific basis and therapeutic applications of these insights.

The Lymphatic Network: Filter and Flow

To honor the elements we begin by honoring the vital healing waters that flow within our seemingly solid forms. The human body as a whole is composed of about 60 percent water; flow and fluid rhythm are essential to our nature.

'Lymph' is from the Latin for clear water, and the lymphatic system has sometimes been referred to as the 'white bloodstream.' It provides continuous cleansing at the cellular level. The lymphatic system allows for drainage of the interstitial fluid that removes metabolic waste products, toxins, and other debris from the tissues. Lymph vessels drain their 'watersheds' inward from the periphery of the body toward the center, returning cleansed fluid to the blood circulation in the upper chest.

The lymph flows slowly through the lymph vessels, mainly propelled by the massaging action of the muscles in action. Numerous one-way valves ensure proper directional flow.

The lymph tissue is protective. The web-like networks we call lymph nodes are considered part of the immune system. The nodes filter bacteria and other foreign matter that has somehow gotten into the circulation and then destroys them with lymphocytes. Swollen nodes are usually an indication that the body is dealing with some sort of infection. Nodes are clustered at the main flexing spaces in the body—the neck, armpits, groin, knees, and ankles.

The spleen is the largest piece of lymphoid tissue in the body. The spleen filters the blood, clearing bacteria and recycling red blood cells. It generates immune response and provides fresh blood when the need arises. In Traditional Chinese Medicine, the Spleen is involved with the Kidneys in the governance of water.

The lymphatics act as a regulating factor in the flow of fluid within the tissues of the body. Blockage of the lymphatics, for whatever reason, can result in fluid accumulating in a given area—which is known as edema, a painful manifestation of stagnation.

Let me quote the inimitable herbalist Michael Moore to sum up lymphatic function. "…lymph tissue, the 'back alley' of blood circulation. Lymph is the alkaline, clear intercellular fluid that drains from the blood capillaries, where the arterial blood separates into thick, gooey venous blood and lymph. It bathes the cells, drains up into the lymph capillaries, through the lymph nodes for cleaning and checking for bad stuff, up through the body, and back to recombine with the venous blood in the upper chest….Lymph nodes in the small intestine absorb most of the dietary fats as well-organized chylomicrons. Lymph nodes and tissue in the spleen, thymus, and tonsils also organize lymphocytes and maintain the software memory of previously encountered antigens and their antibody defense response. Blood feeds the lymph, lymph feeds the cells, lymph cleanses the cells and returns to the blood."[1]

Botanical Support for Lymphatic Function

There are numerous plants with well-earned reputations as lymphatic remedies, known simply in the herb world as 'lymphatics' or 'lymphatic drainers." These include red root [*Ceonothus* spp.], burdock root [*Arctium* spp.], calendula blossoms [*Calendula officinalis*], red clover blossoms and leaves [*Trifolium pratense*], echinacea root, leaves and seeds [*Echinacea* spp.], figwort herb [*Scrophularia* spp.], violet leaves [*Viola* spp.], as well as some potentially toxic plants that are used by means of carefully titrated single-drop dosing. Cleavers, a magical plant that lives wildly among us, is discussed in detail below. It is a delight of woodswalking children and ageless others who still abide in a state of wonder and imagination. May its healing energy enliven us.

Cleavers [*Gallium aparine, and the like*]: Whole above-ground plant. In the Pacific Northwest we find several species of these medicine allies. Here is one to look for— *Gallium aparine* is a taprooted annual with leaves arranged in whorls of six to eight. Cleavers are found clinging to and sprawling over neighboring greenlings. They have square stems festooned with hooked bristles; the sharp-tipped leaves are also bristly on the edges [with *G. aparine* the leaf bristles point backwards]. They are sometimes teasingly called 'velcro plant' or 'tangleweed' because of their propensity to hook onto whatever they touch. One British countryside name is 'sticky-willie.' Cleavers can be found rather abundantly along ditches, in moist clearings, in forests, along streambanks, and such. When gathering, walk extremely gently among them as they are easily trampled. Take care not to disrupt their easily disturbed root systems as you harvest; mindfully clip off most of the above-ground plant in such a manner as to prune the stand. In some cases it will be nearly impossible *not* to cut several stems at the same time as the plants become so wildly intertwined and easily matted. They express a wonderfully vibrant energy.

Cleavers is a mild but effective medicine with an affinity for the urinary tract and lymphatics. It is an excellent tonic for the lymphatic system, possessing alterative and diuretic properties. Cleavers is useful for enlarged lymph nodes in children and adults, as well as in lymphedema [either congenital or as a consequence of radiation scar tissue or surgical removal of lymph nodes] or fluid congestion conditions in general. In the case of lymphedema, it is often used in combination with other supportive agents such as red root, horsechestnut [*Aesculus hippocastanum*] and the bioflavonoid rutin.[2] It is especially relevant in nodal swellings in the neck and armpit regions. Cleavers facilitates removal of metabolic wastes. As a lymphatic tonic, the doctrine of signatures may be at play with this plant—In Scandinavia, masses of the tangled cleavers were used to strain impurities from fresh milk. Cleavers is also indicated in irritation or inflammation of the urinary tract, painful urination, benign prostate enlargement, and nodular deposits under the skin associated with poor elimination.

Once cleavers is dried, it loses much of its healing potency. There are several ways to work with it: an infusion of the fresh or recently dried plant; an expression of the fresh plant juice; or a tincture prepared from the fresh plant. For the **infusion**, use about 2 tablespoons of the fresh plant or 1 tablespoon of the freshly dried plant for each cup of brew. Steep in boiled water for about 15 minutes. When using the **juice**, ingest anywhere from 1 tsp.-1 tablespoon to up to 1-2 ounces several times a day. Fresh juice can be preserved for later use as a *succus* with the addition of pure grain alcohol [3 parts juice by volume to 1 part 190-proof alcohol by volume], or by freezing freshly pressed juice into ice cubes. To make a 1:2 **tincture**, cut up the fresh plant and macerate in a menstruum composed of 100 percent alcohol [190-proof]. Whiz the cut plant and alcohol briefly in a blender. Be sure to do a gazing meditation on the outrageous green color that immediately extracts into the menstruum. What a vibration!

Dietary Support of Lymphatic Drainage

* Follow **a cleansing, anti-inflammatory diet** to give all tissues of elimination a break. Focus on fresh fruits and/or fresh green vegetables.

* **Fresh vegetable juice**, mixed well with saliva when ingested, is deeply cleansing. Always choose organically cultivated produce. Choose veggies that gently promote urination such as carrots, celery, dandelion greens, chickweed, parsley, burdock root, ginger…Start gently and in small quantities to assess how this feels in the body.

* **Limit or avoid** red meats, fatty or fried foods, anything containing partially or fully hydrogenated oils, dairy products, alcohol, sugar and sugar-laden foods and, of course, artificial flavorings, colorings, preservatives, and the like.

* Nosh on **sea vegetables**. Regular consumption of seaweeds helps to detoxify the body, soften hardened masses in the body such as swollen lymph nodes, act as lymphatic drainers, and alkalinize the blood. As with all food and plant medicine, take care in choosing seaweeds that have been harvested from unpolluted environments [and, unfortunately, that is certainly a relative assessment these days].

* **Enjoy pure water liberally** throughout the day. Figure about eight ounces for each 20 pounds of body weight. Carry a bottle filled with delicious unchemicalized water that you enjoy sipping. It is the most vital fluid to consume for a vibrant human life.

Aromatherapy

These essential oils may be diluted into any fixed oil such as jojoba or coconut oil and applied over the affected area. Be sure to test a small area such as the inner elbow to ensure that sensitive skin can tolerate the oils. Always choose high quality base oils that have not been extracted with toxic solvents.

* **Bay Laurel** [*Laurus nobilis*]: distilled from leaves. Apply on swollen lymph nodes to relieve congestion. Improves concentration, uplifts the mind, and promotes mental clarity. The ancient Greeks esteemed this plant and worked with it to stimulate dreams and inspire divination. It is also used for protection against dense energy and disease. Extended therapeutic daily use [for more than three weeks] may result in

sensitivity and irritation of the skin. Use common sense with any powerful substance. Ritual application once a week would not likely be excessive.

- **Birch** [*Betula* spp.]: distilled from bark. Helps drain accumulation of fluids or toxins. A sweet, woody scented oil that is also used to relieve the pain of sore muscles, joints, tendons, and sprains. Lovely in lotion or massage oil or diffused in the bath.

- **Lemon** [*Citrus limonum*], **Lime** [*Citrus aurantifolia*], **Orange** [*Citrus aurantium*]: distilled from peel. These citrus notes can be used alone but their energies are very synergistic when combined. They are anti-infective and improve circulation. They are considered valuable in lymphatic drainage. They each have fresh, clean, bright scents and have a refreshing and uplifting effect on the psyche and mind. Use the citruses mindfully, as sun exposure following application may be overly sensitizing to some skin types; always dilute—undiluted application may be irritating as well.

Body/Spirit Play

- **Dry brush** with a natural bristle brush. Before bathing, brush your whole body to improve circulation and detoxification. Stroke the skin repeatedly in one direction— always toward the heart—until color is gently raised and circulation is increased. Continue until your whole body has been brushed.

- **Move your body!** Lymph flow is dependent in muscle movements, so be deliberate in staying active. Yoga, tai chi chuan, stretching of all sorts is wonderful. Jumping on a mini-trampoline or 'rebounder' is considered an excellent way to stimulate lymph flow and remove wastes from the matrix in which the cells reside.

- **Therapeutic massage** is so helpful in health maintenance. Any professional massage results in increased lymph circulation, and some therapists specialize in lymphatic drainage techniques. Ask your practitioner.

- **Regular use of the sauna** supports lymphatic and kidney function by enhancing detoxification via the skin. Using diaphoretic herbs that open the pores and encourage sweating amplifies the benefit. One classic sweat tea combines equal parts yarrow flower and leaves, elder flowers, and peppermint. *Caution*: Be sure the heat and circulatory stimulation of a sauna is suited for your health circumstances. Saunas are contraindicated in lymphedema.

---

[1] *Medicinal Plants of the Pacific West*—Michael Moore [Santa Fe: Red Crane Books, 1993]

[2] See the section on *Lymphedema* in the **Healing Repertoire** for more information.

Ocean of Mercy, Ocean of Tears: On Water and Electrolytes

I had the assignment to write about hydration, electrolytes, and the kidneys, but when first sitting down, my attention seemed to be divided. The subject of cancer showing itself in our community had captured my awareness and I found my focus wandering there.

Cancer is such a multifaceted subject, and I had attempted to explore what I term "the cancer matrix" holistically in several previous articles[1]. This time, though, the confluence of themes brought my attention to the role of hydration (and mineral status) in cancer manifestation—and in overall well-being, in general.

This is a tricky subject because, on the one hand, pure water imbibed in sufficient quantities is the rarely mentioned essential nutrient for assisting the body in functioning in an orderly, healthy fashion. Rarely mentioned in pharmaceutical medicine, that is. On the other hand, water may also be a vehicle for introducing toxic, cancer-causing substances into our homes and bodies. Both realities are true and in play in our world. Yet, we continue to allow this precious, sacred elixir to be tainted. Whether this ongoing desecration stems from ignorance, apathy or cynical disregard depends on one's point of view.

Water is the most crucial nutrient our animal bodies require to survive. Water accounts for approximately 50-60% of an adult's body weight, relative to the percentages of fat and muscle—and more than 75% of our brains.[2] Sufficient water in our systems is essential for optimal cellular function, and by extension, proper tissue function. Without sufficient water, our physical bodies rather quickly cease to be enlivened with life-force.[3]

Water is involved in a host of metabolic processes, beginning with nutrition and detoxification at the cellular level. In various ways, water is involved with proper blood building, cardiovascular health, joint cushioning, maintenance of cerebrospinal fluid, digestive juice formulation, intestinal waste elimination, renal function, and more. Through moving heat to the surface and via perspiration, water helps maintain balanced body temperature.

Adult bodies contain about 10 gallons of water and it is understood that we lose, on average, about 48 ounces, or six cups, of water each day through the normal processes of breathing, sweating, and urinating. It is easy to see, then, that we need to replenish at least these 48 ounces each day with the purest, freshest water we can find. In fact, it is usually recommended that we drink between 48 and 64 ounces per day. A useful rule of thumb is a minimum of eight ounces of water for each 20 pounds of body weight; for example, at least 56 ounces of water for a person weighing 140 pounds.

Most people need something other than their sense of thirst to remind them to drink this amount of water. Keeping a glass or stainless steel water bottle with you at all times is a convenient and simple way to keep track of the need for water throughout the day.

It is also important to note that beverages such as coffee and alcohol promote dehydration. For health, we must either reduce their consumption or at least replenish water stores. However, we must think of not only replacing an equal amount of water for each cup of java or alcohol we consume—that simply takes us back to zero—but being sure to drink our additional daily requirement.

Insufficient water in our cells slows down metabolism and has even been shown to cause weight gain. Drinking water helps the body burn fat more efficiently and also helps us satisfy the thirst signal we often confuse as a message to eat more food. When we think we are hungry, having a drink of water should be the first response.

Because it alters metabolism, even mild dehydration has been associated with numerous physiological imbalances—impacting mood, energy levels and mental performance. Mild dehydration has been associated with headaches, fatigue, difficulty concentrating, dizziness, lightheadedness. There has been clinical association observed between chronic low fluid intake and cardiovascular disease, diabetes, asthma, and some cancers. Severe dehydration is a medical emergency, effecting cardiovascular and renal function. Symptoms can include rapid heartbeat, rapid breathing, and lowered blood pressure.

Additional clinical research is needed to more fully understand all the ways and means that chronic dehydration can set the stage for disease process such as cancer. In lab research, scientists have observed that the water sheath surrounding cellular DNA influences its very structure, varying the helix shape when water content is lower or higher. Thus, DNA itself—the genetic code for proper cell growth and function—has been shown to be directly responsive to changes in hydration.[4]

Ocean of Tears

Tragically, the source of our drinking water can be cause for concern in its own right. Ground water and municipal water systems are often contaminated with toxic, carcinogenic substances—including fluoride, chlorine, heavy metals, radioactive minerals, rocket fuel, industrial solvents, agricultural pesticides and herbicides, and pharmaceutical drugs [both via urine and drug disposal]. Prescription drugs such as antibiotics, hormones, chemotherapy agents, antidepressants, cardiovascular meds, pain medication…all these and more have been detected in U.S. drinking water.

Public health warnings have been articulated for decades but this contamination has become a political and allegedly economic issue rather than a commonsense medical emergency. Political will in the U.S. has all too frequently been subverted by powerful special interests such as the well-funded chemical lobby—with cynical disregard for epidemiologic data and demonstrated harm to wildlife and humans. It is only through concerted citizen outrage at dramatic, devastating circumstances such as Love Canal that awareness seems to heighten. How many tragedies do we need to wake us up? Are we not experiencing unnecessary suffering and loss of life every day? The European Union has shown more backbone in banning some of the problematic chemicals and reorienting the regulatory landscape to better protect biological life.

Meanwhile, testing for contaminants and effective home-filtering and purification is strongly advised with most drinking water—whether sourced from the municipality or home well.[5] Reverse osmosis and active carbon filtration are two techniques used to remove many toxins. Unfortunately, these are not end-all, be-all solutions and present issues of their own. Be sure to review benefits and limitations when considering any water purification system and match the system to the water you are dealing with.

Purchasing water bottled in plastic is no sustainable solution either. The source of such water must always be questioned and the plastic bottles themselves present significant challenges to our personal health and the health of the environment. Often, the bottles leach cancer-causing, endocrine disrupting chemicals such as bisphenols into the seemingly pure water. And the manufacturing and disposal issues for *millions of tons* of single-use plastic bottles are an enormous factor in earth, stream, and ocean pollution.

Awareness, vigilance and clear-eyed action seem clearly called for if this contamination is to be redressed—both as to sources of pollution and remediation. The vast majority of municipal water systems were not engineered to handle these sorts of substances. We can be health activists first and foremost by being mindful of what we purchase, what products we utilize in our homes and landscapes, what we pour and flush down our drains. It is easy to lay the blame on corporate culpability—where it is certainly deserved—but, as we know so well in this bioregion, change begins with the power of our dollars, our choices, our own awakening to the power of how we direct and allocate our energy. Our broad economic voice—added to local activism in our communities— lends a powerful message and impetus for change.

Ending contamination of our global water supplies—starting with our own complicity then codifying it as the crime against the commons that it is—is perhaps one of the most sane and honorable things we can do in this lifetime. The integrity of our watersheds— the habitats they define and the water they supply—is fundamental to healthy biological existence. Intact, unpolluted watersheds are essential, common treasures that demand all measure of protection we can afford them. Despoiling the waters should be, and is, the most egregious of crimes against the collective.

Electrolytes

Electrolytes are minerals dissolved in the watery plasma of the bloodstream that carry an electric charge. Examples include calcium, magnesium, potassium, phosphorus, sodium, and chloride. Once they dissolve, they break into ions that are either positively or negatively charged. These ions can conduct electrical current in watery media.

Electrolytes regulate fluid distribution in the body, particularly the passage across cell membranes. They transport nutrients into cells and remove waste from them. Their electrical dynamics are involved in nerve transmission, muscle contraction and relaxation, blood pressure regulation, and more. They are involved in scores of enzymatic activities and used in the maintenance and repair of all tissue.

Balance among these electrolytes is key to homeostasis and thus to health—particularly the balance between sodium and potassium. Too much or too little sodium in relation to potassium can contribute to high or low blood pressure, respectively. Also, excess sodium has been seen in association with immune challenges such as cancer manifestation.[6,7]

There are numerous reasons electrolyte imbalances may occur: inadequate hydration; loss of body fluids through prolonged vomiting, diarrhea, sweating [including fever]; inadequate nutrition from daily diet; malabsorption; endocrine disorders; kidney disease; complications of chemotherapy; side effects from pharmaceutical drugs such as diuretics, certain antibiotics, and corticosteroids.

When balance among electrolytes is perturbed, cellular charge is diminished and the osmotic equilibrium between the inside and outside of a cell is less able to protect the cell from invasion by pathogens such as viruses and bacteria. Additionally, electrolytes are responsible for maintaining the correct pH [alkaline/acid measure] in the intracellular fluid so that invading organisms cannot survive. This defense, too, is altered when electrolyte balance is askew.

Electrolyte imbalances may be associated with cardiovascular, gastrointestinal, genitourinary, musculoskeletal, and neurological dysfunctions. Dizziness, irregular heartbeat, leg cramps, muscle weakness or twitching, fatigue, confusion, blood pressure changes, bone health, depression and irritability may all be related to whether one is sufficiently hydrating with water and ingesting minerals in a balanced way during the course of the day.

Properly digesting a diet rich in fresh fruits, vegetables and nutritive herbs is the foremost way to maintain beneficial balance among electrolytes. For instance, the minimum health-promoting ratio of potassium [K] to sodium [Na] in the bloodstream is 5:1. Commercially prepared or overly salted foods often invert this, being high in sodium and low in potassium. In contrast, most fresh fruits and vegetables provide at least a 50:1 potassium-to-sodium ratio. [Carrots are 75:1; apples, 90:1; etc.]

Coconut water provides an assortment of electrolytes in a readily usable form. It supplies potassium, calcium, magnesium, phosphorus, and sodium. The sodium content [252 mg. per cup] is almost half that of its potassium—still on the healthy end of the spectrum but something to watch in light of the rest of one's dietary choices and circumstances. Coconut water can be of great benefit during chemotherapy and dehydration, but is otherwise best used as a replenishing drink after sweating, which is why this beverage is naturally provided to us in tropical regions.

Mineral-Rich Plants

Between writing sessions, I paused to process the red raspberry leaves that had been hanging from the rafters, drying. As I was stripping leaves from stems in preparation for storage for winter teas [*garbling*...I love that word], I thought of the glory of this plant in the growing season, and the joy I feel in living with it and appreciating its many gifts. And, writing this article as I was, I especially gave thanks for the minerals contained within these beautifully preserved leaves—feeling appreciation for all the many ways they nourish and strengthen my body.

The minerals provided by plants connect us directly with the element of earth. Plants take up minerals into their systems that soil microbes have first remodeled into more usable forms. The green alchemists then use the energy of the sun to further transform nutrients and make them more bioavailable to our human organisms. In our daily ingestion of green leaves and plant bodies we undertake an essential, physical communion with the cosmos that charges our systems with lifespark. With mindfulness, every meal we are blessed to consume can be an affirmation of our aliveness and our conscious interdependence with the elemental forces and all living beings.

Many of the edible, mineral-rich plants are common weeds that surround us daily. Many are perceived as nuisance plants, when in reality they freely offer some of the most concentrated nutrition available, without our need to sow and cultivate. Their presence can remind the appreciative soul of the blessedly wild garden we inhabit in this bioregion and can feed us deeply of that knowing. Other regions, too, of course, offer wild sustenance and it is only about awakening our vision to see what is around us, wherever we make our home.

Some mineral-rich plants have specific affinity for the kidneys and the urinary tract, and we will explore that relationship in some detail next month. For now, experience the nutrition of the new plants coming on and those you have preserved from earlier in the Spring: stinging nettle leaves, dandelion [all parts of the plant], chickweed, smooth sow thistle leaves, burdock root, horsetail, blackberry/thimbleberry/raspberry leaves and fruit, wild mustards, chicory leaves and roots, plantain leaves, sheep sorrel leaves, yellow dock roots and leaves [in moderation], lambsquarters, purslane, etc.

Other nutrient-dense plants, such as parsley and sage, are easy to have around you in even the smallest garden space. And, of course, sea vegetables are wonderful providers of a wide array of minerals and trace elements. But that is a story for another day.

Body / Spirit Play

Water is a remarkably impressionable medium. Our thoughts, our emotions, our words, our intentions all influence its internal structure and the purity of its vibration. This is another powerfully meaningful place for us to direct our attention.

Our ancestors knew this, and we connect with deep earth wisdom when we step into the power to choose our ways with care. We can choose to love and bless this element water, to direct our most heartfelt gratefulness to its role in the wheel of all life. We can be mindful of each sip we take, blessing it. We can celebrate each running stream, blessing it. We can notice, in wonder, the magic of turning on a tap and receiving the sacred fluid of the earth. We can feel the grace of each drop of rain upon our skin.

As we each entrain, so the blessing ripples out. Orienting our beings toward the precious purity of water's essential nature vibrates our own inner water with light and creates a focused beacon to purify the waters of the land. May it be so.

[1] Please contact me at nettlelove@gmail.com if you wish to purchase one or more of these articles.

[2] http://faculty.washington.edu/chudler/facts.html. **Eric H. Chudler, Ph.D.** Executive Director, Center for Sensorimotor Neural Engineering, University of Washington Seattle, WA

[3] Please see "The Ways of Water" in the December 2012 edition of *Plants & Planets* for a more complete discussion.

[4] Hassan Khesbak, Olesya Savchuk, Satoru Tsushima, Karim Fahmy. **The Role of Water H-Bond Imbalances in B-DNA Substate Transitions and Peptide Recognition Revealed by Time-Resolved FTIR Spectroscopy.** *Journal of the American Chemical Society*, 2011; 133 (15): 5834 DOI: 10.1021/ja108863v

[5] County well-water testing services will typically test for bacteria and nitrates; in Washington state, search the Department of Ecology website for accredited labs in your area that test for heavy metals and toxic chemicals.

[6] Jansson B. Dietary, total body, and intracellular potassium-to-sodium ratios and their influence on cancer. *Cancer Detect Prev.* 1990;14(5):563-5

[7] Jansson B. Potassium, sodium, and cancer: a review. *J Environ Pathol Toxicol Oncol.* 1996;15(2-4):65-73.

For additional discussion of minerals, please see "Catalysts for Life" in the November 2012 edition of *Plants & Planets*.

May We Abide in the Ocean of Mercy

Lessons from Bacteria

Four laws of ecology: (1) everything is connected to everything else,
(2) everything must go somewhere, (3) nature knows best,
(4) there is no such thing as a free lunch.
— Barry Commoner[1]

Checking on rosehips after the first frost, I followed an animal trail to the edge of a wet meadow. A dense community of thorny rose tribe marked the boundary between the bright grassy open and the cool damp of the autumn forest. Hawthorn, wild rose, blackberry. Within this fruit-laden transition zone, a low arching gateway led into an inviting space. I paused, quieting into my leading. Yes. Bowing gently, I entered an elegant hazel grove that opened like a vaulted cathedral winding expansively between towering old firs and maples. The earth rose sweet with all manner of life-form. Arisal and decay: the ever-turning wheel, the visible pulse of infinity. Around me, sign of four-footed movement and rest was everywhere—and my own animal self sighed deeply to be offered such sanctuary.

Many have come to understand that—for all the complexity and diversity it expresses—the Earth biosphere is one interrelated, indivisible whole. We cannot sustainably seek solutions to human health challenges by limiting our view to human physiology or genetic coding. We cannot view contamination of our soils and waters and air as somehow separate from the poisoning of our animal bodies, which depend on these basic elements for life. We cannot devastate brilliantly balanced systems in our "outer" environment and think there is no consequence for the elegant, interdependent, dynamic systems that maintain the health of our "inner" ecology.

It seems increasingly obvious that when we speak of earth health or human health we must take a systems view. This is holistic medicine expanded to a wide aperture. Deterioration of earth's balance of systems equals deterioration of human health-supporting systems. It doesn't take much imagination to realize the truth of this, and yet there has been huge resistance within our medical and scientific communities to embrace this as so. Our sciences, for the most part, have continued to view the world through restricted viewfinders, even as those exploring fields such as quantum physics and psychoneuroimmunology and evolutionary microbiology are showing us the way toward seeing the dazzling, unified whole.

But collectively we have not yet made the shift toward this understanding. We still argue among ourselves as to the truth of inter-relatedness, as to whether consequence follows action. We still make the question of *how* this remarkable planet came to be a social litmus test—intelligent design or evolution? So much of our attention gets bound up in these polarizing intellectual debates. Meanwhile, we're busy poisoning and killing each other and deconstructing our life-support systems at a feverish pace. As disease processes rage—both physical and psychological—we wonder at their prevalence and await the next pharmaceutical "cure."

Of course, all the while, we take pride asserting the primacy of human "intelligence" and invention over other forms of life.

And, indeed, our human minds and hearts *are* capable of perceiving the truths that underlie the incredible miracle of life on planet Earth. But an essential humility and gratitude takes us there. Many have opened to the exquisite beauty of the mutable equilibrium that pervades our nature. To do so, we must dissolve the membrane of separation into the saturating light of awe and wonder. From this, *any* possibility may emerge, including continued survival of the human species—although this assuredly seems unlikely from a purely rational point of view.

Meanwhile, as humans struggle so mightily to resist the fact of their interpenetration and mortality—perceiving "health" in a blindered, piecemeal manner—other kingdoms of life continue to demonstrate basic strategies and principles that underpin organism survival and evolution. There is much we might learn, should we open to the truth of what they teach.

Human life is not a given, but a miracle of symbiosis with the whole. Human existence is dependent upon favorable circumstances and functioning systems of regulation and adaptability, detoxification and renewal—both within and without. The very idea that some boundary exists is, perhaps, the ultimate pathogen. The whole of the planet embodies a unity, a dynamic relationship of self-regulating systems. As conditions change, species either adapt or die.

The details keep presenting themselves to our understanding—but the collective awakening to what is possible when we comprehend our place in things awaits the critical mass to take group mind to the next wave of potential. Our capacity to shift our awareness is the medicine we have been seeking. Surely, clear awareness will wonder what has taken so long to recognize what is in plain sight.

Systems Within Systems

As many within the deep ecology community have been urging for decades, thinking in systems is essential to understand the complex self-regulating dynamics that govern the possibility of biological life within the earth's living matrix. Disease is a predictable and observable consequence when organisms overpopulate or spoil their habitat. It can be a mechanism for restoring more sustainable dynamics within an ecosystem. "Runaway populations of bacteria, locusts, roaches, mice and grass always collapse."[2]

The impact of rainforest and other old-growth forest devastation echoes throughout layers of systems: on planet-wide systems of self-regulation and restoration; on patterns of air, water and migration; on the diverse communities of biological life integral with that habitat; on the teeming jungle of symbiosis within the soil. The full consequence of such wide-scale soil disturbance has not yet been felt. Erosion, loss of fertile topsoil, choking of rivers—yes, this. But such vast habitat destruction also liberates potential pathogens into the larger planetary system.

Climate changes obviously also play a role. A recently published report by The Wildlife Conservation Society listed 12 diseases and pathogens that may spread to new regions as a result of changing temperatures and precipitation patterns. Some of the diseases and pathogens on the WCS list include: avian influenza, Ebola, plague, parasites, cholera, Lyme disease, tuberculosis, and yellow fever.[3]

Such news is coming steadily now. We have ignored simple truths at our peril.

It is easy to become numb or paralyzed at the extent of what we are facing. Yet, still other principles evidenced by nature show us that change can happen rapidly when enough are ready.

Bacteria as Ancestor and Progeny

We live in a world dominated by microbes. They populate our soils, our waters, our animal bodies. Without their ubiquitous presence, life as we know it would not exist. We are dependent upon bacteria for our nutrition, immunity, adaptability, detoxification, recycling and waste management.

Some bacteria prove pathogenic, for sure, but even in this it can be said that they are serving a role within the whole. And this is to say nothing about viruses and fungi—their potential virulence as well as contributions.

Fear or phobia toward disease-causing bacteria or other pathogens only serves to dampen our innate aliveness and immune capacity. Our efforts should aim to achieve peaceful co-existence with the microbes, to engage some version of right relationship. Through this, we shall strengthen our own vitality.

A sterile world is a barren world.

The oldest fossils known are interpreted to be remains of bacteria. Found in southern Africa, these "microspheres" are dated as over 3.5 billion years old. According to renowned scientist Lynn Margulis: "Neither plant nor animal appeared on Earth until bacteria had undergone at least 2000 million years of chemical and social evolution."

"We animals, all thirty million species of us, emanate from the microcosm. The microbial world, the source and well-spring of soil and air, informs our own survival. A major theme of the microbial drama is the emergence of individuality from the community interactions of once-independent actors."

"The more balanced view of microbe as colleague and ancestor remains almost unexpressed. Our culture ignores the hard-won fact that these disease 'agents,' these 'germs,' also germinated all life. Our ancestors, the germs, were bacteria."[4]

Some Basic Understandings

Our Resident Bacteria

The human body is host to a world of bacteria. As is also true of the soil and forest and other natural systems, bacteria are an essential part of a healthy human ecosystem. They are symbiotic to human life.

It has been estimated that the human body contains approximately a hundred times more microbial genes than human ones. The skin hosts an estimated 100 billion resident bacteria, with 100 trillion in the colon alone.[5]

From 400-500 different types of bacteria line the human digestive system, distributed over its entire length from the mouth to the anus in predictable geographic arrangements. About 99% of the body's microflora populate the digestive tract. Researchers believe that they have co-evolved with us over time.

Our resident bacteria generally exist in a state of ecological balance, which when disturbed, can lead to distress—such as colon inflammation [*Clostridium difficile*], stomach ulceration [*Heliobacter pilori*], or other health challenges. Potentially pathogenic bacteria do not manifest as disease in everyone.

Gut and skin bacteria provide our first level of interface with external environment. By incorporating DNA from their environment into themselves, bacteria assimilate genetic traits and evolve. This is their way of responding fluently to changing circumstances. This is one of the mechanisms pathogenic bacteria use to develop drug resistance. Because the gut is so rich with microflora, and because so much bacterial information travels through with our food, it is a place of both communication and literal internalization of new information.

Microscopic bacteria and fungi are ubiquitous. Everything we touch, every breath we take, every food we eat contains microorganisms. These organisms are masters of transformation; without them, the arisal and decay of form would not transpire.

Like their relatives the soil rhizobacteria, the gut microflora are alchemists—able to transform inorganic substances into organic, bioavailable nutrients [for plant or animal assimilation, respectively], and able to interact with toxins to render them more benign.

This is a remarkable contribution. Healthy populations of intestinal flora provide a first level of detoxification and immune defense, promoting resistance to infectious disease, modulating immunity, and reducing or preventing cancer process.[6]

Friendly flora such as *Lactobacillus acidophilus* and bifidobacteria prevent the establishment or overgrowth of disease-causing microbes such as *Candida, Salmonella, E. coli, Helicobacter pylori, Yersinia pseudotuberculosis*; manufacture nutrients such as the B complex and vitamin K; improve the absorption of minerals such as calcium, magnesium, iron, etc.; maintain the integrity of the intestinal mucosa thus preventing the syndrome known as 'leaky gut' which can lead to sensitivity to certain foods; and more.

Disruptors of Ecology: Both Inner and Outer

At the level of the individual, maintaining the health and integrity of the microbiota, the mucosal lining of the gut, and diverse skin ecology is foremost toward supporting the health and resilience of the body as a whole.

Regular use of non-steroidal anti-inflammatory drugs [NSAIDs] can damage the intestinal lining. Medications such as aspirin, ibuprofen and naproxen are in this category. Other substances that are detrimental to the digestive tract and its inhabitants include: alcohol, chlorine and flouride in water, grilled meats, oral contraceptives, steroid drugs, tobacco smoke, and a wide array of manufactured chemicals.

Antibiotics in the food supply. Animals and fowl are routinely administered antibiotics on industrial animal farms, providing a flow of resistance genes into the human milieu. This, plus the troubling consequences of antibiotic-tainted runoff from these factory farms into groundwater and streams.

Indiscriminate or prophalactic use of broad-spectrum pharmaceutical antibiotics effectively sterilizes the gut and stresses the liver, leaving the host vulnerable to pathogens from foods and environment—and compromises basic strategies for survival. On both the individual and collective levels this practice manifests as loss of diversity and promotion of bacterial mutation toward resistance. Bacteria can evolve far faster than we ourselves have demonstrated thus far.

Widespread use of antibacterial soaps and germ-free toys can ultimately weaken immunity and promote resistant strains of pathogens. Triclosan, the chemical often added to soaps, toothpastes, mouthwash, etc., can trigger multi-drug resistance in *E. coli, Salmonella, Shigella,* and other intestinal bacteria. Triclosan and related chemicals persist in treated wastewater and, over the past 20 years, have become pervasive in groundwater, well-water, and fresh water lakes and streams across the United States.[7]

The "hygiene hypothesis" being explored by researchers suggests that it is our constant exposure to microbes as babies and in childhood that promotes a healthy and responsive immune system as adults—and that our current *lack* of early exposure to diverse bacteria because of hyper-antimicrobial practices in our food/water supply and home environments contributes toward the dramatic increase in asthma, allergies, and eczema.

Proliferation of childhood vaccine mandates. This is a complex topic well beyond the scope of this article. Opinions differ greatly as to the wisdom of expanding this prophylactic approach. The following recent development illustrates just one aspect of the challenge in this realm.

A highly drug-resistant strain of the *Strep* bacteria has emerged [Serotype 19A], perhaps as a consequence of immunization against other variants of the bacteria. Since 2000, American toddlers have been vaccinated against *Streptococcus pneumoniae*, or *pneumococcus*. This organism is a cause of meningitis, pneumonia and other life-threatening conditions, generally impacting children under five years and the elderly. *Pneumococci* exist in 91 forms, while the vaccine, Prevnar, is aimed at seven of these. While infection by these seven strains has declined, infection by 19A—not addressed by the vaccine—is rising as the competition has vanished.[8]

Lessons from Bacteria

Here are some lessons from our bacterial teachers, in a nutshell: What doesn't kill you makes you stronger. Change can happen rapidly. Group mind will light up when sufficient numbers are awake. Evolution requires adaptability. Don't be attached to what's worked in the past. There is strength in diversity. Together, anything is possible. In fact, peace is possible, but it ain't static.

Oh, and: Don't kill the messenger.

Quorum sensing: Group Communication

In the late 1960s, researchers discovered that a marine bacterium [*Vibrio fischeri*] produced light, or bioluminescence, when its population reached a critical mass. Somehow, the bacteria were able to sense others of their kind and turn on this particular activity when sufficient numbers were present in a given vicinity. This phenomenon became known as quorum sensing.

Then in the 1990s, molecular biologist Bonnie Bassler and her research team at Princeton showed that a pathogenic *Vibrio* species [*V. cholerae*] released toxins via quorum sensing. The bacteria were able to defer expression of their virulence until enough had gathered to overwhelm the efforts of host immune response. Quorum sensing has been seen to control gene expression in dozens of bacterial species, including *Bacillus anthracis, E. coli, Salmonella, Staphylococcus aureus*, and many other pathogens known to promote human distress.

Quorum sensing, then, involves the production, release, and subsequent detection of signaling molecules that allows bacteria to regulate gene expression in response to changes in population density. When a threshold is reached, the group responds with a collective alteration of what it can do. It's the hundredth monkey principle on the micro scale! In addition, other species mixed into a soup with the transforming group have been seen to express the adaptation.[9]

Bassler, *et al* found that every bacterium they tested had its own chemical signaling molecule to communicate with others like it—a sort of dialect for a given species. In addition, studies show that other signaling molecules allow bacteria to communicate *between* species—a universal bacterial language Bassler calls "bacterial Esperanto."[10]

Quorum sensing allows bacteria to coordinate their behavior to survive and thrive in their activities. It allows them to change their behavior in unison to adapt to changing circumstances or to carry out processes that require many cells acting together to be effective. It allows them to adapt to availability of nutrients, defend against competing microorganisms, avoid compounds potentially toxic to them, and coordinate their virulence so to overwhelm the immune system of the host. Bassler's work shows that quorum sensing allows bacteria to act as multi-cellular organisms.

Diversity promotes survival and health of systems.

It has been shown that the diversity of species required for healthy human microflora depends on a continual introduction of new bacteria into the body. This is hardly an endorsement for the sterilization mentality in our modern psyche: antibacterial soaps, surfaces, and so on. Experiments have shown how germ-deprived study animals became sick and died when later introduced into a normal bacterial-rich colony of fellow rats.

Without bacteria, the intestinal tract cannot develop appropriately. In addition, in the 1960s, NASA studies showed that a steady diet of dehydrated and irradiated space food resulted in altered intestinal microflora and immune depletion in astronauts.[11,12] This affirms the global traditions of naturally fermented foods and drinks, discussed more fully later.

Interdependent co-existence describes the whole.

Once again, nature's models point us toward understanding health and wellness as cultivation of dynamic co-existence and adaptation among diverse organisms within an ecological whole, the indivisible web of relationships. Within the body, as with microscopic life in the soil of intact ecosystems, everything has its role and its place. It is when these ecosystems are ravaged or distorted that untold consequences ensue as the web responds.

Healthy ecosystem is defined as a state of dynamic equilibrium, not as a static state.

Information is constantly circulating within the biosphere as well as human physiological systems. The ability to adapt nimbly and effectively to this information and respond to feedback is a basic feature of living systems and a requirement for their persistence.

Collaboration, [genetic] communication and sharing of resources promote survival.

Once resistant strains of disease-causing microbes appear, their resistance seems to spread rapidly. In fact, the presence of antibiotics have been seen to *stimulate* DNA transfer. Bacteria have an assortment of ways for picking up new traits. Genetic material from survivors—drug-resistant bacteria—literally begins to circulate even across species and genera, promoting multi-drug resistance. Bacteria can swap genetic material, collect new genes from the environment, or have them delivered by a type of virus called a phage. Bacteria, in this way, relate as one organism with shared focus and resources toward survival.

Vivid Consequences of Ignorance

MRSA and beyond

The rampant and ill-considered prescribing of pharmaceutical antibiotics—and the excessive use of antibacterial agents in daily life and in agriculture—has contributed to the rapid evolution of some bugs quite determined to survive. MRSA is a clear example of this.

MRSA refers to a strain of *Staphylococcus aureus* that has become resistant to the broad-spectrum antibiotics that have commonly been used to treat it. The acronym stands for methicillin-resistant *Staphylococcus aureus.* It can be fatal.

Staph bacteria are typically found on the skin or in the nose of an estimated one-in-three people; a person can be "colonized" without manifesting symptoms. Healthy people who are colonized can pass the *Staph* on to others, however.

In the past, *Staph* could be successfully treated with antibiotic drugs. But for an assortment of reasons, Staph has become resistant to its pharmaceutical nemesis, methicillin. This occurred first in settings such as nursing homes and dialysis centers, and was dubbed HA-MRSA for healthcare-associated MRSA. It has been found that treatment with flouroquinolones [ciprofloxacin, ofloxacin, or levofloxacin] or cephalosporin antibiotics can increase the risk of HA-MRSA.

Elders, with potentially less vigorous gut microbiota and immune function, are particularly at risk in this. Ditto others with weakened immune systems. Hospital infections are said to affect one out of every 22 patients, totaling 1.7 million infection cases each year in hospitals and 99,000 deaths subsequent to infection [though there may be other contributing causes], according to the federal Centers for Disease Control and Prevention.

More recently, another form of MRSA has shown up on the screen, this among otherwise healthy people in the community. This form is called CA-MRSA, or community-associated MRSA. It has shown up among younger people, particularly athletes involved in contact sports where the bacteria spreads through cuts, skin-to-skin contact, and sharing towels, uniforms or equipment. In addition, it is expressing among those living with HIV/AIDS, in prisons, and among those in close contact with healthcare workers.

MRSA can manifest as serious skin and soft tissue infection, as well as a challenging form of pneumonia—any of which can evolve into a life-threatening situation.

An extremely toxic antibiotic, vancomycin, has been used against MRSA successfully in some cases. Its toxicity itself, however, is concerning as it can cause kidney damage and hearing loss. Beyond that, some hospitals are already observing bacteria that are resistant to vancomycin—so-called VRE, vancomycin-resistant *Enterococcus*, which first showed up in U.S. hospitals in 1988. Of course, the next level of fear involves the offspring of VRE and MRSA—vancomycin-resistant *Staphylococcus aureus,* which first showed up in Michigan in 2002. VRSA manifests as unstoppable *Staph* pneumonia, blood infection, meningitis, and so on.[13]

Every new antibiotic seems to be an agent promoting bacterial evolution toward resistant strains.

Additional Food for Thought

Cannabinoids found active against MRSA and extremely drug-resistant *Mycobacterium tuberculosis* [XDR-TB].

Investigators at Italy's Universita del Piemonte Orientale and Britain's University of London, School of Pharmacy assessed the antibacterial properties of five cannabinoids against various strains of multidrug-resistant bacteria, including MRSA.

"All compounds showed potent antibacterial activity; activity was exceptional against some of these strains," the researchers determined. In their recently published study, they noted that cannabinoids demonstrated "potent" antibacterial activity against EMRSA-15 and EMRSA-16, the major epidemic MRSA strains occurring in U.K. hospitals.

The authors concluded: "Although the use of cannabinoids as systemic antibacterial agents awaits rigorous clinical trials…their topical application to reduce skin colonization by MRSA seems promising. *Cannabis sativa*…represents an interesting source of antibacterial agents to address the problem of multidrug resistance in MRSA and other pathogenic bacteria."[14]

Honey has been used for thousands of years as an antiseptic wound dressing.

Its antibacterial activity is due mainly due to its delivery of hydrogen peroxide. The antibacterial potency of honey of average level activity is "well in excess of that needed to stop the growth of MRSA and VRE."[15] Additionally, New Zealand **Manuka honey** [*Leptospermum scoparium*] contains plant-derived antibacterial components. In this study, the antibacterial activity of manuka honey proved about twice as great as the hydrogen peroxide activity of other honey against VRE, but was similar in activity to other honeys against MRSA.

Strengthening the Terrain

Just as the health of the soil and the diversity of the lifeforms it supports influences the health of the plant that draws its substance from it, so also the vitality of our inner ecology is key to our own well-being. This brings us to the understanding that even germ-warrior Louis Pasteur was said to have expressed on his deathbed: that it is less the microbe that is the cause of disease than the state of the host, "le terrain."

Bolstering our innate resilience, vitality and immunity is the place to focus our attention. Healthful living foods, such as cultured dairy, grain and vegetable products, can support immunity and encourage proper intestinal ecology. Beneficial botanical allies such as adaptogens and medicinal mushrooms can deeply strengthen our regulatory and immune functioning. Other supportive foods are described below.

Probiotics are living microorganisms in fermented foods which, when eaten regularly, encourage equilibrium of the intestinal flora and hence have assorted positive effects on the host. Probably the best known probiotics are the lactic acid bacteria and bifidobacteria, which are used to culture dairy products such as yogurt and kefir. Probiotics inhibit the growth of pathogenic bacteria in the intestines. For instance, healthy populations have been shown to successfully compete with *Clostridium difficile* for necessary nutrients such as simple carbohydrates. They fill an ecological niche by adhering to intestinal walls. Probiotics in cultured dairy products generally lessen symptoms of lactose intolerance.

These foods or supplemental strains can be purchased ready made and, well prepared, these confer benefit. Even better yet is the home preparation of such foods, an ancient tradition across the globe to preserve both food and health. This offers profound communion. Author and noted fermentationist Sandor Katz describes it elegantly:

"By fermenting food and drinks with wild microorganisms present in your home environment, you become more interconnected with the life forces of the world around you. Your environment becomes you, as you invite the microbial populations you share the Earth with to enter your diet and your intestinal ecology."[16]

Feeding friendly flora. What have been termed prebiotics provide sources of energy for the gut microflora. These are non-digestible carbohydrates sourced from certain foods that selectively encourage the growth of beneficial intestinal bacteria. They may be found in burdock root, dandelion root, Jerusalem artichoke, onion, garlic, endive, leek, asparagus, beans and peas.

Even small amounts of such foods have been shown to increase populations of colonic bifidobacteria, with a resulting decrease in pathogenic bacteria such as *Clostridia*.[17]

Fermented soy food—such as tempeh, natto, miso—is sometimes termed synbiotic, in that it is created when probiotic bacteria ferments prebiotic-rich [oligosaccharide-rich] soybeans.

Other implications of regular consumption of foods considered prebiotic include improvement of calcium absorption, improved cholesterol metabolism, and chemical dynamics that support disease prevention, particularly of the colon and liver.

Sufficient hydrochloric acid in the stomach provides a deadly barrier to pathogenic bacteria, while acid-loving friendly flora remain intact. Routine ingestion of antacid medications is a questionable practice. Plant medicines such as dandelion root, when taken before meals, encourages secretion of HCl.

Coda

At some point, perhaps, humans shall be wise enough to unhesitatingly enlist the intelligence of the bacterial [and fungal] world to guide us toward balance and healing. Bacteria are clearly inventive and nimble in responding to changing circumstances and environments. They seem to be infinitely adaptable, and able to communicate these adaptations across apparent barriers of space and kind.

Their strategies toward promoting success of the group point us toward the evolutionary imperative for humankind. Recognizing that we are "individuals by incorporation" and recognizing this algorithim vibrating infinitely through the manifest world is the magical key to break open our heads and awaken the group mind to its true nature.

"The tendency of 'independent' life is to bind together and reemerge in a new wholeness at a higher, larger level of organization. I suspect that the near future of *Homo sapiens* as a species requires our reorientation toward the fusions and mergers of the planetmates that have preceded us in the microcosm...Now and throughout Earth's history, symbioses, both stable and ephemeral, have prevailed."[18]

---

[1] *Closing the Circle* by Barry Commoner [New York: Knopf, 1971]

[2] *Symbiotic Planet: A New View of Evolution* by Lynn Margulis [New York: Basic Books, 1998]

[3] "Wildlife Group Lists Diseases that Global Warming May Spur" reported 8 October 2008 by the Center for Infectious Disease Research & Policy [CIDRAP], University of Minnesota. CIDRAP noted: "The list does not include some other mosquito-borne diseases that have often been mentioned as candidates to increase their ranges in a warming world, such as dengue fever, malaria, and chikungunya fever."

[4] Margulis, *op.cit.*

[5] *Good Germs, Bad Germs: Health and Survival in a Bacterial World* by Jessica Snyder Sachs [New York: Hill and Wang, 2007]

[6] "Probiotics and Prebiotics: Can Regulating the Activities of Intestinal Bacteria Benefit Health?" *BMJ* 1999;318:999-1003

[7] Sachs, *op.cit.*

[8] "Worrisome Infection Eludes a Leading Children's Vaccine," Laura Beil, *The New York Times*, 14 October 2008.

[9] The Hundredth Monkey principle refers to a phenomenon whereby when a critical mass or tipping point is reached, a perceptual and behavioral shift occurs within the group consciousness, both locally and non-locally. Evolutionary biologist Rupert Sheldrake explores these organizing principles as "morphic fields" and "morphic resonance." See his book *A New Science of Life* for examples of such evolutionary shifts as demonstrated by animal experiments.

[10] "Talking Bacteria," *Scientific American*, February 2004.

[11] Sachs, *op.cit.*

[12] This same dynamic occurs on the level of larger systems, such as rainforests. Virgin rainforests are estimated to contain almost 62% of all the biological diversity on Earth. As forests are destroyed at a dizzying rate, species are extinguished to the tune of one

every two minutes and thirty-three seconds, or about 560 species per day, according to some estimates. It does not require scientific study to understand that enormous consequences must follow from this dramatic alteration of natural order.

[13] Sachs, *op.cit.*

[14] "Antibacterial Cannabinoids from *Cannabis sativa*," *Journal of Natural Products* 2008, 71, 1427-1430

[15] "The Potential for Using Honey to Treat Wounds Infected with MRSA and VRE," paper presented at the first World Wound Healing Congress, September 2000, Melbourne, Australia

[16] *Wild Fermentation: The Flavor, Nutrition, and Craft of Live-Culture Foods* by Sandor Ellix Katz [White River Junction, VT: Chelsea Green Publishing Co., 2003]

[17] "Intestinal Warfare: The Role of Short-Chain Fructooligosaccharides in Health and Disease," *Nutrition in Clinical Care*, Vol. 3 Issue 5, pgs. 266-273, 9 Oct 2008.

[18] Margulis, *op.cit.*

I refer you to the work of James Lovelock, Terence McKenna, Lynn Margulis, Rupert Sheldrake, Candace Pert, E.O. Wilson, Amory Lovins, Bill Mollison, and others who have blasted wide our perceptual framing from various points of entry.

May All Beings Co-Exist in Peace

On Depression:
Finding Our Way Home

"The more clearly you understand yourself and your emotions,
The more you become a lover of what is."

— ***Baruch Spinoza***

What is it that we have come to term depression? What is this state of mind and being? Is it an endogenous issue, a matter of biochemical imbalances? Is it situational, a response to obvious disappointments, chronic illness, or traumas such as loss of a loved one? Is it seasonal, a contraction evoked by relentlessly dim skies? Is it a spiritual matter, a death and potential rebirth? Is it a transient state or one that describes life-long emotional tone? Is it a symptom of an overlighting cultural disharmony? It is well beyond the scope of this short article to explore this question fully but I wish to offer some ideas for consideration.

Seventeen million Americans are characterized as clinically depressed; more than 28 million ingest either anti-depressant or anti-anxiety prescription drugs. These numbers stagger the imagination and provoke questions of all kinds. Some observers have offered blistering critiques of this free-flowing chemical pipeline. The pervasiveness of these statistics is certainly alarming.

Yet, in some circumstances, these pharmaceutical substances certainly can be life saving and life changing. They may help a person navigate difficult terrain with sufficient energy to make the shifts required to resume living *without* these drugs. They may help those dealing with chronic or untreatable disease, long-term caregiving, or the dying process make their way through with more grace. They surely have a role to play.

What is the larger cultural context within which such numbers turn to drugs for aid? Why do so many experience a sense of isolation and shame and failure in dealing with feelings or circumstances which are obviously so widely shared? What does this say about our ability to support each other in community, during times of personal struggle as well as celebration?

Without casting judgment on anyone who relies on the aid of pharmaceuticals, there are some questions we might explore collectively concerning what we call depression.

First of all, how might we—within group, in community—create space for those undergoing deep emotional process so that drugs are less needed as a way to reframe the experience, so the person challenged might have an alternative to drugs when compelled to satisfy the needs of our families and co-workers? How do we make space for these dark nights of the soul, these periods of emotional intensity? How do we create a shared appreciation for individually-timed retreats from group responsibilities and expectations to allow for personal reflection, release, and renewal? How do we support extended periods of convalescence from life-changing illness? How do we help cultivate alternative views of depression that give more honor to the deep, earth-shifting, spiritual work of transformation? How do we support each other in reconnecting deeply with the gifts and blessings of the greenworld on a regular basis?

Feeling stuck personally, how do we break out of the energy pattern we find ourselves in? How do we recognize we are stuck in the first place? How much of what we label 'depression' is really incongruence between our soul purpose or soul promptings and the way we are currently living? How much of a role do fear, anxiety, and inhibition play in our lives? Are we making choices from a place of love or from fear?

This one life is so precious and fleeting. Do we allow space to regularly reflect on the truth of impermanence and allow realization of this truth to heal our lives? Within such open witness, we can experience how everything changes. We can learn to become still enough to watch the flow of thoughts streaming through our awareness. We can observe what beliefs, perceptions, and emotions run our inner programming. We can see mental constructs, how they have served us, and those to which we are attached. Surrendering layer upon layer of these filters, we might know vast freedom and compassion. We can experience such overwhelming gratitude…. When we are sick, overburdened, or in the midst of feeling depressed, however, it can feel difficult to even consider such reflection as an option.

Meditation teacher and author Stephen Levine offers another approach to contemplating impermanence. In his book *A Year to Live* he poses the title's premise: given one last year to live in this body, what would you do with that time? How would you re-align, readjust, recalibrate your life? What would you give away and what would you take on? How would you live your heart's desire? If the answers to these questions feel so right given the idea of 365 days in which to live fully, we can explore further: why am I not living in this way now? Why and how do I hesitate to act on this knowing today? Why do I hesitate to make this so? What holds me back—what circumstances, what beliefs, what fears, what expectations? If we recognize a withholding, a hesitation, a limiting construct, can we release it—with tender compassion for oneself? In what ways can the present moment be reimagined?

Living each day true to our calling, true to our nature, true to our vision, true to our most heartfelt inclinations is a purifying path—no matter when we undertake it. Continually we are faced with letting go of what no longer serves our highest purpose—both on the inner and outer planes. As we are able to release our attachments and ideas of ourselves, our substance becomes increasingly refined. We resonate increasingly with our truth as a bell cast from finely blended metals resonates clearly with vibration.

It takes great courage to examine our lives in this way and to act on what we find. In depression, as in any intense journey, we may ask: "Will I ever come out of this? Will this chapter have an ending or is this the narrative of my life evermore?" All constructed things being impermanent, then surely *this* state of mind will change as well. It is for us to trust, surrender, and allow. Some Buddhist teachers speak of "taking the one seat." It is about finding our calm center, riding the breath, and staying put in our meditative frame—not just when we are sitting quietly but in all of our activities, as well. We can cultivate the view of curious observer, engaged with life yet with a broad view. The dance of life continues within us and around us and as we keep our seat, so to speak, we witness the turbulence and the tranquility. And ultimately we see it to be the same fabric. No matter the chaos, pain, confusion, or ecstasy: "Even this is something I can work with." From this place we move and act in our lives.

May we trust that all that comes to us, all that comes to our attention—is a teaching, a gift from the most exquisitely compassionate healing master who sees us thoroughly. Receive even the most difficult realities as temporary, as transitory, as an opening—to feel our shared fear, our shared anxiety, our shared sadness, our shared experience of isolation. It is a gift, though sometimes a seemingly terrible one, to share this intense fullness of our humanity. It can be a gift for deepening our compassion and our patience. We each take our turns expressing life force in its myriad manifestations. We each give voice to aliveness in many ways throughout this lifetime. So, let us be kind to ourselves. Let us be kind to others. Let us soften around 'what is.' We each take a turn, holding energy for each other. In this we hold energy for the group, for the many.

Body / Spirit Play

- Move your body in some way every day, even if to crawl. If you feel you simply cannot motivate, imagine yourself moving in some way in your mind's eye. Eventually find a way to stretch, to walk, to unfurl your muscles, to dance. Be gentle with yourself and grateful for every inspiration.

- Find music that you love to hear echo inside of your being. It can be music that makes you weep, music that calms you, music that makes you smile. Music that moves you to stretch, to meditate, to dance. Music you choose as the soundtrack for your life.

- Touch the healing green earth with your body every single day: your bare feet on the soil, your hands in the dirt, your back against tree, your belly on the earth, even simply gazing upon a tree through a pane of glass….Give away your pain and your confusion. Take in the life force with every breath. Allow the vibrant energy of green life to fill you. You deserve it. You are alive.

- Depression may be about being stuck in our identification with ego, personality, or grief itself….Bless the grief as a teacher, as part of what is. Ask for help in finding your way home. Have compassion for yourself, gentle tenderness for this moment of struggle. Open to the luminous Spirit behind all form. Open to the suffering of others. Recognize their pain as expression of the collective pain. Send love and blessing to those who suffer. Open to this love and blessing as it vibrates within you. Rest in the breath of the divine Mother. Rest deeply in the heart of what is. Relax around any mental chattering that arises. Note how thoughts separate, create a barrier, how they impede communion with the divine. You are one with this, this ocean of compassion.

Trust it. Dissolve as a drop into the deathless ocean of being, the peace beyond thought...love, compassion, tenderness, space...home.

Some Biochemical Considerations

- **Underactive thyroid function** is often associated with affective disorders. Iodine-rich sea vegetables, such as dulse, hijiki, arame, alaria, wakame, kelp, bladderwrack —in the diet or as supplement—may offer benefit here.

- **Stress affects adrenal function**. Increased levels of endogenous cortisol can manifest as depression, mania, nervousness, anxiety, insomnia, and other challenges. Adaptogenic plants and nervine herbs can be remarkable in their benefit, especially when used in skillful combinations based on constitution. Such blessed botanicals include: Bacopa, ashwagandha, eleuthero, codonopsis, reishi, gotu kola, holy basil, rosemary, damiana, St. Johnswort, kava, oatstraw, and many more...

- **Environmental toxins** such as heavy metals, solvents, pesticides, herbicides have an affinity for nerve tissue; associated toxicity symptoms include depression, confusion, mental illness, other signs of impaired nervous system function. Here we look to protect and promote liver detoxification function via plant medicines such as milk thistle seed, schisandra berry, dandelion root. Further support cellular protection and detoxification with sodium alginate-rich sea vegetables and lignan-containing foods such as flax seeds, ground and added to foods.

- **Nutrient deficiencies** are common in clinically depressed individuals: most common are B vitamin deficiencies, especially folic acid, B_{12}, and B_6. To ensure adequate supply of essential nutrients, eliminate refined carbohydrates and alcohol from the diet. Emphasize whole, organically cultivated, unprocessed foods—fruits, vegetables, grains, beans, nuts, seeds. Lightly sprout what you can for optimal benefit. In addition, ensure that digestion and assimilation are functioning well in the first place.

- **Omega-3 fatty acids**: Insufficiency linked to depression. These essential substances affect the ability of cell membranes throughout the body to respond optimally to chemical messengers such as hormones. They allow neurological cell membranes, especially in the brain, to remain properly fluid and responsive to neurotransmitters and the activity of monoamine oxidase—factors implicated in depression. Daily intake of high quality marine-sourced or organic seed oils is recommended.

- **Food allergies**: Depression and fatigue may be associated with food allergies or sensitivities, and may also include symptoms of muscle and joint aches, drowsiness, difficulty in concentrating, and nervousness. Identify and work with food challenges; improve digestion and assimilation with appropriate herbs; tonify the integrity of a gut that may have been chronically compromised.

Engaging with Pain

I received the assignment to write an article about pain while visiting with my extended family. We were immersed in assorted therapeutic dealings regarding skeletal, ligament, knee, and foot function. While absorbed in unconditional love and compassion with them always, their respective health statuses nonetheless proved rich material for reflection. I offer a grateful bow in their direction.

My elder relations have consistently been profound teachers for me: sometimes through the transmission of hard-won life wisdom, sometimes through the practice of their particular realms of mastery, sometimes through their capacity to love and to help others, sometimes through their reflection of universal tendencies. This last vehicle comes into play regarding the various approaches to health I have witnessed. One finds comfort in medical labels to describe various symptoms or physical experiences and feels a vague unease when a physician concludes that little is essentially wrong; another assumes nothing is really wrong even when prudence would suggest diagnostic information might be in order. One has defined themselves as over-the-hill athletically since middle age; another continues to stretch and train in their mid-eighties. One perceives aging as a progressive and predictable loss; another is unwilling to acknowledge lessened function. Beginning in childhood, I began observing how an individual's language, assumptions, and expectations seemed to inform their distinct experiences—and this observation has deeply motivated my own ongoing investigations of subtle and not-so-subtle perceptual frames of reference. What role does mindset play in our lives?

One of the associations I have come to recognize exploring my own life is that how we perceive our experience, how we cast it or frame it, how spaciously we allow it, significantly influences the vibratory impact it has. We can become consumed and agitated over injury or physical distress—or we can acknowledge our circumstances without identifying with them, and become more skillful at resting in change and impermanence because of it. We can practice opening to the death of expectation.

The nature of pain itself is worthy of extended consideration and experimentation. It can feel so solid and enduring at times. And yet when we penetrate the seeming solidity with the warmth of compassion and a merciful willingness, a precious jewel may be found within. Pain can be a guide into primal or deeply held material that awaits our acceptance. It can show us the cost of resistance.

Certainly, Buddhist teachings speak at length of this—particularly the relationship between pain and suffering. These vivid sensations cannot ultimately be avoided; it is our mental and psychological relationship to them that may be profitably addressed. It is said that locating our attention inside the experience of pain amplifies the experience of suffering, and surely many of us have found that to be true in our personal stories. If we allow pain to be, just as it is—for it, too, is part of the wholeness that we seek—movement and transformation are free also to be.

It can be useful to ask ourselves how our bodies and minds behave in the presence of pain, either physical or emotional. We may find that we "clench" or constrict around the pain, perhaps reflexively. Clenching or contracting can be felt almost as a holding of the breath, a waiting for something to pass. This instinctive response may be an effort at resistance, avoidance, protection, containment, flight, fear—fill in the blank for yourself. Try noticing the consequences of these involuntary reactions to pain, either chronic or acute. Notice if your reaction lessens or heightens the sensation, if it restricts or enhances movement. Relax judging mind in this—our unconsidered responses are just that, neither good nor bad. Just notice.

What I notice for myself is that if I constrict around pain—for instance, pain in my knee when hiking steep trails in the mountains—that very constriction concentrates my awareness into the pain; I come to anticipate it with each downhill step. That anticipation, combined with my contracted body holding, further restricts my movements and in turn restricts the possibilities of movement without pain. I notice a decidedly decreased lyricism and flow in my walking..

What I also notice is that when I play with this sensation of pain and my reactivity to it, my experience is quite different. When I first notice the relatively quiet twinges arise in my awareness of my knee moving down the slope, I become more mindful of my gait. Instead of focusing on the initial signals of pain, I allow them to be a cue. I turn my attention to opening my body more with the rhythm of the breath, relaxing the skeletal muscles, feeling the shoulders drop, deepening the connection with the earth. Opening my body, relaxing my mind, keeping my attention focused within the whah! of being where I am—in this I find my stride changing and the movement shifting. Now, the flow of life-in-motion is motivating the body, rather than the body moving of its own efforts, steered by a brain that is expecting pain or limiting possibility. This is challenging to express in words; interesting and transformative to experience.

Here, once again, we are presented with the encouragement to open around our sensation—expanding our perceptual aperture, making more space for the whole of what is—rather than fixing our awareness within a particular sensation or experience. Constriction of our perception, like constriction of our bodies, tends to constellate patterns of conditioned response.

Related to this is the crystallization that occurs when we locate our identity within a particular medical diagnosis. "I'm a diabetic." "I'm bipolar." "I'm an insomniac." "I'm arthritic." "I'm dyslexic." "I'm a cancer patient." "I have attention deficit disorder." Every time a person identifies with such a medicalized label they are affirming that identity for themselves. They are solidifying the flow of bodymind experience into a conclusion of pathology. They are declaring the definition they accept as enduring. How does this labeling by self and society influence our journey and our perception of available choices?

The organizing power of Logos, of the Word, to craft our experience and our sense of possibility is profound. Where do we place our attention?

Rather than narrowing our view by collapsing into such self-identification, what might we allow to flower if instead we rest in the knowing that all is in flow, all is in motion, all is change and vibration, all is a field of limitless possibility?

Instead of holding tight, gripping an idea of ourselves as limited and fixed, subscribing to a linear view of life...instead of this, what if we cultivate a more relaxed and open bodymind attitude that allows for sensation and experience to freely arise—and, also, by its nature, to recede and transform into the always fresh potential of the moment. What then?

What About Essiac?

Surely, if you or your loved one is dealing with some form of cancer, a friend or relative has suggested trying an herbal formula called Essiac tea. Essiac is well-known within natural healing circles for its purported benefits for folks dealing with cancer. The name is taken from spelling backwards the last name of Rene Caisse, a Canadian nurse who worked with this formula for many years in her practice. Caisse's story is an interesting one in the annals of alternative medicine, and contains all the usual themes of health claims, accusations of quackery, repression, and persecution. For details of her story, see Ralph Moss' *Herbs Against Cancer* listed in the recommended reading section.

The basic Essiac formula contains four herbs: Burdock root [*Arctium lappa*], slippery elm bark [*Ulmus fulva*], sheep sorrel leaves [*Acetosella vulgaris*], and Turkey rhubarb root [*Rheum palmatum*]. Burdock has a history of inclusion in herbal formulas intended to address tumor activity. It is one of the constituents in Harry Hoxsey's infamous cancer treatment [see Moss and *Cancer Salves* by Ingrid Naiman]. Burdock is a deep body cleanser—supporting lymphatic flow, as well as kidney and liver function. It has a mildly laxative effect, and the constellation of its benefits makes it a fine choice for overall detoxification support.

No matter what the formula's effect on the progression of cancer itself, it may have a useful role to play. The ingredients promote the body's more efficient elimination of metabolic waste matter—and constipation and stagnation can be painful problems for someone bedridden or dealing with cancer. For that matter, simply working with burdock root alone or burdock combined with yellow dock root (in the same genus as sheep sorrel) would be an option as well. These herbs will help to keep things moving, supporting a body whose detoxification mechanisms are being overly taxed by disease processes. In this way, the Essiac formula or its variants may serve to give ease and lessen suffering. In many situations, this gift is enough.

I would not recommend Essiac to be used as a tonic to prevent cancer, however. There are many other approaches that are much more gentle and which support optimal health by building vital energy, tonifying our inherent capacities to stay in balance and live vibrantly. Adaptogenic herbs, immune system modulators, antioxidant nutrients, vibrant organic foods, meditation, prayer, daily movement and breathing practices, and sufficient water, rest and play are some of these approaches. For more information about vitalization as prevention, see **Recommended Reading**.

Toward Preventing Cancer
Being Here Now: Finding Our Way Through

"Natural forces are the healers of disease."

*— **Hippocrates***

Meditations on an evening walk—The question of "preventing" of cancer is playing within me...I don't know what the future may hold in terms of my own health, but what I do know now as my body moves along this path is that I am alive and joyful, that this breath is an awe-inspiring gift, that my feet touch the earth with rhythm, that the foxglove are bursting into fullness, that honeysuckle trumpets punctuate the green, that my lungs are full of the sweet cool breeze, that the greenworld shimmers all around, that these woods pulsate with life...

I am not moralistic about cancer—that if one is "good" or "clean" or "correct" in choice and habit, one will never be visited by this disease. I believe that the conditions surrounding the manifestation of cancer are much more random, indifferent, and complex. And yet, having said that, I also perceive that there are behaviors, attitudes, herbs, and foods that can help to optimize our feeling of wellness and aliveness day to day—approaches which may enhance our sense of vitality and enthusiasm as we explore all that This Great Life offers to us.

If one of cancer's most profound gifts is to remind us of what is truly important and essential—to remind us to freshly meet each new moment—then let us live now with no regrets as to what we have allowed ourselves to feel or to be. Let us invite the greenworld to open and to sustain our hearts, to energize our wonder and appreciation, to fill us with our own possibilities, to inspire our living as largely and lovingly as we may.

News item — "Often the best way to prevent cancer is also the most wrenching. Researchers report that women with the so-called breast-cancer gene can cut their risk of breast and ovarian cancers 75% if they have their ovaries and Fallopian tubes removed....Removing the ovaries helps prevent breast cancer by stemming the flow of estrogen, which spurs tumor growth; the procedure helps prevent ovarian cancer by eliminating the organs, though tumor cells may still exist nearby. Doctors think ovary removal may be an easier choice—especially for women who have completed childbearing—than the other surgical alternative: a prophylactic double mastectomy." *[Time Magazine citing the New England Journal of Medicine, June 3, 2002]*

Why does it seemingly make more sense in our medical culture to cut into human flesh "preventatively" than to explore for broader causative factors—for instance, to examine the role that industrial / chemical contamination and ecological disruption play in the incidence of disease? When considering the concept of "preventing" cancer from a wholistic perspective, we must go far beyond surgical excision of threatening body parts. Let us first of all look at the web of life in which cancer plays its part. Let us look at the basic health of our life-supporting systems—our water, our air, our soil, our food. This simple truth cannot be stated overly often. To explore approaches that optimize our potential for maintaining wellness, we must first look at the complex matrix of biological relationships that either support or undermine the basic possibility for health. Might we one day acknowledge as a culture that human health cannot be considered apart from environmental and ecosystem health? Nature teaches us that when a given species expands its impact beyond the capacity for its environment to sustain it, some sort of remedy manifests so to collapse the population back to manageable numbers.

This conversation is necessarily lengthy and complex, although so exquisitely simple at its essence—at least, from my admittedly biased point of view. It is clearly beyond the scope of this article to explore this perspective much farther, but let this be the larger context for what follows.

Optimizing well-being in the midst of a desecrated paradise

Here are some brushstrokes of a vision for the world I hold with many who are reading this. What experience do we create through this interdependent life we share and craft?

Remember and celebrate that into which we were born. Breathe deeply of the life-enhancing vibrations of nature. Give thanks for all that surrounds us and of which we are a part. What an amazing vision planet earth manifests! What an intricate perfection the web of life evidences. Decay as well as renewal is inherent in natural life. This law turns the wheel around and around.

Cultivate a sense of perspective as to what truly matters in your life. Seek to avoid dissipation of precious life force through needless worry and anxiety. What is available to experience in this sacred moment? Experience it fully.

Perceive the divine in yourself and in all whom you encounter. Bow in recognition of that luminescence.

Honor your body and the bodies of others. It is the same body. Nourish it well, bless whatever you take in, allow true relaxation and rest. Soothe yourself and extend compassion and nurture to those you touch.

Love freely and exuberantly. Breathe softer our own open hearts. Feel the ocean of love in which we abide.

Make of your living an art and a spiritual practice. Express your understanding as skillfully as possible in dealings with others. Make your way sacred.

Celebrate physicality. Dance, stretch, move, lift, reach, dig, fly, float, connect. Fully inhabit the vehicle your spirit animates. If you are not here, now, when might you be?

Lavish appreciation and compassion on those you love, especially on the difficult teachers you encounter. Each and any moment holds the possibility of being the reason you took birth.

Dream, serve, make beauty.

No matter what particulars appear on our individual healing journeys, may we each do our best to live fully and freely and in love. Perhaps then there will be little to regret as yet undone when we stand at each threshold of physical transformation.

Some biochemical considerations in optimizing wellness

There is so much that could be said on this topic. Please accept this outline of some selected areas on which to place our attention. Our collective understanding is a work-in-progress; may it expand as our capacity to honor the exquisite wisdom of life on earth expands.

Constitutional tonification. Support optimal vitality through a personalized evaluation. Individually appropriate herbs and foods can amplify one's inherent capacity to express vibrancy and aliveness.

Sufficient hydration. Adequate consumption of pure water is essential to promote proper cellular metabolism, cleansing, and homeostasis. Water is basic to life. Cravings for food might often be a cry for water—Choose water first. It is in many ways more vital.

Adequate mineralization. Numerous researchers note a correlation between the incidence of malignant tissue and mineral deficiencies. Note that many traditional healing plants are rich in minerals: Stinging nettles, horsetail, oatstraw, thimbleberry, red raspberry, red clover, dandelion, yellow dock, parsley, sea vegetables, lambsquarters, amaranth leaves, mustard, purslane, chickweed, burdock.

Basic resistance to detrimental effects of stress. Adequate rest and relaxation; meditation; restorative physical activity. Adaptogenic plants [which support stamina and resiliency] and nerve tissue allies: Stinging nettles, ashwagandha, schisandra, astragalus, codonopsis, He shou wu, *Panax ginseng, Panax quinquifolium*, eleuthero, oatstraw, passionflower, skullcap, rosemary, kava, St. Johnswort, damiana, linden, lemon balm, chamomile, vervain.

Alterative herbs to assist intercellular cleansing, effective elimination, and re-establishment of overall nutrition and homeostasis. These plants are the traditional foundations of natural healing approaches for chronic disease. They are best selected in tandem with personal research or herbal consultation. Burdock, cleavers, yellow dock, red clover, nettles, *Echinacea*, Oregon grape, red alder, sarsaparilla…

Maintenance of collagen/ground substance integrity. Breaking down the structure of connective tissue and changing the resistant consistency of ground substance is a strategy used in the proliferation and metastasis of some cancerous cells. Preventive nutrition seeks to maintain connective tissue integrity and inhibit inappropriate enzymatic destruction. Vitamin C, other antioxidants, L-lysine, horsetail, hawthorn, gotu kola, rose hips, green tea, turmeric, various medicinal mushrooms.

Minimizing voluntary exposure to toxins. Choose organically cultivated foods, especially those with high fat content such as oils, nuts, seeds, dairy products. Avoid industrially farmed animal foods. Avoid commercially cultivated tropical fruits, which are often sprayed with chemicals banned for use in the States. Avoid artificial sweeteners. Avoid or minimize exposure to: newly built structures, newly carpeted or tiled surfaces, composite building material and furnishings, typically available fresh paint and printing inks, chemically treated fabrics, pharmaceutical drugs, unnecessary diagnostic radiations, electromagnetic radiation from communication devices, horticultural pesticides, household chemicals, smoke, vehicle emissions. Tragically, the list is longer still.

Exercise. Breathe deeply and mindfully. Stretch, leap, run, roll, row. Expand, contract, activate, strengthen, balance, loosen, release. Putting the body deliberately into motion can improve circulation, detoxification, and benefit emotional poise. Essential medicine.

Immune system support. Numerous lifestyle factors decrease immune function. For instance, it has been found that three ounces of sugar in any form provokes a 50% reduction in white cell activity for one to five hours. Other causes of immune suppression or overload include: food allergies, stress, excessive alcohol, nutrient deficits, drugs [aspirin, acetaminophen, ibuprofen, corticosteroids, etc.], inadequate rest, toxic chemicals, heavy metals, pesticides, air pollution, degraded gut flora, and so on. Natural substances which support proper immune response include: Reishi, shiitake, maitake, cordyceps, astragalus, schisandra, dandelion, milk thistle, probiotics…Some potent allies used in cooking: thyme, oregano, rosemary, garlic, onions, mushrooms, pumpkin seeds…

Antioxidant supplementation, herbs and foods. Combining antioxidant herbs and nutritional supplements seems to produce a synergistic effect capable of inhibiting cancer and protecting healthy cells from damage. Antioxidants help to regulate oxygen activity in the body and promote the balance between healthful oxygenation of cells and damaging effects of excessive oxidative activity. Vitamins C & E, beta-carotene, selenium, green tea, rooibus, rosehips, grape seeds and skins, rosemary.

Recommended Reading

Cancer & Natural Medicine: A Textbook of Basic Science and Clinical Research—John Boik [Princeton, MN: Oregon Medical Press, 1996]

Herbal Medicine, Healing & Cancer: A Comprehensive Program for Prevention and Treatment—Donald R. Yance, Jr. [Chicago: Keats Publishing, 1999]

Natural Compounds in Cancer Therapy—John Boik [Princeton, MN: Oregon Medical Press, 2001]

Dr. Gaynor's Cancer Prevention Program—Mitchell L. Gaynor, MD and Jerry Hickey, RPh [New York: Kensington Books, 1999]

The Tibetan Book of Living and Dying—Sogyal Rinpoche [New York: HarperCollins, 1992]

Total Wellness: Improve Your Health by Understanding the Body's Healing Systems—Joseph Pizzorno, ND [Rocklin, CA: Prima Publishing, 1996]

Your Body's Many Cries for Water: You Are Not Sick, You Are Thirsty!—F. Batmanghelidj, MD [Falls Church, VA: Global Health Solutions, 1995]

The Impact of Stress on Memory: Overview

"Consciousness is the ground of memory....
It includes not only the ordinary memory of information but what we really remember in
our hearts, those things that most deeply affect us for good or ill....
Memory can give us either bondage or liberation. True memory is self-remembrance,
remembering our Divine nature in consciousness. False memory is memory of personal
joys and sorrows, the history of the ego."[§]

— David Frawley

Observing my elder family members and friends has offered great insight into some of the factors surrounding memory loss associated with aging. It is abundantly clear that stress and anxiety play a key role in provoking confusion and forgetfulness. When the atmosphere is calm and quiet and the energy in flow, clarity dominates; when the television is on or multiple people are speaking at once or contention is in the air or there is an appointment to be met or it is late in the day, anxiety arises—soon followed by confusion or forgetting, which then heightens the agitation and amps up the challenge. If some memory lapse occurs even within a calm setting or state, the spaciousness can allow for clarity to breach the emergent choppy seas and still them.

The more that relaxation can be induced—through deep breathing, biofeedback, botanical calmatives, physical retreat from the circumstance, exercise, sleep, and so on—the sooner clarity returns. In the moment, this is dependent, of course, on the individual being able to recognize that they are caught in an energy spiral. Potential for such recognition seems most possible when habits are quite entrained. Somehow, that mental patterning and bodily memory may spark awareness of what is transpiring within the heat of it, can at times shine a light through the confusion.

Establishing more predictability in the day is also of great benefit in stabilizing the bodymind—mealtime rhythms, systems for organizing daily supplies, times for spiritual practice, exercise, and regimens of all sorts.

This all points, once again, to the lifelong benefits of establishing routines early in our lives that regularly help clear the bodymind of stress and its attendant biochemical messengers; that help us regularly access spacious clarity. Not only does this help us navigate the flow of daily life with more grace, awareness, and ease but it sets up patterns of cellular/cognitive behavior that our bodyminds may more readily default to when under duress.

Body, mind and spirit—and biosphere—are one, as we are now so fortunate to recognize. Yet, we are just beginning to understand the full implications of this truth—how this unity influences health, a sense of well-being, and the overall nature of experience. And, of course, by definition, this reverberates from the individual throughout the collective.

One fascinating area of investigation is the impact of stress on memory. Rather than look immediately outward into the medical research that is being done in this regard, perhaps we can first look inward and investigate how stressors in our lives impact our ability to think clearly, impact our sense of poise in moments of challenge and decision making, impact our capacity to make mental connections, to learn, to retain, to recall.

Most of us can relate to stressful situations in which we could not remember important information, like our phone number or address: in response to the shock of an accident, the sudden death of a loved one, or a distressing medical diagnosis. Many people experience the so-called "white coat syndrome" in which their blood pressure is elevated simply while sitting in their doctor's office, anticipating the visit.

Stress impacts our lives in ways other than through our emotional bodies—and those sources of stress may seem more subtle because they are largely unseen. Cellular membranes, DNA, and endocrine glands respond to these invisible 'external' information bits, much as they do to direct internal signals. Our bodily perception of such stressors, whether recognized consciously or not, influences physiology.

There is the stress conveyed by ambient noise, artificial lighting [both day and night], proximity to electronic or microwave equipment, radiation from diagnostic imaging, electric and cellular communication grids, and the stress inherent to our slavish relationship with "time."

Additionally, there is the significant stress to our delicately calibrated systems due to the ubiquitous presence of human-made chemicals contaminating our environments. These powerful chemicals can and do disrupt endocrine function, among other consequences, in humans and other forms of life. We are stressed through our daily contact with plastics, polystyrene, chlorine, and more; artificial scents in household and bodycare products; toxic preservatives; dental compounds; hormones, antibiotics, pesticides, herbicides, and pharmaceuticals in our foods and waters.

Another stress factor has to do with our level of social involvement. As with so many things, there is a continuum at play. Too much engagement with others can create stress just as social isolation does. Neither extreme is desirable, from the point of view of well-being. A balance of being with others and being in solitude seems to be the ticket for a healthy life. This may come as no surprise, yet in our social-media culture, it requires mindfulness to see the full import of this. We may think ourselves alone, quietly tapping into our social network via computer screens, yet our systems are being flooded not only with the life details of others, but also the light and other vibratory emanations from the electronic devices themselves.

Aging itself, the very fact of aliveness, creates stress on the bodymind as the normal consequences of physiological activity and metabolism take a toll over time. Our capacity to adapt to changing circumstances—both inner and outer—can become less nimble, with a cascade of corollary effects. Our ability to reset, to restore, to renew, to replenish can become less efficient. Inflammation and oxidative stress can become more dominant at the cellular level. Chronic mental stress, of course, adds to these phenomena—as the realms of mind and body are utterly interwoven.

Not all of the factors mentioned above may be perceptible to some people's awareness as contributing to their stress levels, yet the bodymind is well aware of them and receives their impact and imprint. They might be understood as silent yet significant stressors. Modern life has created layers of stress that the human organism is not equipped to handle without mindful engagement. We need to be aware of such stress promoters—and appreciate their range of health consequences—in order to be motivated to limit our exposures to the best of our ability.

The more we do this as an ongoing lifestyle practice early in our lives, the more we support ourselves on all levels going forward. There is no time like the present, regardless of our current age, to begin to be more mindful.

A Brief Look at the Physiology of Stress

Stress, from whatever factors, has a broad range of impact on health and well-being, well beyond the aim of this article to explore. Essentially, stress influences the production of hormones of various types and subsequently causes changes in immune, cardiac, and gastrointestinal function. Other consequences derive from these. Before we look specifically at how stress may impact memory, let's review some basics.

Within the body's orchestration, stress is essentially managed by endocrine glands [the HPA axis] and the autonomic nervous system [particularly the sympathetic nervous system]. The dynamic communication among these players—how they perceive, how they respond, how they offer feedback, and how sensitive they are to chemical messages—influences the body's overall responses and state of being at any given time.

The HPA axis is composed of key endocrine glands: The hypothalamus, the pituitary, and the adrenals. The hypothalamus, located in the head, manages homeostasis, temperature and metabolism. It is called the keeper of internal balance. Perceiving stressors, the hypothalamus sends signals to the pituitary and adrenals, as well as to the sympathetic nervous system. Through this signaling process, the thyroid and reproductive glands are also informed that the organism is being stressed.

The adrenal glands respond to the distress signal by producing hormones—cortisol [from the adrenal cortex] and adrenaline and noradrenaline [from the adrenal medulla]. These hormones prepare the body for whatever physical and mental response may be necessary to survive the perceived threat.

For instance, heightened adrenaline in the bloodstream increases concentration, breathing and heart rates, blood sugar levels, oxygen consumption, and nervous system activity.

Cortisol stimulates the liberation of nutrients from tissue to promote more efficient muscle and brain function. It also regulates cardiovascular function, especially blood pressure, and supports immune system responses to infection and inflammation. Ultimately, both too little and too much circulating cortisol can have deleterious impacts on health.

All this, ideally, is intended to be a short-term mobilization of a human organism's resources to respond to an immediate threat to its continued existence. If these hormones are not expended by physical activity in response to the stressor, there are numerous physiological consequences.

It is now generally understood that living in a state of heightened physiological arousal from chronic and ubiquitous stressors challenges the body to a degree it was not natively designed to handle.

The Effect of Stress on Memory

Let's focus on cortisol for a moment. With cortisol, as with all endogenous chemicals, proper balance is key. We need sufficient quantities circulating in our bloodstream to allow for adequate physical, metabolic, and emotional motivation; chronic high levels, though, have been associated with premature aging, bone loss, cancer, Alzheimer's Disease, and much more.

Cortisol levels naturally tend to increase with aging, though not for everyone. Stress seems to be a major influence, including the stress of chronic inflammation and persistent or repeated infection. Too much cortisol can manifest as anxiety, insomnia, suppressed immunity, insulin resistance, obesity, osteoporosis, and more. Over time, chronic elevated cortisol can cause brain cells to shrink, impairing cognitive function. Then again, too *little* cortisol can also express as mental confusion and lethargy.

Appropriate cortisol secretion is critical for maintaining healthful levels of glucose in the bloodstream, providing energy for metabolic activity of all types, including brain function for which it is the primary fuel. In balance, maximum levels of secretion occur in the morning between 7-9am; cortisol levels have typically dropped by mid-afternoon, reaching their nadir by 1am. Then secretions progressively increase through the early morning.

Normally, cortisol levels are held within a tight range by the neuroendocrine dynamic. When subjected to constant stress or imbalance, cortisol levels can build and damage sensitive endocrine and nerve cells, thus thwarting proper regulation and exacerbating the challenge.

Elevated cortisol levels have been shown to contribute to age-related memory loss and cognitive decline through numerous mechanisms. Excess cortisol can damage: the hypothalamus, which coordinates appropriate body responses to stressors in the first place; and the hippocampus, the part of the brain where cognitive maps are stored, the deterioration of which is thought to be associated with much of the memory loss of Alzheimer's Disease. Additionally, elevated cortisol impacts insulin and glucose metabolism, and destabilizes the central and autonomic nervous systems by promoting nerve cell degeneration.

Not surprisingly, research suggests that increased or chronic levels of stress, along with high levels of cortisol and inflammatory process, is associated with increased risk of developing Alzheimer's Disease.[‡]

Managing the Stress Response

Our sensitive bodyminds possess an inherent capacity to adapt appropriately to stressors and restore homeostasis when the stress has passed. However, as we've noted, life in the current era bombards our systems with stress both obvious and not.

Pioneer stress researcher Hans Selye, in first elucidating his General Adaptive Syndrome in 1936, concluded that stress was a major cause of disease because chronic stress generates long-term chemical changes within the body and mind. He described a predictable biological pattern of response by which the body attempts to restore homeostasis when challenged. Yet, he also observed that there is a limited supply of this adaptive energy, a supply that declines under the influence of continuous stress.

In traditional systems of botanical medicine such as Traditional Chinese Medicine and Ayurveda, certain revered plants have a long history of use as longevity or rejuvenative tonics for enhancing the bodymind's capacity to restore equilibrium and thereby maintain proper function with aging. In recent times, these ancient "harmony" or "rasayana" remedies have come to be known as adaptogens. In botanical medicine, adaptogens are often used in combination with soothing, calming nervine plants.

Additionally, there are many practices to deepen our capacity to meet the stress of life with more grace and resiliency. The benefits of t'ai chi chuan, qi gong, yoga, breathwork, chanting/singing/toning, dance, meditation, prayer, ceremony and such practices are increasingly understood for the beneficial role they play on all levels of our being. It is perhaps no coincidence that these practices, too, have been carried forward by ancient traditions of holistic well-being.

Plant Allies

Once again, nature illustrates its healing brilliance. Numerous plants with traditional applications for supporting cognition and memory are calming to the bodymind. Each in its own way, these allies may influence the HPA axis and/or the nervous system directly.

In general, adaptogenic plants possess various compounds that are antioxidant, anti-inflammatory, renewing and stabilizing to the neuroendocrine system, especially HPA axis. They assist the body in maintaining homeostasis for longer periods, improve its ability to be less reactive to stressors, and enhance the capacity to recover with a minimal expenditure of energy. They optimize the process of adaptation—increasing function where it is insufficient and decreasing it where it may be excessive. All of this helps to minimize the consequences of stress on the bodymind.

In addition, many of these plants—as well as some of the others listed below—can help normalize neurotransmitter levels in the brain or improve circulation and oxygenation, directly enhancing cognitive function and mental clarity. They also tend to promote physical energy, endurance, and stamina. Some have been shown to have a protective effect against ionizing radiation.

Adaptogenic plants to consider include: Ashwagandha, both Asian and American ginsengs, sacred basil, eleuthero, rhodiola, and schisandra. Additional plants that have been shown to enhance cerebral function include the nervines bacopa, gotu kola, rosemary, sage, lavender, and kava kava. The mushrooms reishi, lion's mane, and cordyceps also have important roles to play, as well as the leaves of the ancient ginkgo tree.

Each plant medicine possesses a distinctive array of energetic properties, chemical constituents and activities, giving them particular affinities for constitutional types and patterns of presenting symptoms. While readers can certainly study these plants and choose those that seem most suited for their own situations, it is also of great benefit to enlist the counsel of a trained holistic herbalist, naturopathic physician, or other knowledgeable practitioner. A skillful formulation of these treasured remedies can work deeply to help restore harmony and balance in a given individual. *These plants will be discussed in more detail in the following chapter.*

Essential Oils for the Mind

Always be sure to dilute pure essential oils with an organic fixed oil such as olive, jojoba, grapeseed, and so on, before applying to skin. It's wise to test a small patch of skin with this mixture, perhaps in the inner elbow, to ensure that it will not cause a reaction.

And please remember: For some people, even the purest essential oils properly used will still be intolerable to their sense of smell and bodily sensitivity. Please be aware and considerate of those around you.

Cinnamon bark [*Cinnamomum verum*] and **Peppermint** [*Mentha* x *piperita*]: Improves attention, working memory, task accomplishment.

Clary sage [*Salvia sclarea*]: Relaxes, refreshes, improves clarity.

Frankincense [*Boswellia carterii*]: Ancient oil for contemplation. Calming, centering, uplifting; aids focus and clarity.

Jasmine [*Jasminum officinale*]: Shown to improve problem solving when diffused into the space one is occupying.

Lavender [*Lavandula angustifolia, particularly*]: Reduces anxiety; improves depression, memory. Has been shown to benefit those with aggressive dementia.

Black pepper [*Piper nigrum*]: Increases alertness and concentration.

Pine [*Pinus sylvestris*]: Invigorates, refreshes, opens the breath. Can be combined with rosemary e.o. to enhance memory, especially in the elderly.

Rosemary [*Rosmarinus officianalis*] and **Peppermint** [*Mentha* x *piperita*]: Stimulate cerebral circulation and activity, memory, alertness, recall. Refreshing.

§Frawley, David. *Ayurveda and the Mind: The Healing of Consciousness* [Twin Lakes, WI: Lotus Press, 1996]

Frawley, David and Lad, Vasant. *The Yoga of Herbs: An Ayurvedic Guide to Herbal Medicine.* [Twin Lakes, WI: Lotus Press, 1986]

Mojay, Gabriel. *Aromatherapy for Healing the Spirit.* [Rochester, VT: Healing Arts Press, 1997]

Pizzorno, Joseph and Murray, Michael. *Textbook of Natural Medicine 4th edition.* [St. Louis, MO: Elsevier/Churchill Livingstone, 2013]

Price, Shirley and Price, Len, editors. *Aromatherapy for Health Professionals, 4th edition.* [London: Churchill Livingstone, 2012]

Williams, J.E. *Prolonging Health.* [Charlottesville, VA: Hampton Roads Publishing Co. Inc., 2003]

Williamson, Elizabeth M. *Major Herbs of Ayurveda.* [London: Churchill Livingstone, 2002]

‡Winston, David and Maimes, Steven. *Adaptogens: Herbs for Strength, Stamina, and Stress Relief.* [Rochester, VT: Healing Arts Press, 2007]

The Impact of Stress on Memory:
~ The Plant Allies ~

"Our deeper consciousness governs memory on an organic level, including the memory that exists in our cells, through which the body functions."

— **Dr. David Frawley**

Brain health is a life-long, whole systems issue—complex and fascinating. The ongoing health of the brain impacts all aspects of our physiological functioning, not merely the memory.

All that we do to maintain physical balance and flexibility in turn helps us maintain clear and supple minds and a spirit more adaptive to change. T'ai chi chuan, yoga, and dance are exemplary practices in this effort. An open, responsive body—and exercise in general—promotes oxygen flow to the brain and throughout the tissues, enhancing function in all regards. A nutrient-rich diet [including specialized medicinal plant nutrients], a sense of purpose, and proper rest and renewal are core factors in living out our days with agility of body, mind and spirit.

Additionally, it is beneficial to continue to learn new things and engage in mentally challenging activities; to stay socially involved with friends, family and community; to balance such activity with regular periods of reflection and solitude. Meditation and mindfulness practices are also allies in the efforts to maintain mental acuity as we grow older.

The previous chapter began the discussion about the physiological impacts of stress of all kinds on memory and cognitive function. Here, we continue by looking in more detail at some of the premier plant allies that can be of benefit addressing this key aspect of healthy aging.

Overview of Relevant Plant Allies

First, a brief review of what was mentioned in the previous chapter:

Numerous plants with traditional applications for supporting cognition and memory are calming to the bodymind. Each in its own way, these allies may influence the HPA axis and/or the nervous system directly.

In general, adaptogenic plants possess compounds that are antioxidant, anti-inflammatory, renewing and stabilizing to the neuroendocrine system, especially the HPA axis. They assist the body in maintaining homeostasis for longer periods, improve its ability to be less reactive to stressors, and enhance the capacity to recover with a minimal expenditure of energy. They optimize the process of adaptation—increasing function where it is insufficient and decreasing it where it may be excessive. All of this helps to minimize the consequences of stress on the bodymind.

In addition, many of these plants—as well as some of the others listed below—can help normalize neurotransmitter levels in the brain or improve circulation and oxygenation, directly enhancing cognitive function and mental clarity. They also tend to promote physical energy, endurance, and stamina. Some have been shown to have a protective effect against ionizing radiation.

Adaptogenic plants tend to be the treasured longevity tonics in their various cultural traditions. They may be used either preventatively—both approaching and during a period of stress—or restoratively, following such a period. They are generally used for a minimum three-month course or longer, and usually in some combination, balanced to address the particular constitution and needs of an individual.

Though stress is our focus in this overview, certainly there are other relevant factors in supporting the health of the mind. Chronic inflammation is another key that is crucial to manage in any program to promote a long and thoughtful life. It is certainly no coincidence that essentially all of the plants traditionally used to support memory possess anti-inflammatory activity. Additionally, anti-inflammatory botanicals such as turmeric and ginger rhizomes, as well as sufficient intake of essential fatty acids, have proven themselves to be supportive allies in this regard.

It is also highly noteworthy that many of the plants described below to benefit memory and mental function also benefit the heart and overall cardiovascular function—helping to protect, calm, harmonize, and strengthen its function. Reishi, rosemary, *Panax ginseng*, ashwagandha, rhodiola, bacopa, schisandra, ginkgo, for instance, all have an affinity with the heart and vascular tissue.

In Traditional Chinese Medicine, the Heart is considered the abode of the Mind; mental activity and consciousness "reside" in the Heart.[10] Supporting the sphere of activity termed the Heart is understood to help preserve long-term memory, and to benefit thinking, sleep, and emotional balance. From this point of view, then, the classic heart tonic hawthorn [*Crataegus* spp.] certainly must also be included in our *materia medica* for supporting mind and memory.

A Selection of Plant Allies

Ashwagandha [*Withania somnifera*]: root. Bitter, warming, drying. One of the most revered plants in Ayurveda. Calming adaptogen, nervine, rasayana [rejuvenative tonic], anti-inflammatory, antioxidant, sedative, hypotensive, cardioprotective, astringent, diuretic, antispasmodic, immunomodulator. Calming, nurturing, clarifying tonic for the mind. Promotes deep, restorative sleep. Builds tissue, energizes muscles, and improves recovery time. Other indications: adrenal exhaustion, sluggish thyroid function, physical depletion, chronic fatigue, anxiety, depression, confusion, impaired memory, hypertension, insomnia, peptic ulcers, impotence, fibromyalgia, rheumatoid arthritis, asthma, multiple sclerosis, anorexia nervosa, iron-deficient anemia, adjunct support in cancer therapies. **Formats**: Traditionally prepared as either a water or milk decoction [honey or raw sugar may be added], mixed with ghee, or eaten as a powder on a daily basis. Also prepared as tincture [1:5, 45% alcohol] or extract or powder in capsules. ***Please note***: Some sources caution against ingesting ashwagandha during pregnancy; in India it is considered appropriate for all ages, including young children and pregnant women—this discrepancy may be related to the dose, format or frequency used. Because of conflicting recommendations, use during pregnancy is suggested only with the guidance of a knowledgeable healthcare practitioner.

Ginseng [*Panax ginseng*]: Sweet/bitter, mild, warming. [The "red" steamed root is considered more warming and stimulating than the raw "white" root.] Adaptogen and tonic to replenish vital energy. Considered anti-fatigue and anti-aging. Qi tonic and adaptogen to replenish vital energy, rejuvenative, demulcent, stimulant, anti-inflammatory, hypotensive, anticonvulsant, blood-sugar regulating. Stimulating and regulatory to both the central nervous system and to the endocrine system. Immune normalizing. Benefits the cardiovascular system. Enhances cerebral circulation. Ginseng has been recognized since antiquity for "quieting the spirit, curbing the emotion, stopping agitation, removing noxious influence, brightening the eyes, enlightening the mind and increasing the wisdom."[1] Clinical study suggests that *Panax ginseng* is effective in enhancing cognitive performance in patients dealing with Alzheimer's Disease.[12] Ginseng has shown protective benefit against radiation exposure and to improve recovery from radiation sickness. Other indications: Poor memory [mostly in the "middle-aged" and older], debility, weakness, fatigue, adrenal depletion, poor appetite and digestion, emaciation, shortness of breath, palpitations. It is typically used in combination with other herbs. Formats: Decoction, tincture, medicated wine, powder in food, capsules. ***Please note***: Use of red ginseng may potentiate the effects of caffeine or other stimulants in sensitive people. False or excess heat conditions; one source lists high blood pressure, though it may be skillfully used clinically for that purpose in appropriate circumstances. Some sources contraindicate use during pregnancy, though that caution is not consistent with traditional use in Asia. Use with guidance of a practitioner conversant with botanical medicine if taking pharmaceutical drugs: ginseng with its complex chemistry and amphoteric nature has been seen to have seemingly contradictory effects on physiology depending on the individual observed. Regarding concurrent use with anticoagulant drugs, Stargrove *et al* conclude that the "weight of the currently available research data suggests that the reported ginseng-warfarin interaction is not clinically significant."

American Ginseng [*Panax quinquifolius*]: root. Sweet, slightly bitter, neutral or slightly cool. Adaptogen, Qi and Yin tonic, demulcent, rejuvenative, stomachic, immune enhancing, anti-tumor, antiviral, antioxidant, metabolic and endocrine enhancement. A true member of the ginseng family native to North America, American ginseng is especially nourishing to the lungs, skin, and stomach. It builds adaptive energy without the warming effects of Asian ginseng; it is typically the ginseng of choice for those who are overly *yang*. Regulates basic metabolism, benefits vital energy, enhances cerebral circulation, improves digestion and assimilation, promotes fluid production, supplements and moistens the Lungs, clears heat. Key plant for those exhausted from overwork. It has been shown to reduce fatigue, strengthen adrenal function, enhance reproductive performance, improve liver metabolism, enhance immunity, may protect healthy tissue from radiation damage. Various ginsenoside constituents have been found to support nerve regeneration and inhibit ß-amyloid peptide, the production of which is associated with progression of conditions such as Alzheimer's. **Formats:** Decoction, tincture, medicated wine, powder in food, capsules. *Please note*: In terms of possible interactions, Gardner *et al* conclude that "concomitant use of warfarin and American ginseng may reduce the efficacy of warfarin and should be under the supervision of a healthcare professional." Related to the comment on Asian ginseng in previous entry, Stargrove *et al* recommend further research into possible differences between American and Asian species as to their influence on blood coagulation and any possible interactions with prescription anticoagulant agents.

Eleuthero [*Eleutherococcus senticosus*]: root and root bark. Bitter/sweet, neutral/warm. Also known as Siberian ginseng, Eleuthero was originally the most clinically studied adaptogenic herb. Also antioxidant and anti-inflammatory. Reinforces the vital force, invigorates the Spleen and Kidney, calms the nerves, stabilizes energy. Many physiological effects of Eleuthero have been demonstrated including blood-sugar regulation, memory enhancement, increased cognitive performance, liver protection, increased resistance to stress, normalization of adrenal response, enhanced immunity, inhibition of carcinogenesis, increased stamina and improved oxygen metabolism, inhibition of platelet aggregation, and protection against ionizing radiation.[2] Used as adjunct support during allopathic treatments for cancer. **Formats:** Decoction, tincture, powder, or extract in capsules.

Reishi [*Ganoderma lucidum*] aka Ling zhi: polypore fruiting body and mycelium. Sweet, neutral. Revered tonic of immortality and spiritual potency. Affinity for respiratory, cardiovascular, immune, liver function. More commonly thought of as an immune system tonic, reishi also nurtures the heart, soothes the spirit, and calms the mind. It is believed to protect the spirit and to nurture the growth of intelligence, wisdom, and spiritual insight. Adaptogen, immune amphoteric, antimicrobial, antioxidant, anti-inflammatory, liver protective, cardiotonic, adjunct treatment for cancer [inhibition of proliferation plus increases activity of some chemotherapeutic agents; reduces adverse effects of chemo and radiation]. Research has shown reishi to protect the brain from ß-amyloid plaque formation, associated with Alzheimer's progression. Inhibits platelet aggregation. *Ganoderma* is used to tonify the blood and vital energy. *Ganoderma* is used in formulas for insomnia, palpitations, anxiety, nerve pain, impaired memory, chronic hepatitis, kidney inflammation, general weakness and debility, heart disease, excess lipids in blood, cancer, allergies, asthma and bronchitis, and hypertension. **Formats:** Dried mushroom decoction as tea or soup base, tincture, extract in capsules. *Ganoderma* beers and wines are produced in China and Japan.

Rhodiola [*Rhodiola rosea*]: root. Aka rose root, arctic root, golden root. Sweet/slightly bitter/spicy, cool, dry. Affinity for lungs, cardiovascular, nervous and endocrine systems. Cooling adaptogen, nervine, neuroprotective, antioxidant, immune enhancing, cardioprotective, anti-inflammatory. Benefits memory, improves physical performance, enhances the body's response to all manner of stress—including chemotherapy and radiation. Likely superior to *Panax ginseng* for acute stress; adaptogens can work well, synergistically, in formulations. Mildly stimulating to the central nervous system, it has been used to lift the spirits. Indications: Physical and mental stress or fatigue, impaired immune response associated with physical or emotional stress, adjunct to cancer prevention and treatment, oxygen deprivation and high altitude sickness, head trauma, depressed mood, Parkinson's disease, memory loss. Rhodiola has been shown to inhibit acetylcholine esterase, which helps explain its use to enhance mental performance and memory.[3] It surely has a role to play in addressing dementia. **Formats**: Light decoction, tincture, extract in capsules. Can be used ongoing as tonic or in higher dose for short-term acute stress [such as exam, athletic contest, etc.].

Gotu kola [*Centella asiatica*]: leaf. Bitter, cooling. Nervine, anxiolytic, mild adaptogen, anti-inflammatory, vulnerary [wound healing]. The heart-shaped leaves of this tender, creeping perennial are highly esteemed in India as a restorative, rasayana tonic particularly for the brain and nervous system. *Centella* is traditionally used to preserve memory and promote intellect. It is a rich source of potassium and B vitamins. Clinically, it is also used to relieve mental fatigue and to address head injuries, such as concussion. Gotu kola is being investigated for its potential benefit in Alzheimer's Disease—among other actions supporting brain function, it seems to inhibit ß-amyloid plaque formation.[12] Additionally, it is the herb of choice for many indications including rheumatism, ulcers, leprosy, varicosities, and to normalize the metabolism of connective tissue. Both externally and internally, it is used to speed the healing of wounds, burns, ulcers, and to minimize scarring after surgery or accident. **Formats:** The properly dried plant may be made into an infusion or, better still, ingested freshly picked or preserved by tincturing or freeze-drying. Can be made into medicated ghee. Grow your own or look for organically cultivated herb as there is much poor-quality gotu kola in the marketplace. It is well suited for sowing in containers.

Bacopa [*Bacopa monniera*]: leaf and stem. Astringent, bitter, cooling. Nervine, neuro-protective, anxiolytic, mildly sedative, antioxidant, anti-inflammatory, antispasmodic, cardiotonic, analgesic, vulnerary, bronchiodilating. Like gotu kola, bacopa is a potassium-rich, water-loving plant—and considered rasayana in Ayurvedic medicine. Both *Bacopa* and *Centella* are sometimes referred to as *Brahmi*. Used to enhance memory, focus and improve sleep; it helps reduce anxiety and nervous exhaustion. Bacopa is mildly anticonvulsant and is used in the treatment of trauma to the head. It has been shown to have a significant effect in the retention of new information[4] and shown to slow the progression of neurodegenerative process. Significantly, Bacopa has been shown to be brain-protective in those taking pharmaceutical anti-seizure medications, such as phenytoin—helping to alleviate drug-related "brain fog" without affecting the drug's anticonvulsant activity.[5] **Formats**: Tea, tincture, capsules of standardized extract. As with gotu kola, it is key to use only organically cultivated herb, as the plant readily absorbs toxins in its environment.

Schisandra [*Schisandra chinensis*]: fruit. "Five tastes fruit": Possesses the five flavors sweet, sour, acrid-bitter, salty—though its dominant tastes are sour and salty, with an overall warm, dry energy. Considered a harmonizing remedy in Asian medicine. Tonic and restorative, nervine, adaptogenic; antioxidant, anti-inflammatory, astringent; liver protective and regenerative. Enhances detoxification. Cardioprotective, antitussive. Schisandra exerts a normalizing influence on blood pressure. Mildly stimulating to nerve tissue, schisandra does not overexcite—it enhances cognitive function and reflexes while also calming the nervous system and soothing anxiety. Used to promote restful sleep, enhance memory, lighten depression, calm palpitations and stress-induced asthma. According to herbalist David Winston, scientists in S. Korea have speculated that schisandra might benefit people with Alzheimer's. **Formats:** Light decoction/infusion, tincture, extract, or capsules. ***Please note***: Schisandra may influence the way the liver metabolizes drugs, therefore avoid concurrent use with pharmaceuticals. Avoid during pregnancy—may stimulate uterine contractions. Traditional Chinese botanical medicine cautions against its use in cases of excess heat in the interior or where an exterior disorder such as rash is lingering. May occasionally cause heartburn in susceptible individuals.

Holy Basil, Sacred Basil [*Ocimum sanctum aka O. tenuiflorum*]: leaf. Aka Tulsi, Tulasi. Pungent, heating. Adaptogenic, nervine, neuroprotective, antispasmodic, antibacterial, antiseptic, anti-inflammatory, antioxidant, diaphoretic, febrifuge. Supports normal cortisol and blood sugar levels. Helps relieve anxiety, mental confusion, inability to focus. Demonstrates significant protection against ionizing radiation.[15,18] In India, it is thought that devotion to this plant cultivates states of higher consciousness. In Ayurvedic medicine, Tulsi is utilized to purify and stabilize the mind, emotions and body—opening the heart and awareness, strengthening clarity and compassion. Recent research has shown that holy basil has adaptogenic properties, enhancing adrenal function and improving the body/mind's response to stress. Studies on patients in India have found that holy basil prevents stress-related conditions such as peptic ulcers, colitis, asthma, and hypertension. It has been used, often in combination with calamus root, to revitalize the mind after a period of psychoactive drug habituation. **Formats:** The leaf tea is lovely, sometimes drunk with honey. Powdered herb or extract in capsules. Tincture. Fresh leaf juice applied topically on wounds or fungus. Tulsi stems are worn as beads around the neck for their protective and energy-clearing qualities. In India, Tulsi tea is often used for pregnant and lactating women as well as for children.

Rosemary [*Rosmarinus officinalis*]: leaf. Pungent/bitter, warm. Nervine with affinities for digestion, cardiovascular, liver. Anti-bacterial, astringent, carminative, circulatory and nervine stimulant, anti-inflammatory. choleretic. A key constituent is rosmarinic acid, a potent antioxidant. A powerful preserver, this compound possesses neuroprotective, antimutagenic, radioprotective, anti-inflammatory, antibacterial, and antiviral properties. The complex chemistry of rosemary seems to prevent the breakdown of the neurotransmitter acetylcholine, thus explaining its storied acclaim as a memory tonic. Tones and calms digestion where psychological tension is present: dyspepsia, headache, depression. Other indications: Feeling dull after eating, especially mentally; tendency toward cold hands and feet and/or varicosities; forgetfulness, brain "fog." **Formats:** Tea, tincture [fresh or dried], essential oil. ***Please note***: The essential oil and concentrated extracts are generally contraindicated during pregnancy; limited use as a tea or culinary herb is not.

Other botanicals that have a role to play in supporting memory include sage [*Salvia officinalis*], kava [*Piper methysticum*], lavender [*Lavendula angustifolia, L. officinalis*] and the mushrooms lion's mane [*Hericum erinaceus*] and cordyceps [*Cordyceps sinensis*].

Though it is technically neither an adaptogen nor a nervine, we cannot omit the following herb in any discussion of memory and brain function:

Ginkgo [*Ginkgo biloba*]: leaf. Neutral. This deciduous tree has survived unchanged for about 150 million years and is able to endure persistent stress and pollutants; a ginkgo tree can live for a thousand years. Affinity for brain and circulation. The cognitive benefits are most observable when decline has been noted, particularly in elders. Inhibits platelet aggregation. Increases tissue oxygenation. Antioxidant, neuroprotective, vasotonic and circulatory stimulant, anti-inflammatory, antispasmodic, anti-allergenic, anti-asthmatic. Indications: Cerebral insufficiency [memory loss, dementia, lack of concentration, dizziness, tinnitis, headache, mood challenges, etc.], asthma, peripheral vascular issues. **Formats**: Tincture, standardized extract. The extract used for clinical response is standardized to contain 24% flavonoid glycosides or more and 6% terpenoids. ***Please note***: Gingko as concentrated extract may potentiate pharmaceutical MAO-inhibitors. Use with caution in combination with anticoagulant or anti-platelet medications, including aspirin. Ginkgo extract is generally avoided for 2-3 weeks preceding surgery. Such potential risks may be overstated; "careful individual assessment and monitoring, with case-by-case therapeutic choices, remain the best practice."[17]

[1] From *Shen Nong Ben Cao Jing* compiled around the 1st century C.E.

[2] Based originally on Soviet-era Russian research and documentation.

[3] Hillhouse, BJ *et al*. Acetylcholine Esterase Inhibitors in *Rhodiola rosea*. *Pharmaceutical Biology* 42(1):68-72,2004. Study authors recommended research into its potential treating disorders such as Alzheimer's disease.

[4] Roodenrys S *et al*. Chronic Effects of Brahmi (*Bacopa monnieri*) on Human Memory. *Neuropsychopharmacology* 27:279-281,2002.

[5] Vohora D, Pal SN, Pillai KK. Protection from phenytoin-induced cognitive deficit by *Bacopa monniera*, a reputed Indian nootropic plant. *J Ethnopharmacology*, 2000 Aug;71(3):383-90. Effect noted within one week of using standardized extract daily.

[6] Bone, Kerry. *Clinical Applications of Ayurvedic and Chinese Herbs* [Queensland, Australia: Phytotherapy Press, 1996]

[7] Chen, John K and Chen,Tina T. *Chinese Medical Herbology and Pharmacology* [City of Industry, CA: Art of Medicine Press, 2004]

[8] Frawley, David. *Ayurveda and the Mind: The Healing of Consciousness* [Twin Lakes, WI: Lotus Press, 1996]

[9] Frawley, David and Lad, Vasant. *The Yoga of Herbs: An Ayurvedic Guide to Herbal Medicine* [Twin Lakes, WI: Lotus Press, 1986]

[10] Maciocia, Giovanni. *The Foundations of Chinese Medicine* [London: Churchill Livingstone, 1989]

[11] McGuffin, Michael *et al*, editors. *Botanical Safety Handbook* [Boca Raton, FL: CRC Press, 1997]

[12] Pizzorno, Joseph and Murray, Michael. *Textbook of Natural Medicine 4th edition* [St. Louis, MO: Elsevier/Churchill Livingstone, 2013]

[13] Powell, Martin. *Medicinal Mushrooms: A Clinical Guide* [East Sussex, UK: Mycology Press, 2010]

[14] Rogers, Robert. *The Fungal Pharmacy* [Berkeley, CA: North Atlantic Books, 2011]

[15] Singh, Narendra and Hoette, Yamuna with Ralph Miller. *Tulsi: The Mother Medicine of Nature* [Lucknow, India: International Institute of Herbal Medicine, 2002]

[16] Stamets, Paul with C Dusty Wu Yao. *MycoMedicinals* [Olympia, WA: MycoMedia Productions, 2002, 3rd edition]

[17] Stargrove M, Treasure J, McKee DL. *Herb, Nutrient, and Drug Interactions* [St. Louis, MO: Mosby/Elsevier, 2008]

[18] Williamson, Elizabeth M. *Major Herbs of Ayurveda* [London: Churchill Livingstone, 2002]

[19] Winston, David and Maimes, Steven. *Adaptogens: Herbs for Strength, Stamina, and Stress Relief* [Rochester, VT: Healing Arts Press, 2007]

Food Combining Strategies

There is no single way to approach healthful eating. What works for one person might not work for another—on an assortment of levels. Often, those with sensitive digestion find that they need to be more mindful of how, what and when they eat. The guidelines that follow are presented as an offering for your experimentation. This approach is suggested by a number of holistic nutritionists as a way of simplifying the demands placed on the digestive tract at any one time. Try the strategy as stated, make note of how you feel, experiment. Listen to your body and trust what you learn.

May your food nourish you and strengthen you and energize the work you are here to do.

1. **Eat fruits alone and on an empty stomach**.

2. **Eat protein foods with non-starchy and/or sea vegetables**.

3. **Eat grains and starchy vegetables with non-starchy and/or sea vegetables**.

Minding the Breath

Breath Awareness

For caregivers, especially…

Make sure that you're breathing deeply, at least once in a while. Life and its circumstances can cause us to almost hold our breath, as if waiting for the other shoe to drop. When we check in with our breathing, we can discover this shallow breathing pattern…or rapid breathing that's fueled by stress hormones. Whatever its quality, noticing our breath and deliberately shifting into a more calming pattern can be profound for our experience of body and mind.

Use common sounds, such as a ringing telephone, someone calling you by name, birdsong, a dog barking, and so on—or common sights, such as red traffic lights while driving to prompt you to check your breathing. At any of the cues you have chosen, stop everything for a moment, tune into your body, and breathe deeply through your nose allowing your belly gently to expand. Do this slowly and consciously five times, softening your belly and filling your torso with life-giving breath as you do so. With each exhalation, feel the breath cleansing you—relaxing and lightening your whole being. With practice, you will bring attention more frequently to the presence of the breath.

Rhythmic Breath

Find a quiet place to sit down, with your feet flat on the floor, spine straight, and head facing forward. Relax hands in your lap or on the top of your thighs, whichever feels more natural. Before beginning the exercise, take a few full breaths and relax your shoulders and jaw, stretch your hands, and open the whole of your body.

Begin by taking in a full breath through your nose to a slow count of five. Once you've reached five, exhale through your nose to the count of 10, at the same pace. This isn't about straining your breath; just allow yourself to find a gentle rhythm with the counting.

This technique can also incorporate sound. While exhaling to the count of 10, place the tip of your tongue on the roof of your mouth, just behind your teeth, and hum until your exhale is complete. Your teeth, face, and the top of your head will vibrate as you're sounding. If that doesn't happen, move your tongue around until you can feel the vibration.

There is no pause in this breath—experience it as a circular wave. As soon as you've counted to five, begin to exhale. And once you reach 10 on the outbreath, begin to inhale again. Repeat this cycle 10 times. Stop or slow down at any point if you feel lightheaded or dizzy. Track the cycles using your fingers, if you like.

Resources

This table offers quick access to select sources of desired products. These are certainly not the only quality sources for these products in the marketplace, but they will point you in a good direction. Company names may be abbreviated in the chart. Details for each manufacturer are in the annotated listing that follows.

PRODUCT	SUPPLIER
Agar agar	Eden Foods, Mountain Rose
***Arnica montana*, homeopathic—internal and topical gels**	Boiron, Heel, Hylands, Topricin [formula]
***Arnica montana* oil**	Gaia, Herbalist & Alchemist, HerbPharm, Life-flo, Mountain Rose, Wise Woman
Arrowroot powder	Mountain Rose
Ayurvedic herbs/formulas	Ayush, Banyan, Planetary, Tattva's
B vitamins, sublingual	Source Naturals
Baby food, organic	Earth's Best, Happy Family, Plum Organics, Yummy Spoonfuls
Baby wipes	Natracare
Bee products	YS Organic Bee Farm
Betonite clay	Mountain Rose, Uncle Harry's
Biofeedback devices/programs	HeartMath, Wild Divine
Bitter digestive tonics	Gaia, Herbalist & Alchemist, HerbPharm, Wise Woman, Planetary
Blackberry root extract	Herbalist & Alchemist
Black cumin seed oil	Mountain Rose
Calendula succus	Wise Woman Herbals
Carob bean powder	Mountain Rose
Castor oil	Heritage Store
Ceremonial plants	Herbalist & Alchemist, Mountain Rose
Charcoal, activated	Source Naturals, Uncle Harry's
Chinese herbs/formulas	Health Concerns, Imperial Elixir, Mayway, Planetary, Pure Essence
Chlorophyll	Herbs Etc.
Chyawanprash	Ayush [AmlaPlex], Banyan, Tattva's
Coconut oil	Barleans, Garden of Life, Life-flo, Nutiva
Corydalis	Mayway, Natura
Diaper rash balm	Motherlove, Weleda
DGL [deglycyrrhizinated licorice]	Enzymatic, Planetary, Source Naturals

PRODUCT	SUPPLIER
D-Mannose	NOW, Source Naturals
Eggwhite protein	NOW Foods
Enzymes	Enzymedica, Flora, Garden of Life, Jarrow, Source Naturals
Essential oils	Simplers, Veriditas
Essential oils, in capsules	Europharma, Enzymatic, Now, Planetary
Essiac-like variations	Flora, Gaia, Herbs Etc., Mountain Rose
Fish oils	Barleans, New Chapter, Nordic Naturals
Flower essences	Flower Essence Services, Healing Herbs
Glutamine powder	NOW, ProHealth, Source Naturals
Goldenseal powder	Mountain Rose, Oregon's Wild Harvest
Greens / fruit powders	Barlean's, Eclectic, Garden of Life, HealthForce, Pure Planet, Source Naturals
Hair / scalp tonics	Banyan, Mountain Rose, Tattva's, Uncle Harry's, Weleda
Herb extracts—single, liquid	Eclectic, Gaia, Herbalist & Alchemist, HerbPharm, Herbs Etc., Wise Woman
Herb extracts—single, in capsules	Eclectic, EcoNugenics, Gaia, HerbPharm, Imperial Elixir, New Chapter, NOW, Oregon's Wild Harvest, Planetary
Herb extracts, solid	Gaia, Herbalist & Alchemist, Wise Woman
Herb oils, infused	Banyan, Gaia, Herbalist & Alchemist, HerbPharm, Tattva's, Wild Carrot, Wise Woman
Herb powders, in capsules	Eclectic, Main Coast Sea Vegetables, Oregon's Wild Harvest
Herb powders, bulk	Ayush, Banyan, Mayway, Mountain Rose, Oregon's Wild Harvest, Tattva's
Herb formulations	EcoNugenics, Enzymatic Therapy, Flora, Gaia, Herbalist & Alchemist, Herbs Etc., HerbPharm, MegaFood, Natura, New Chapter, Pure Essence, NOW, Wise Woman
Homeopathic remedies	Boiron, Heel, Hylands, Liddell, Similasan
Hoxsey-like alterative formulas	Gaia, Herbalist & Alchemist, HerbPharm
Hyaluronic acid and lozenges	Hyalogics
Hydrosols, rose or lavender	Simpler's, Veriditas
Incontinence pads	NatraCare
Iron, plant-based	Flora, Gaia, MegaFood
Iron, heme	Europharma

PRODUCT	SUPPLIER
Kudzu root starch	Eden Foods
Licorice solid extract	Wise Woman
Lip balms	Weleda, Wild Carrot, many natural brands
Lysine, topical	Planetary, Wise Woman Herbals
Manuka honey	YS Organic Bee Farms
Marrow Plus	Health Concerns [Natura has version of this]
Medicinal mushrooms	Fungi Perfecti, Health Concerns, Mushroom Science, New Chapter, Planetary
Mineral powders	NOW, Pure Essence, Source Naturals
Mineral liquids	Flora, Gaia, Pure Planet, Source Naturals
Modified citrus pectin	EcoNugenics, NOW, Source Naturals
Mouth rinses and sprays, herbal/otherwise	Herbalist & Alchemist, HerbPharm, Herbs Etc., Heritage Store, Hyalogic, Thayer's, Uncle Harry's, YS Organic Bee Farms
Multivitamins	MegaFood, New Chapter, NOW, Pure Essence, Source Naturals
Myrrh gum powder	Mountain Rose, Oregon's Wild Harvest
Neem oil	Banyan, Tattva's, NOW
Neti pots	Banyan, Himalayan Institute
Nutrients, single	Jarrow, MegaFood, NOW, Source Naturals
Oils, essential	Simpler's, Veriditas
Oils, infused	Banyan, Gaia, Herbalist & Alchemist, HerbPharm, Tattva's, Wild Carrot, Wise Woman
Oils, pressed [nut/seed]	Flora, NOW, Mountain Rose
Oregon grape root, powder	Mountain Rose, Oregon's Wild Harvest
Powdered fruits/vegetables	Barlean's, Eclectic, Garden of Life, HealthForce, MegaFood, Mountain Rose, Pure Planet
Probiotics	Flora, Garden of Life, Jarrow, NOW
Propolis	Gaia, Herbalist & Alchemist, HerbPharm, Wise Woman, YS Organic Bee Farm
Protein powders	Garden of Life, HealthForce, NOW, Nutiva
Rosehip seed oil	Life-Flo, Mountain Rose, NOW
Royal jelly	Imperial Elixir, YS Organic Bee Farm
Saccharomyces boulardii	Jarrow, NOW
Salves, herbal healing	FES, Gaia, Herbalist & Alchemist, HerbPharm, Hyalogic, Wild Carrot, Wild Woman

PRODUCT	SUPPLIER
Seabuckthorn oil, topical	Life-Flo, Mountain Rose, Weleda, Wild Carrot [soap]
Seabuckthorn oil, internal	Eclectic, Europharma, New Chapter
Seaweeds	Island Herbs, Maine Coast Sea Vegetables, Maine Seaweed, Modifilan, Pure Planet
Silica, horsetail-sourced	Europharma, Flora; bulk herb: Mountain Rose, Oregon's Wild Harvest
Silver hydrosol	Sovereign Silver/Natural-Immunogenics
Slippery elm	Mountain Rose, Oregon's Wild Harvest, Planetary [lozenges], Thayers [lozenges/sprays]
St. Johnswort oil	Gaia, Herbalist & Alchemist, HerbPharm, Mountain Rose, Wise Woman
Sulfur powder	Heritage Store
Sulfur soap	Enzymatic Therapy, Heritage Store
Suppositories—rectal, vaginal	Wise Woman Herbals
Tongue scraper	Banyan, Uncle Harry's
Triphala	Ayush, Banyan, Planetary Herbals, Tattva's
Turmeric, bio-available	EcoNugenics, Europharma, Gaia, Jarrow, New Chapter, Tattva's
Vitamin E oil, dropper bottle	Freeda, Life-flo, NOW
Whey protein formulas	Natura, ProHealth
Whey protein isolate	NOW
Zinc [without copper]	MegaFood
Zinc lozenges	Source Naturals

The Suppliers

Numerous reputable growers, suppliers, medicine makers, and manufacturers are listed here. This is certainly not all-inclusive, simply a starting point to help you access what you are looking for in a time-sparing way.

Although contact information is given—and some products can *only* be purchased directly—most sell via bricks-and-mortar retailers. Please consider purchasing or ordering through your local health food store or herb shop, if at all possible. In this way, we can help support community health and well-being in addition to our own. Most of the company websites offer a wealth of information—providing background on their missions, quality commitments, and specific product details.

The list is broken out to highlight certain categories of suppliers. Suppliers are listed alphabetically within sections. *Please note*: I have no financial interest in any of these companies; I simply appreciate what they have to offer.

Hand-Harvested Sea Vegetables, aka Seaweeds

These are all small businesses, run by premier North American seaweed wildcrafters—those respected teachers from whom other herbalists and natural healers often first become intimate with these amazing healing plants.

Island Herbs—Ryan Drum. Sustainably wildharvested by hand. Seaweeds in bulk. Address: PO Box 25, Waldron Island, WA 98297-0025. Online: www.ryandrum.com.

Maine Coast Sea Vegetables—Linnette and Shep Erhart. Seaweeds in bulk, capsules, sprinkles, snacks. Sustainably wildharvested by hand and certified organic. Address: 3 George's Pond Rd., Franklin, ME 04634. Phone: 207-565-2907. Online: www.seaveg.com.

Maine Seaweed—Larch Hanson. Seaweeds in bulk. Sustainably wildharvested by hand. Address: PO Box 57, Steuben, ME 04680. Phone: 207-546-2875. Online: www.theseaweedman.com.

Strictly Herbal Preparations / Bulk Herbs

At the time of this writing, most of these companies are owned and run by highly respected herbalists or other natural health practitioners. Those designated with an asterisk [*] produce the majority of their products from plants grown on their own organically certified herb farms. Most also use certified organic alcohol in their water/alcohol-extracted preparations.

Eclectic Institute*—Ed Alstat, ND. Specializing in freshly freeze-dried organic herbs in capsules or loose-powder form. Capsules: e.g. cornsilk, cranberry, nettles, dandelion leaf and root, ginger, hawthorn, yellow dock, broccoli sprouts, wasabi, hops, oats, passionflower, more. Wide selection of individual or combination powders to easily add concentrated nutrition to water or smoothies: e.g. Black Raspberry, Beets, Celery, Kale, Lemon Greens, Mushroom Espresso, Nettles, Nutrigenomic Berry, etc. Source of Larix, in liquid or capsules. Liquid extracts made with organic alcohol or glycerine. Children's line. Address: 36350 SE Industrial Way, Sandy, OR 97055. Phone: 800-332-4372; 503-668-4120. Online: www.eclecticherb.com.

Gaia Herbs*—Rick Scalzo, herbalist. Wide selection of single herbs and formulas as both liquid extracts and in liquid phytocaps: Ashwagandha, astragalus, black elderberry, cinnamon bark, cranberry concentrate, eleuthero, Asian ginseng, green tea, hibiscus, holy basil, kava kava, milk thistle, olive leaf, passionflower, rhodiola, St. Johnswort, etc. Herbal infused oils, salves, hawthorn solid extract, liquid plant-based iron, Hoxsey Red Clover Supreme, children's line. Address: 101 Gaia Herbs Dr, Brevard, NC 28712. Phone: 800-831-7780. Online: www.gaiaherbs.com.

Herbalist & Alchemist*—David Winston, herbalist. Extensive selection of single plant liquid extracts, including many not generally available—e.g. blackberry root bark. Formulations [DW's Alterative Compound, etc.], glycerites [alcohol-free]. Salves, infused oils [including poke root, hypericum, thuja], solid extracts [blueberry, cranberry/blueberry, elderberry, hawthorn, pomegranate/goji]. Immune Adapt capsules. Children's line. Ceremonial plants for clearing. Address: 51 South Wandling Ave, Washington, NJ 07882. Phone: 908-689-9020. Online: www.herbalist-alchemist.com. I ever honor David as one of my foundational teachers of plant medicine.

Herbs Etc.—Daniel Gagnon, herbalist. Chloroxygen concentrated chlorophyll [liquid and caps]. *Herbs Etc.* manufacturers what I consider to be the finest chlorophyll concentrate available in the herbal marketplace. Sourced from stinging nettles [*Urtica dioica*], their **ChlorOxygen** needs no refrigeration, and has a simple water/glycerine base. Available in three forms: original, with peppermint and spearmint essential oils, or in gelcaps; Lymphatonic [caps]; Essiac formula in capsules; wide assortment of high quality herbal formulations in non-alcohol formats. Address: 1345 Cerrillos Rd, Santa Fe, NM 87505. Phone: 888-694-3727. Online: www.herbsetc.com.

HerbPharm*—Ed Smith, Sara Katz, herbalists. Pioneer botanical extract company. Wide selection of single-herb liquid extracts [e.g. propolis, dragon's blood, lemon balm, skullcap, Oregon grape, passionflower, hops, usnea, yellow dock, spilanthes, andrographis, cleavers, and dozens more], formulas [Herbal Detox, etc.], glycerites [alcohol-free], herbal oils and salves, herbal extracts in capsules [e.g. Super Echinacea, Anxiety Soother, eleuthero, Asian ginseng, kava, milk thistle, rhodiola, St. Johnswort, etc.]. Address: P.O. Box 116, Williams, OR 97544. Phone: 800-348-4372; 541-846-6262. Online: www.herb-pharm.com.

Mountain Rose Herbs—Certified organic bulk herbs and herb powders, fixed oils, herbal oils, salts, waxes, bottles and jars. Betonite clay, agar-agar, arrowroot powder, carob powder, black cumin seed oil [*Nigella*], Oregon grape root/goldenseal powder, slippery elm powder, sliced reishi, jojoba oil, more. Address: P.O. Box 50220, Eugene, OR 97405. Phone: 800-879-3337. Online: www.mountainroseherbs.com.

Oregon's Wild Harvest*—Pamela Martin-Buresh, Randy Buresh. Farm also Demeter® Certified Biodynamic. Bulk herbs [slippery elm powder, Oregon grape/goldenseal powder, ; wide selection of capsules [e.g. American ginseng, ashwagandha, astragalus, bladderwrack, burdock, cascara sagrada, chaste tree, true cinnamon, dandelion root, Eleuthero, ginger, gymnema, hawthorn, holy basil, kava, slippery elm, stinging nettles, Oregon grape, schisandra, wormwood, etc.]. Small children's line. Address: 39831 Hywy 26, Sandy, OR 97055. Phone: 800-316-6869; 503-668-7713. Online: www.oregonswildharvest.com.

Wise Woman Herbals*—Suppositories, hemorrhoid salve [Bottoms Up Balm], Calendula Succus, Licorice Lysine Plus [topical goo], Licorice Solid Extract [other solids: Eleuthero, hawthorn, mixed berry, rosehips, green tea, passionflower], botanical oils, salves including the antifungal Tea Tree Salve, UTI Formula, syrups, Essiance Elixir, G.I. Capsules [aka Robert's Formula], assortment of herbal glycerites, and more…Address: P.O. Box 279, Creswell, OR 97426. Phone: 541-895-5172. Online: www.wisewomanherbals.com.

Other Manufacturers and Suppliers

Companies that exclusively produce Ayurvedic products, medicinal mushrooms, essential oils, homeopathic remedies, enzymes, and flower essences are listed later in their own separate sections.

Barleans*—Dedicated to organic cultivation and non-GMO supply. Flax oils and ground seed, fish oils, greens powders, extra-virgin coconut oil [fair-trade], evening primrose oil, borage oil, chia seeds, etc. Address: 800-445-3529; 360-384-0485. Online: www.barleans.com.

EcoNugenics*—Isaac Eliaz, MD, MS, LAc. Clinical-grade products: Modified citrus pectin [PectaSol], honokiol [magnolia bark extract], detoxification formulas, metabolic support formulas, immunity, etc. Address: 396 Tesconi Ct, Santa Rosa, CA 95401. Phone: 800-308-5518, 707-521-3370. Online: www.econugenics.com.

Eden Foods*—Large assortment of foods: Organic kudzu root starch, umeboshi paste and whole plums, ume plum balls and concentrate, tekka miso condiment [carrots, burdock root, lotus root, sesame oil, hacho miso], organic seeds and nuts, much more. Address: 701 Tecumseh Rd, Clinton, MI 49236. Phone: 888-424-3336. Online: www.edenfoods.com.

Enzymatic Therapy*—Numerous iterations of DGL [deglycyrrhizinated licorice], enteric-coated peppermint oil, IP6 and inositol formulas, Petadolex [Butterbur/*Petasites*], asparagus extract, Better Bladder [pumpkin seed extract], Yeast Balance, Laxative-3

Blend [magnesium and non-habituating herbs], Derma-Klear sulfur soap, etc. Address: 825 Challenger Dr, Green Bay, WI 54311. Phone: 800-783-2286. Online: www.enzymatictherapy.com.

Europharma—Numerous high quality products, some imported from Europe. CuraMed [BCM® curcumin: well-studied, highly absorbable form of turmeric. One 750-mg softgel equivalent to 10 500-mg caps of curcumin 95%.]; anti-inflammatory, analgesic Curamin; DGL; Hair Renew; Healthy Feet and Nerves; Liver Fractions [heme iron in caps]; black currant seed oil; silica; sea buckthorn oil caps; strontium; tri-iodine; numerous specialized formulas for bone, bladder, brain, gut, thyroid health, etc. Some essential oil formulas in caps for internal use. Address: 955 Challenger Dr, Green Bay, WI 54311. Phone: 866-598-5487; 920-406-6500. Online: www.europharmausa.com.

Flora—Numerous high quality products, primarily in glass bottles, some imported from Europe. FlorEssence detoxification formula; enzymes; probiotics [including oral-specific]; certified organic flaxseed oil, pumpkin seed oil, sesame oil; liquid food-based minerals [calcium, magnesium, iron]; multiple grades of manuka honey; FloraLax bulking laxative blend [organic flaxseeds, oatbran, and psyllium seed husks]; silica, more. Address: 805 East Badger Rd, Lynden, WA 98264. Phone: 800-446-2110. Online: www.florahealth.com.

Garden of Life—Emphasis on organically certified, non-GMO foods and supplements. Probiotics [Primal Defense, five-day intensive, etc.]; enzymes; Superseed [sprouted grains, seeds and legumes]; extensive line of supplementary protein formulas [including goat milk protein], greens, and fruit formulas; flax and chia seeds; immune support; extra-virgin coconut oil; omega fatty acids; wholefood nutritional bars; multivitamins, more. Address: 5500 Village Blvd, Suite 202, West Palm Beach, FL 33407. Phone: 866-465-0051. Online: www.gardenoflife.com.

Health Concerns—Andrew Gaeddert, herbalist. Offers practitioner lines based on traditional Chinese herbal formulas. Marrow Plus, Astra 8, Power Mushrooms, GB-6, Schisandra Dreams, etc. Address: 8001 Capwell Dr, Oakland, CA 94621. Phone: 800-233-9355; 510-639-0280. Online: www.healthconcerns.com.

HealthForce Nutritionals—Offers extensive line of nutrient-dense powders: green blends, raw fruit juices, protein formulas, spirulina, chlorella, and other foods. Flagship product: VitaMineral Green. Address: 1835A S Centre City Pkwy #411, Escondido, CA 92025-6504. Phone: 800-357-2717; 760-747-8822. Online: www.healthforce.com.

Hyalogic—High molecular weight hyaluronic acid products. Pure HA, plus products for dental hygiene, lip and skin support, lozenges, eye health. Address: 610 NW Platte Valley Dr, Riverside, MO 64150. Phone: 866-318-8484; 913-422-9395. Online: www.hyalogic.com.

Imperial Elixir Products—Ginco International. All products made from quality *whole* roots; *Panax* spp. products made from six-year-old roots. Capsules: e.g. royal jelly [two strengths], Siberian Eleuthero [5:1 or 10:1 extracts], American ginseng, Asian ginseng,

Tienchi ginseng [from Yunnan Province], etc. Address: 725 Cochran St, Unit C, Simi Valley, CA 93065. Phone: 800-284-2598. Online: www.gincointernational.com.

Jarrow—Quality line of many single and compound nutrients: bile acid factors, probiotics [including vaginal-specific], *Saccharomyces boulardii*, antioxidants, ubiqinol, enzymes, bone health, joint health, much more. Address: 1824 South Robertson Blvd, Los Angeles, CA 90035-4317. Phone: 800-726-0886. Online: www.jarrow.com.

Life-flo—Emphasizing certified organic [not all products], cruelty-free, paraben-free bodycare products: Magnesium oil, seabuckthorn oil, rosehip seed oil, calendula oil, an array of nut and seed oils, betonite clay, etc. Address: Phoenix, AZ 85029. Phone: 800-258-8337. Online: www.life-flo.com.

Mayway—Purveyors of traditional Chinese patent medicines such as Curing Pills, Calm Stomach, Great Corydalis, etc. Their own Plum Flower line, plus other a few other manufacturers. Sulfur-free bulk herbs, tested for heavy metals and other contaminants: *Corydalis, He shou wu, Poria cocos* [Fu ling], etc. Address: 1338 Mandela Parkway, Oakland, CA 94607. Phone: 800-262-9929; 510-208-3113. Online: www.mayway.com.

MegaFood—High quality food-sourced supplemental nutrients and formulas: Zinc, selenium, iron, chromium, multivitamins. Address: 8 Bowers Rd, Derry, NH 03038. Phone: 800-848-2542. Online: www.megafood.com.

Modifilan—Alginate-rich detoxifying product extracted from *Laminaria*, a brown seaweed harvested from the north Atlantic Ocean [40 lb. raw *Laminaria* = 1 lb. Modifilan]. Address: PO Box 2606, Kirkland, WA 98083-2606. Phone: 866-434-4039; 206-274-0008. Online: www.modifilan-seaweed-extract.com.

Natura Health Products—Donald Yance, MH, CN, RH (AHG). Yance is an herbalist's herbalist, a clinically focused master teacher. He is the founder of the Mederi Centre for Natural Healing in Ashland, OR [clinic: 541-488-3133]. Much of his Natura line is only sold through practitioners, while some formulas are available to the general public. These are exceptional formulations that combine cutting-edge botanical knowledge with ancient principles for supporting optimal health. Beyond Whey, ImmuneCare, Vital Adapt, Power Adapt, Cell Guardian, Inflammaway, etc. Address: 125 Clear Creek Dr, Ashland, OR 97520. Phone: 888-628-8720; 541-488-0210. Online: www.naturahealthproducts.com.

Natural-Immunogenics—Sovereign Silver brand [colloidal] silver hydrosol: high quality, well-tested product. See website for wealth of background information. Address: 3265 W. McNab Rd, Pompano, FL 33069. Phone: 888-328-8840. Online: www.natural-immunogenics.com.

New Chapter—High quality food-sourced supplemental nutrients and formulas: Non-GMO and certified organic. Multivitamins; CO_2-extracted individual herbs [holy basil, lemon balm, St. Johnswort, turmeric, ginger, rhodiola, sea buckthorn, cinnamon, etc.]; salmon oil; targeted formulas [including Tranquilnite to benefit sleep]; wild salmon-sourced fish oil; medicinal mushrooms, more. Address: 90 Technology Dr, Brattleboro, VT 05301. Phone: 800-543-7279. Online: www.newchapter.com.

NOW Foods—Huge selection of high-quality nutritional supplements: Non-GMO lecithin granules; micro-filtered whey protein concentrate powder, egg white powder; modified citrus pectin; CoQ10 [Ubiquinol]; amino acids [L-carnosine, L-lysine, L-glutamine, acetyl-L-carnitine, L-tyrosine, L-tryptophan, etc.]; D-mannose; vitamin D3; lutein, astaxanthin, rutin; *Saccharomyces boulardii*; grapeseed extract; oils, foods, much more. Address: West—575 Vista Blvd, Sparks, NV 89434; Midwest—395 S. Glen Ellyn Rd, Bloomingdale, IL 60108. Phone: 888-669-3663. Online: www.nowfoods.com.

Nutiva—Premium non-GMO and certified organic products. Extra-virgin coconut oil [fair trade], pureed coconut butter ["Manna"], coconut flour, hempseed and protein, chia seeds, red palm oil, etc. Address: 213 West Cutting Blvd, Richmond, CA 94804. Phone: 800-993-4367. Online: www.nutiva.com.

Planetary Herbals—Michael Tierra, Roy Upton. Herbalist-run supplier of Ayurvedic and traditional Chinese tonic herbs and formulations—in tabs and liquids. Triphala, holy basil, Coleus forskohlii, amla, ashwagandha, bacopa, codonopsis, DGL, dong quai, forskohlii, ginseng, guggul, loquat syrup, lysine lip balm, medicinal mushrooms, Myelin Sheath Support, oil of oregano, pumpkin seed oil, schisandra, stevia liquid, wasabi, much more. Address: PO Box 1760, Soquel, CA 95073. Phone: 800-606-6226; 831-438-1700. Online: www.planetaryherbals.com.

ProHealth—Wide selection of single nutrients and formulations. Glutamine powders, immune formula powders, thymus glandular, ubiqinol, high-dose vitamin D3, much more. Extensive focus on nutrients for fibromyalgia and chronic fatigue syndrome. Address: 2040 Alameda Padre Serra, Santa Barbara, CA 93103. Phone: 800-366-6056. Online: www.prohealth.com.

Pure Essence—Jery Cochern. Cochern originated the concept of food-based nutritional supplements when he previously founded pioneer-brand Rainbow Light. Pure Essence formulas are based on a synthesis of Western herbal understanding and traditional eastern tonic formulating principles. Well-designed formulas to support liver function, energy, brain health, eye/vision, stress/mood, joints and bones, more. Address: PO Box 95397, Las Vegas, NV 89193. Phone: 888-254-8000. Online: www.pureessencelabs.com.

Pure Planet—Spirulina, chlorella, red marine algae, liquid trace minerals, aloe concentrate, organic carrot juice powder, tart cherry concentrate, more. Address: 1542 Seabright Ave, Long Beach, CA 90813. Phone: 562-951-1124. Online: www.pureplanet.com.

Source Naturals—Huge selection of high-quality nutritional supplements: CoQ10 [Ubiquinol]; alpha-lipoic acid, R-lipoic acid; sublingual B vitamins; pine bark extract, amino acids [L-lysine, L-tryptophan, L-theanine, L-glutamine, etc.]; FOS; propolis in capsules; zinc lozenges and sprays; chlorella, spirulina, much more. Address: 23 Janis

Way, Scotts Valley, CA 95066. Phone: 800-815-2333; 831-438-1144. Online: www.sourcenaturals.com.

Thayers—Slippery elm lozenges in several flavors. Dry mouth sprays and lozenges. Witch hazel products. Address: P.O. Box 56, Westport, CT 06881. Phone: 888-842-9371. Online: www.thayers.com.

Topical BioMedics—Producers of homeopathic **Topricin** pain-relieving creams and lotions. Three formulas. Original Topricin [joints, nerves, muscles]; foot therapy [neuropathy, *plantar fasciitis*, etc.]; children's formula. Free of parabens and petroleum. Address: 6565 Spring Brook Ave #207, Rhinebeck, NY 12572. Phone: 800-959-1007; 845-871-4900. Online: www.topricin.com.

Uncle Harry's—Assortment of eclectic products. Mouth care [spray breath freshener, mouthwashes, tooth powders, tongue cleaner; products for gum/canker sores, sensitive teeth]. Footcare [antifungal spray, heel salve, oatmeal/salt soaks]. Hair and scalp [oils, dry shampoo]. Bath [Epsom salts, detox bath—clay, sea salt, seaweed]. Raw Northwest honey. Activated charcoal powder. Address: 6975-176th Ave NE, Ste 360, Redmond, WA 98502. Phone: 866-781-0815; 425-558-4251. Online: www.uncleharrys.com.

Weleda—Some **especially gentle bodycare products**. A pioneering company, providing holistically conceived bodycare products—made from plants grown via organic and biodynamic methods. Inspired by the visionary philosophy of Dr. Rudolf Steiner. A full line of calendula-based babycare products, ideal for sensitive skin—Calendula diaper rash cream, soap, cream bath, bodywash, shampoo. Also richly nourishing Skin Food cream; gentle toothpastes [salt, plant gel, etc.]; rosemary conditioning hair and scalp oil; products based on sea buckthorn oil; lavender bath; much more. Address: 1 Bridge St, Suite 42, Irvington, NY 10533. Phone: 800-241-1030. Online: www.weleda.com.

Wild Carrot Herbals—Jody Berry, herbalist. Exquisite line of artisan-crafted products mainly sourced from organic family garden and wildcrafting. Selection of healing salves [turmeric, anti-fungal, hemorrhoids, sore muscle, general wound-healing support]; body lotions; massage oils; more. Address: PO Box 348, Enterprise, OR 97828. Phone: 800-988-4491; 541-263-5539. On-ine: www.wildcarrotherbals.com.

Y.S. Organic Bee Farms—Pioneers in certified organic beekeeping in North America. Royal jelly [fresh, in honey, in capsules], bee pollen, propolis, raw manuka honey, manuka honey + propolis lozenges, ginseng honey, more. Available only through distributors and quality natural health stores. Address: 2774 N 4351 Rd, Sheridan, IL 60551. Phone: 800-654-4593. Online: www.ysorganic.com.

Ayurvedic Herbs and Formulations

Ayush Herbs—Herbal formulations composed by practicing Ayurvedic and naturopathic doctors using certified organic herbs. Capsules and bulk powders of single herbs. Veterinary formulas, as well. Address: 2239 152nd Ave NE, Redmond, WA 98052. Phone: 800-925-1371; 425-637-1400. Online: www.ayush.com.

Banyan Botanicals—Certified organic Ayurvedic herbs and formulations in tablets, powders, and liquid extracts. Also hair/scalp oils, body oils, salves, neem soap, food oils, chyawanprash, tea blends, kitchari kits, tongue scraper, neti pots, books, more. Address: 6705 Eagle Rock Ave NE, Albuquerque, NM 87113. Phone: 800-953-6424; 541-488-9525. Online: www.banyanbotanicals.com.

Tattva's Herbs—Certified organic Ayurvedic herbs and supercritical [CO_2] extracts in capsule form; some bulk herb powders: Triphala [caps/powder], amla/amalaki, gotu kola, holy basil [tulsi/tulasi], ashwagandha [caps/powder], neem [caps and oil], ginger, bacopa, boswellia, turmeric, shilajit [moomiyo], mucuna. Also hair/scalp oils, body oils, chyawanprash, coconut oil, more. Address: 9634 Roosevelt Way NE, Seattle, WA 98115. Phone: 877-828-8824; 206-568-3169. Online: www.tattvasherbs.com.

Homeopathic Remedies

Boiron—Full line of classic homeopathic individual remedies in a range of dosages. Tiny pellets in familiar blue tubes. *Arnica montana, Arsenicum album, Belladonna, Chamomilla, Gelsemium sempervirens, Hypericum perforatum, Nux vomica, Symphytum officinale, etc.* Also, combination formulas. Plus classic Arnica gel for external application. Address: 6 Campus Blvd, Newtown Square, PA 19073. Phone: 800-264-7661. Online: www.boironusa.com.

Heel—Traumeel gel or tablets; homeopathic formulas for throat relief, mental focus, tension, detoxification kit, more. Address: 10421 Research Rd, SE, Albuquerque, NM 87123. Phone: 800-920-9203; 505-293-3843. Online: www.heelusa.com.

Hylands—Calms, Calms Forte; Restless Legs; Leg Cramps and Leg Cramps PM, much more. Address: Los Angeles, CA. Phone: 800-624-9659. Online: www.hylands.com.

Liddell Laboratories—Line of water-based remedies formulated by a homeopathic physician based on his 25 years of clinical practice. Products include: Anxiety, Appetite Increase, Back Pain/Sciatica, Bladder/UTI, Canker/Cold Sore, Detox line [EMFs, metals, chemicals], Herpes Simplex, Incontinence, Overwhelm, more. Address: 201 Apple Blvd, Woodbine, IA 51579. Phone: 800-460-7733. Online: www.liddell.net.

Similasan—High quality homeopathic eyedrops: Irritated Eye Relief [pink eye], Allergy Eye Relief, Dry Eye Relief, and other products. Children's line also. Address: 1805 Shea

Center Dr, Suite 270, Highlands Ranch, CO 80129. Phone: 800-240-9780. Online: www.similasannaturalremedies.com.

Medicinal Mushrooms

Fungi Perfecti—Paul Stamets, mycologist. Certified organic Host Defense line of freeze-dried mycelium/fruitbody extracts in both vegetarian capsules and liquids: Agaricon, chaga, cordyceps, coriolus/turkey tail, lion's mane, maitake, mesima, reishi, shiitake, combination formulas. Address: P.O. Box 7634, Olympia, WA 98507. Phone: 800-780-9126; 360-426-9292. Online: www.fungi.com.

Mushroom Science—Prepared from traditional hot water extractions primarily from mushroom fruiting bodies grown on wood. In vegetarian capsules: Agaricus, chaga, cordyceps, Coriolus PSP and PSK, lion's mane, maitake, Maitake Gold [liquid], reishi, shiitake, Tremella, Immune Builder blend. Same products sold to practitioners under alternate labeling as ***JHS Natural Products.*** Address: Eugene, OR. Phone: 888-283-6583; 541-344-8753. Online: www.mushroomscience.com.

Enzymes

Enzymedica—Wide assortment of well-formulated digestive enzyme products plus specialized formulas such as Acid Soothe, MucoStop, Natto-K [nattokinase], ViraStop, LypoGold [designed to aid in fat digestion], Candidase, etc. and the high-potency proteolytic enzyme blend SerraGold [serratiopeptidase aka serrapeptase]. Address: Venice, FL 34392. Phone: 888-918-1118, 941-505-5565. Online: www.enzymedica.com.

HCP Formulas—Manufacturers of Fibrenza, a formulation of 14 proteolytic enzymes—including serrapeptase and nattokinase—to provide systemic activity when taken away from food. Address: 2221 W Baseline Rd, Ste 101, Tempe, AZ 85283. Phone: 800-710-2585. Online: www.fibrenza.com.

Essential Oils

Simplers Botanicals—Therapeutic quality, certified organic essential oils and herbal extracts. In addition to an extensive line of essential oils, Simplers offers carrier oils such as argan oil, jojoba oil, rosehip oil as well as oils infused with healing plants [arnica, calendula, comfrey, St. Johnswort]; hydrosols. Address: Sebastopol, CA 95473. Phone: 800-229-2512. Online: www.shopsimplers.com.

Veriditas—Melissa Farris, herbalist and certified aromatherapist. Therapeutic quality, certified organic essential oils. Artisanal line of single oils, condition-specific formulations, hydrosols. Website is great source of use and safety guidelines for essential oil applications. Address: Wisconsin. Phone: 952-831-6776. Online: www.veriditasbotanicals.com

Flower Essences

*There are numerous wonderful flower essence lines, prepared from plants that flourish in various geographic regions and habitats—such as California, the southwest desert, Alaska, Columbia Gorge, vegetable- and rose-garden essences, and others. I encourage you to explore these lines as well. Those listed below provide ready access to the particular flower remedies noted in the **Flower Essences** chapter of this book.*

Flower Essence Services—Patricia Kaminski and Richard Katz. Premium flower essences, sprays, oils prepared in traditional manner, primarily from plants growing on FES's Terra Flora wildflower preserve and garden sanctuary [certified organic + Demeter biodynamic]. Address: PO Box 1769, Nevada City, CA 95959. Phone: 800-548-0075. Online: www.fesflowers.com. Great source of information on flower essences, their history and applications.

Healing Herbs—Julian Barnard. English flower essences prepared from the same plant species and according to methods used by pioneer Dr. Edward Bach in the 1930s. Distributed in North America by Flower Essence Services [see above]. Online: www.healingherbs.co.uk.

Miscellaneous Supplies

Heritage Store—Lots of useful products, many inspired by the Edgar Cayce readings: Cotton flannel for castor oil packs, organic and standard castor oil, Alka-Thyme mouth rinse, sulfur soap, baking soda bar soap, witch hazel bar soap, Sulflax Powder [sulfur and salts], fig syrup, black seed oil, Aura Smudge [spray with juniper and sage essential oils], and much more. Address: Virginia Beach, VA 23451. Phone: 800-862-2923. Online: www.heritagestore.com.

Natracare—**Baby wipes** made from certified organic cotton infused with organic essential oils to soothe tender bottoms. **Dry + Lite Incontinence Pads**: Pure cotton next to the skin, with no petroleum-derived absorbents or plastics. Award-winning company pioneering environmental ethics, with product line made from chlorine-free, biodegradable materials. Online: www.natracare.com.

BioFeedback Devices/Programs

HeartMath—An outgrowth of the non-profit Institute of HeartMath. Since 1991, the Institute has conducted research into the heart-brain connection in health and disease, and how emotions and thoughts influence physiology overall. The **EmWave2** is a portable, hand-held biofeedback device that translates pulse rate into visual and auditory cues—these help guide the user into a relaxed, meditative state. There are also computer-aided biofeedback programs available. Address: 14700 West Park Ave, Boulder Creek, CA 95006. Phone: 800-450-9111. Online: www.heartmath.com.

Wild Divine—Creative computer programs that use game-like interfaces to train the mind to relax. This biofeedback system monitoring the pulse demonstrates how different thoughts, emotions, breathing and postures affects peace of mind and the ability to accomplish certain tasks. Numerous software/game options. Address: PO Box 61072, Boulder City, NV 89006. Phone: 866-594-9453. Online: www.wilddivine.com.

Yoga / T'ai chi chuan / Qi gong demonstrations

Ideally, one learns these practices working directly with a teacher. If that is not possible, the next best thing is to access the many excellent resources that exist both in DVD format and on the internet. Below are just a couple of suggestions.

Gaiam—Large selection of instructional DVDs and digital downloads: Yoga, fitness, meditation. Yoga supplies, organic cotton bedding, much more. Address: 833 W South Boulder Rd, PO Box 3095, Boulder, CO 80307-3095. Phone: 877-989-6321. Online: www.gaiam.com.

Smiling Chi—Teacher Gene Dryer, who has been practicing martial arts for more than 35 years, offers a very generous offering of instruction on his freely accessible website. Instructions for simple chi kung [qi gong] and t'ai chi practices are offered in both written and video formats. He also discusses and demonstrates simple ways to access the Relaxation Response, perform AcuTouch stimulation of the body's energy pathways, and more. This site is a wonderful gift. Gene also has a DVD for sale: *Basic Movement for Health*, a gentle program particularly suited for those who must be sedentary for much of the day. www.smilingchi.com.

Local Health Food Store / Natural Lifestyle Shop

Foods, bulk herbs, supplements. Wrist bands to prevent nausea, wool flannel for castor oil packs, tea-making gear [strainers, etc.], natural fiber brushes for dry brushing, essential-oil based hand and room sanitizers, eye mask for sleep, organic aloe vera gel or juice, rose or lavender hydrosols, organic baby wipes, organic baby foods, books, uplifting images [cards], soothing music, meditation cushions, DVDs [qi gong, t'ai chi chuan, yoga, pilates…], miso, non-toxic candles [from beeswax, soy or sustainably sourced palm oil], small glass bottles, spray bottles, sheepskin fleece…

Local Full-Service Drugstore

Thermometers, wrist pulse/blood pressure monitors, bedpans, sitzbath basins, shower benches, home nursing gear—walkers, crutches, canes, commodes, transport chairs, wheelchairs [some equipment may be available for rent], ear plugs, hot water bottles, heating pads, Epsom salts, boric acid, eyewash cups, enema bags, suppository molds [may need to order], nursing gloves, pads, gauze, and supplies....

Living Will / Financial and Legal Affairs

Living Wills: A Guide to Advance Directives, Health Care Power of Attorney, and Other Key Documents—Harvard Medical School [Boston: Harvard Health Publications, 2013]. Protect your right to make crucial health decisions. This 44-page document is a comprehensive overview to the questions, preferences, and gray areas that require consideration. Though each medical institution may offer their own abbreviated forms that suffice for legal purposes, this thorough resource can guide families through the difficult conversations that need to be had in the process of decision-making. Available for immediate purchase/download online: www.health.harvard.edu.

If Something Should Happen: How to Organize Your Financial and Legal Affairs— Marla Brill [Great Barrington, MA: American Institute for Economic Research (AIER), 2010]. Handy, very useful 50-page document outlining considerations regarding the topics in subtitle. Its workbook-style design provides a one-document overview of personal details regarding liabilities, assets, personal and professional contacts, life insurance and pension details, medical insurance and health history, where to find personal papers and records, safe deposit location, internet passwords, and more. Contact: AIER, 250 Division St, PO Box 1000, Great Barrington, MA 01230. Phone: 888-528-1216. Email: info@aier.org. Online: www.aier.org.

The Language of Herbalism

Actions: The nutritional and therapeutic energies of a plant.

Acute: Presenting symptoms typified by severity, sudden onset, and generally short duration.

Adaptogen: Substance that improves the body's resistance and response to stress and—in the presence of stress—helps return body processes to normal with minimal impact.

Aerial: Referring to the parts of a plant that grow above the ground.

Alterative: A substance that tends to gradually restore health and well-being; alters existing processes and promotes normal functioning.

Amphoteric: Appearing to be indicated for contradictory symptoms in a given system.

Analgesic: A substance that relieves pain.

Anesthetic: A substance that decreases sensitivity to pain.

Anodyne: A substance that relieves pain, usually with an accompanying sedative effect.

Anthelmintic: A substance that expels or kills intestinal worms or parasites.

Antibacterial: A substance that specifically destroys or prevents the growth of bacteria.

Anti-emetic: A substance that eases nausea and relieves vomiting.

Anti-inflammatory: A substance that helps counteract or diminish inflammation.

Antimicrobial: A substance that destroys or inhibits the growth of micro-organisms—ranging from bacteria, fungi, viruses.

Antipruritic: A substance that relieves itching.

Antipyretic: A substance that reduces or dispels fever. Also known as *febrifuge*.

Antiseptic: A substance that prevents sepsis (putrefaction of tissue) by inhibiting the growth of causative bacteria on contact.

Antispasmodic: A substance that relieves or prevents muscular spasms, convulsions, or cramps. Can sometimes be applied externally as well as ingested internally.

Aperient: (Latin: "*opening*") A gentle laxative agent, promoting easy evacuation of the bowels.

Aphrodisiac: Increases sexual appetite and vitality. In herbal medicine, plants known as aphrodisiac often act by promoting overall energy levels and circulation of vital force.

Aromatic: Spicy, often fragrant herbs containing volatile essential oils which aid in digestion and relieve flatulence.

Astringent: A substance that causes the contraction of tissues; can reduce secretions and diminish swelling.

Atonic: Lack of tone or vital energy; weakness of an organ or system.

Bile: A bitter digestive secretion from the liver, usually greenish in color. An aid in the digestion of fats, bile is stored in the gall bladder and excreted into the small intestine as needed. Acts as a laxative and a detoxifying medium.

Bitter/bitter tonic: A substance or combination having a bitter taste which stimulates the flow of saliva and gastric juices; used to increase a deficient appetite, improve the acidity of stomach secretion, improve assimilation.

Blood purifier: A somewhat vague traditional reference to those herbs that seem to accelerate excretion of metabolic waste products through the blood stream, especially when skin eruptions are present. Term usually applied to herbs that stimulate lymphatic drainage, liver function, bile excretion, and normal evacuation of the large intestine.

Bolus: A suppository inserted into the vagina or the rectum.

Bronchial dilation: The relaxation and opening of the upper lungs, thereby easing the breath and relaxing spasms.

Calmative: A substance that nourishes the nervous system and promotes relaxation.

Cardiac tonic: A substance that nourishes and strengthens heart metabolism.

Cardiovascular: Relating to the heart and the blood vessels.

Carminative: A substance (usually a volatile oil) that reduces and eliminates gas from the stomach and intestines, helping to relieve pain and distention. Promotes peristalsis and relaxes the stomach.

Catarrh: An inflammation of any mucous membrane—especially the respiratory tract— usually accompanied by congestion and increased secretion of mucus.

Cathartic: A harsh substance causing vigorous evacuation of the bowels, often accompanied by cramping or griping pains.

Cholagogue: A substance that promotes the flow of bile into the intestine.

Choleretic: A substance that promotes bile secretion by the liver.

Chronic: Referring to disease, imbalance, or habit that continues for a long period of time, with seemingly little change occurring. The opposite of acute.

Compress: A hot, wet external application used on painful, inflamed areas. Cotton towel, cloth or flannel is soaked in a strong tea and applied directly. The process is repeated when the material cools. Also known as *Fomentation*.

Constitution: The fundamental physical and emotional makeup of a person, including inherent strengths and weaknesses.

Cooling: That which reduces heat (in the form of inflammation, fever, etc.).

Counterirritant: An irritating substance deliberately applied externally to relieve pain in a deep-seated area of the body or to increase circulation and thereby speed healing.

Decoction: A preparation made by gently simmering plant parts in water for a minimum of 20 minutes or longer. In general, the harder, denser parts of plants are prepared this way—roots, barks, seeds—in an approximate proportion of ¼ -½ cup of herb to one quart of water. Soak the plant material in the water for 15 minutes to overnight prior to cooking, if time and memory allows.

Demulcent: A substance that will soothe mucous membranes or protect them from irritation, either by direct contact or via reflex mechanisms.

Diaphoretic: A substance that promotes perspiration and elimination through the skin.

Digestive system: Relating to the stomach and intestines.

Diuretic: A substance that increases the formation and flow of urine.

Emetic: A substance that induces vomiting.

Emollient: A substance that soothes, softens and protects the skin.

Empirical: Knowledge dependent upon experience or observation alone, rather than scientific theory, logic, or proof.

Enzyme: An organic catalyst that accelerates the speed of chemical reactions, as in spurring the breakdown of other substances.

Expectorant: A substance that promotes the expulsion of mucus from the respiratory tract via various mechanisms of activity.

Febrifuge: A substance that reduces or dispels fevers. Also known as *antipyretic*.

Fixed oil: An oil that does not easily vaporize, in contrast with volatile essential oils. Examples are common seed, nut, and vegetable oils.

Flower essence: A non-aromatic preparation containing the vibratory qualities of a plant's flower at its peak of bloom. Primarily used therapeutically to address spiritual and emotional issues.

Fomentation: Compress.

Fungicide: Agent that kills fungus.

Gastro-intestinal: Pertaining to the stomach and intestines.

Genito-urinary: Pertaining to the genitalia and the urinary organs.

Glycerin: A sweet, syrupy alcohol that can be produced synthetically from propylene alcohol or naturally—and preferably—derived from vegetable oils. Used as a solvent, lubricant, emollient, and humectant.

Glycerite: An herbal extract that uses glycerin as the principle solvent or preservative. Vegetable-sourced glycerin is, of course, preferred.

Hemostatic: A substance that slows or stops bleeding, internally or externally.

Hepatic: A substance which nourishes and strengthens the liver and its functioning.

Homeostasis: A dynamic equilibrium within a system, a state of balance, orchestrated by an interplay of feedback and regulation.

Homeopathy: A system of healing based on the premise that "like cures like." Remedies employed are vibrational in nature, administering in minute doses the same substances that in larger amounts would induce sickness. Therapy addresses specific symptom pictures rather than disease categories.

Humectant: A compound used topically to prevent water loss and drying of the skin.

Hypo-/Hyperchlorhydria: Respectively, insufficiency or excess of hydrochloric acid in gastric secretion.

Infusion: An herbal extract in which the plant is steeped in water. This method is generally used for leaves and flowers, and roots containing highly volatile constituents. A therapeutically beneficial infusion generally involves both more quantity of herb and more steeping time than a more casual beverage tea (although certainly a plant is healing by its very nature, irrespective of human 'processing' traditions.). Typically, about ¼-½ cup of herb is steeped in one quart of boiled water—from one hour to overnight.

Laxative: (Latin: "to *loosen*") A substance which promotes evacuation of the bowels via these main actions: increasing the bulk of the feces, softening the stools, lubricating the intestinal walls, or increasing peristalsis by irritating the intestinal mucosa.

Lithotriptic or **anti-lithic**: An agent which dissolves kidney and bladder stones or what is referred to as gravel.

Lymphatic: Pertaining to the lymph tissue or lymph system.

Materia Medica: A compilation of information on plants [or other drugs] used in the treatment of dis-ease, including a detailed physical description, listing of relevant species, chemical constituents, and information about their properties, preparation, dosage and use.

Medical Herbalism: An application of using plants for healing, or phytotherapy, which may or may not employ a holistic view of health and disease. Some medical or clinical herbalists view the body solely through a physio-medical lens, simply addressing discreet disease entities using plant medicine/chemicals rather than pharmaceutical ones. Other clinical herbalists embrace a more holistic view and attempt to work with a more comprehensive constitutional or bodymind approach to the symptom picture that a client is presenting.

Menstruum: A solvent used in the preparation of herbal extracts, usually consisting of some plant-specific ratio of alcohol to water, glycerin to water, or vinegar to water.

Mucilaginous: Mucus-like, gelatinous, sticky substance. Mucilaginous herbs soothe and heal the skin as well as mucous membranes within the body.

Musculo-skeletal: Referring to the muscles, skeleton, and connective tissue.

Narcotic: A substance that depresses central nervous system function, thereby relieving pain and promoting sleep.

Naturopathy: A system of medicine that employs many methods to assist the body's natural mechanisms for maintaining health. Therapies include herbs, nutrition, homeopathy, nutritional supplementation, massage, hydrotherapy, and others.

Nervine: A substance that soothes, restores, and strengthens the functioning of the nervous system. Nerve-influencing plants can be stimulating or tonic or sedating.

Nephritic: A substance useful for the kidneys.

Nutritive: That which promotes growth and repair by providing nourishment via vitamin complexes, minerals, amino acids, sugars, starches, chlorophyll, inherent vibrancy.

Palliative: A substance that relieves/masks symptoms without addressing their underlying cause.

Pectoral: A substance that treats imbalances in the chest and lungs.

Peristalsis: Contractions of smooth muscle tissue that are rhythmical and wave-like. Term usually refers to the activity of the intestinal tract.

Phytotherapy: The therapeutic use of plants. Please see *Medical Herbalism* entry.

Poultice: A mass of substance heated and applied to any part of the body, usually held between two pieces of muslin and changed when substance cools. Used to alleviate pain, reduce inflammation, and heal tissue damage (bruises, sprains, and inflammations).

Prophylactic: An agent that prevents disease or imbalance.

Pulmonary: Pertaining to the lungs.

Purgative: A strong laxative/cathartic, which relieves constipation by stimulating the bowel to rapidly evacuate.

Qi: (or Chi): Expression representing vital force in traditional Chinese medical thought. As with other TCM concepts, it is best perceived as function rather than substance. Consider also ki (Japanese), prana (Vedic), bioenergy, etc.

Refrigerant: A cooling agent; reduces body temperature.

Renal: Referring to the kidneys and their function.

Resin: A gummy, oily secretion of a plant.

Respiratory: Referring to the lungs and air passages.

Restorative: A substance that promotes a return to normal functioning; often used following an illness to support convalescence.

Rhizome: A creeping horizontal underground stem that gives rise to several roots and shoots. What are commonly called ginger and turmeric "roots" are examples of rhizomes.

Root: The part of the plant which usually resides below ground level—holding it in place, drawing water and nutrients from the soil, and storing nourishment. Also, that connection we experience with source when our beings are vibrant and in balance.

Rubifacient: A substance that—when applied locally—dilates capillaries, increasing superficial circulation and causing a reddening of the skin.

Salve: Topical preparation of herbs infused via heat or time into a fatty base such as oil and then solidified, typically with beeswax or cocoa butter.

Secondary action: Refers to those actions of an herb that enhance and support its primary activity or activities.

Sedative: A substance that calms or tranquilizes the nerves and often induces sleep.

Seed: The fulfillment of the plant's cycle. The promise of return—the part of the plant that contains the embryo and the potential to grow into a new plant if sown.

Somatic: Referring to the physicality of the body as distinguished from mental, emotional, or spiritual aspects.

Specific: A remedy having a reliable, particular effect on a symptom or pattern of imbalance.

Steep: Extracting the essence from plants—usually leaves, flowers, and soft roots—by infusing them into water, most commonly after the water has been boiled.

Stimulant: A substance that increases and enhances the functioning of the body; increases internal heat. For instance, an herbal stimulant such as ginger rhizome promotes peripheral circulation and increases digestive fire.

Styptic: An agent used externally to slow or staunch bleeding by contracting the tissue and blood vessels.

Succus: Freshly expressed plant juice preserved with at least 20% alcohol. Typical ratio is 3 parts plant juice by volume to 1 part alcohol by volume. Plural, *succi*.

Suppository: A substance or substances of therapeutic value introduced into the rectum or vagina, usually via a solidified fatty agent such as cocoa butter which melts at body temperature.

System affinity: The relatedness that the actions of a plant evidence for a particular system, tissue, or function in the body.

Systemic: That which affects the body as a whole.

Tea: A simple infusion made by pouring 1 cup of hot water over 1-3 teaspoons of herb and letting it steep in a covered container for 10-15 minutes.

Tincture: A solution of medicinal plant substances in a menstruum consisting of water and another solvent—typically alcohol or, in some cases, apple cider vinegar or glycerin. The ratio of water to alcohol varies from plant to plant, specific to the constituents being extracted. Especially indicated when a plant's active constituents are not water-soluble or best preserved fresh.

Tonic: A substance or combination that invigorates, nourishes, strengthens.

Toxins: Poisonous substances of exogenous or endogenous origin. Examples include: environmental pollutants; agricultural chemicals; waste products from intestinal parasites; metabolic waste, etc.

Tuber: A thick, underground stem or root of certain plants, often presenting buds.

Urinary tonic: A substance that nourishes and strengthens the functioning of the urinary organs and membranes.

Vasoconstrictor: A substance that causes a narrowing of blood vessels.

Vasodilator: A substance that causes relaxation and widening of blood vessels.

Venous: Pertaining to the veins.

Vermifuge: An agent that expels intestinal worms, without necessarily killing them. Also known as *anthelmintic*.

Volatile: Evaporates readily.

Volatile oil: An oil which vaporizes readily as contrasted with a fixed oil which does not. An essential oil is a volatile oil while the oil extracted from nuts or seeds is fixed.

Vulnerary: A substance that promotes the healing of wounds and abrasions—protects against infection and stimulates cell growth.

Wise Woman/Green Wisdom Tradition: The practice of herbalism in which knowledge and the wise and appropriate application of that knowledge is transmitted through relationship—through apprenticeship, teaching circles, dreams and direct contact with the plant themselves. The goal is to empower the seeker to reawaken their inherent connection with the Greenworld and trust the vast treasure of healing wisdom available through that relationship. It is a holistic tradition in which the bodymind health and well-being of a human individual is not seen as separate from or more important than the health and well-being of the community and the ecosystem. It honors the web of life, which expresses Great Mystery. "Wise Woman" is often used to describe this approach and that term has been a very healing affirmation for the collective consciousness. The term "Green Wisdom" embraces kindred folk of all genders working in this manner and places the focus where it ultimately belongs—on the blessed Greenworld where this wisdom and healing resides.

References

Helping Repertoire

[1] Levi E Fried and Jack L Arbiser. Honokiol, a Multifunctional Antiogenic and Antitumor Agent. *Antioxid. Redox Signal*. Vol.11, No.5, 2009, 1139-1148.

[2] Sumit Arora, *et al*. Honokiol: A Novel Natural Agent for Cancer Prevention and Therapy. *Curr Mol Med*. 2012 December: 12(10):1244-1252.

[3] http://faculty.washington.edu/chudler/facts.html. **Eric H Chudler, Ph.D.** Executive Director, Center for Sensorimotor Neural Engineering, University of Washington Seattle, WA

[4] Anupum Haksar, *et al*. *Zingiber officinale* exhibits behavioral radioprotection against radiation-induced CTA in a gender-specific manner. *Pharmacol Biochem Behav*. 2006 Jun;84(2):179-88. Epub 2006 Jun 21.

[5] Sharma A, *et al*. *Zingiber officinale* Rosc. modulates gamma radiation-induced conditioned taste aversion. *Pharmacol Biochem Behav*. 2005 Aug;81(4):864-70.

[6] Zhiqiang Meng, M Kay Garcia, Chaosu Hu, Joseph Chiang, Mark Chambers, David I Rosenthal, Huiting Peng, Ying Zhang, Qi Zhao, Genming Zhao, Luming Liu, Amy Spelman, J Lynn Palmer, Qi Wei, Lorenzo Cohen. Randomized controlled trial of acupuncture for prevention of radiation-induced xerostomia among patients with nasopharyngeal carcinoma. *Cancer*, 2011; DOI: 10.1002/cncr.26550

[7] Choose a high molecular weight (at least 1 million Daltons), purified (protein free) version that matches the hyaluronic acid natively produced. Native HA weighs between approximately 800,000 and 6 million Daltons). Two types of this are available in the commercial marketplace: HA from microbial fermentation (vegetarian) or HA from rooster combs. The purified HA from microbial fermentation has published evidence of uptake following oral ingestion—HA absorbed into the bloodstream was seen to localize in joint and salivary glands.

[8] Narayan A, Mendon C. Comparing the effect of different mouthrinses on de novo plaque formation. *J Contemp Dent Pract*. 2012 Jul-Aug;13(4):460-3

[9] Shobha Tandon, Kunal Gupta, Sugandhi Rao, KJ Malagi. Effect of Triphala Mouthwash on the Caries Status. *International Journal of Ayurveda Research*, Apr-Jun (2010): 93–99. NCBI. Web. 16 Oct. 2013

[10] Lee MJ, Lambert JD, Prabhu S, *et al*. Delivery of tea polyphenols to the oral cavity by green tea leaves and black tea extract. *Cancer Epidemiol Biomarkers Prev*. 2004;13:132-137.

[11] Suresh Rao, *et al*. The Indian Spice Turmeric Delays and Mitigates Radiation-Induced Oral Mucositis in Patients Undergoing Treatment for Head and Neck Cancer: An Investigational Study. *Integrative Cancer Therapies*, 2013 October 31.

[12] Choose a high molecular weight (at least 1 million Daltons), purified (protein free) version that matches the hyaluronic acid natively produced. Native HA weighs between approximately 800,000 and 6 million Daltons). Two types of this are available in the commercial marketplace: HA from microbial fermentation (vegetarian) or HA from rooster combs. The purified HA from microbial fermentation has published evidence of uptake following oral ingestion—HA absorbed into the bloodstream was seen to localize in joint and salivary glands.

[13] Kelesidis T and Pothoulakis C. Efficacy and safety of the probiotic strain *Saccharomyces boulardii* for the prevention and therapy of gastrointestinal disorders. *Therap Adv Gastroenterol*. 2012 March; 5(2): 111-125.

[14] Sanchez A, Reeser JL, *et al*. Role of sugars in human neutrophilic phagocytosis. *Am J of Clin Nut* 26: November 1973:1180-1184.

[15] Laïd Boukraâ, editor. *Honey in Traditional and Modern Medicine*. [Boca Raton, FL: CRC Press, 2014.

[16] G Appendino, S Gibbons, A Giana, A Pagani, G Grassi, M Stavri, E Smith, and M Mukhlesur Rahman. "Antibacterial Cannabinoids from *Cannabis sativa*," *J Nat Prod* 2008, 71, 1427-1430

[17] Shelley S Magill, MD, PhD, *et al*. Multistate Point-Prevalence Survey of Health Care-Associated Infections, *N Engl J Med* 2014; 370:1198-1208, March 27, 2014. The survey results were also posted by the Center for Disease Control in April of 2014.

[18] Kelesidis, T and Pothoulakis, C. Efficacy and safety of the probiotic strain *Saccharomyces boulardii* for the prevention and therapy of gastrointestinal disorders. *Therap Adv Gastroenterol*. 2012 March; 5(2): 111-125.

[19] Michael Murray, ND *et al. How to Prevent and Treat Cancer with Natural Medicine.* [New York: Riverhead Books, 2002, p244-245]

[20] Mitchell Bebel Stargrove, ND, LAc Jonathan Treasure, MNIMH, Dwight L McKee, MD. *Herb, Nutrient, and Drug Interactions: Clinical Implications and Therapeutic Strategies* [St. Louis, MO: Mosby/Elsevier, 2008]

[21] Wu X, Hu H, Guo L, Wang H. Clinical observation of post-herpetic neuralgia treated with TCM herbal cupping therapy. *Zhongguo Zhen Jiu.* 2013 Feb;33(2):141-4

[22] Sanchez A, Reeser JL, *et al.* Role of sugars in human neutrophilic phagocytosis. *Am J of Clin Nut* 26: November 1973:1180-1184.

[23] Costagliola M, Agrosi M. Second-degree burns: a comparative, multicenter, randomized trial of hyaluronic acid plus silver sulfadiazine vs. silver sulfadiazine alone. *Curr Med Res Opin.* 2005 Aug;21(8):1235-40

[24] Voigt J, Driver VR. Hyaluronic acid derivatives and their healing effect on burns, epithelial surgical wounds, and chronic wounds: a systematic review and meta-analysis of randomized controlled trials. *Wound Repair Regen.* 2012 May-Jun;20(3):317-31.

[25] Choose a high molecular weight (at least 1 million Daltons), purified (protein free) version that matches the hyaluronic acid natively produced. Native HA weighs between approximately 800,000 and 6 million Daltons). Two types of this are available in the commercial marketplace: HA from microbial fermentation (vegetarian) or HA from rooster combs. The purified HA from microbial fermentation has published evidence of uptake following oral ingestion—HA absorbed into the bloodstream was seen to localize in joint and salivary glands.

Repairing the Garment: Surgery and Beyond

[1] Avadhani A, Miley H. Probiotics for prevention of antibiotic-associated diarrhea and Clostridium difficile-associated disease in hospitalized adults--a meta-analysis. *J Am Acad Nurse Pract.* 2011 Jun;23(6):269-74. doi: 10.1111/j.1745-7599.2011.00617.x. Epub 2011 Apr 27.

[2] Hickson M. Probiotics in the prevention of antibiotic-associated diarrhoea and *Clostridium difficile* infection. *Ther Adv Gastroenterol* [2011] 4[3]:185-197.

[3] Mitchell Bebel Stargrove, ND, LAc Jonathan Treasure, MNIMH, Dwight L McKee, MD. *Herb, Nutrient, and Drug Interactions: Clinical Implications and Therapeutic Strategies* [St. Louis, MO: Mosby/Elsevier, 2008]

[4] Eliaz I, Hotchkiss AT, Fishman ML, Rode D. The Effect of Modified Citrus Pectin on Urinary Excretion of Toxic Elements. *Phytother Res* 20, 859-864 (2006)

[5] Michael Murray, ND *et al. How to Prevent and Treat Cancer with Natural Medicine.* [New York: Riverhead Books, 2002]

[6] Stargrove, *op.cit.*

[7] ***Please note***: Use propolis with caution if prone to allergy or hypersensitivity to bee stings, bee products, or tree resins.

Chemo / Radiation Considerations

[1] KM Skubitz and PM Anderson. Oral Glutamine to prevent chemotherapy induced stomatitis: A Pilot Study. *J of Lab & Clin Med,* 1996; 127(2)223-228.

[2] MA Ciorba, TE Riehl, MS Rao, C Moon, X Ee, GM Nava, MR Walker, JM Marinshaw, TS Stappenbeck, WF Stenson. Lactobacillus probiotic protects intestinal epithelium from radiation injury in a TLR-2/cyclo-oxygenase-2-dependent manner. *Gut,* 2011; DOI: 10.1136/gutjnl-2011-300367.

[3] Hiromitsu Watanabe. Beneficial Biological Effects of Miso with Reference to Radiation Injury, Cancer and Hypertension. *J Toxicol Pathol* 2013; 26: 91–103

[4] Eliaz I, Hotchkiss AT, Fishman ML, Rode D. The Effect of Modified Citrus Pectin on Urinary Excretion of Toxic Elements. *Phytother Res* 20, 859-864 (2006)

[5] Michael Murray, ND *et al. How to Prevent and Treat Cancer with Natural Medicine.* [New York: Riverhead Books, 2002]

Additional references accompany individual sections.

Bibliography

Alschuler, Lise ND and Gazella, Karolyn. *The Definitive Guide to Cancer: An Integrative Approach to Prevention, Treatment, and Healing* [Berkeley, CA: Celestial Arts, 2010]

Austin, Steve ND and Hitchcock, Cathy. *Breast Cancer: What You Should Know (But May Not Be Told) About Prevention, Diagnosis, and Treatment* [Rocklin, CA: Prima Publishing, 1994]

Balch, Phyllis A and Balch, James F MD. *Prescription for Nutritional Healing* [New York: Avery Publishing Group, 3rd edition, 2000]

Batmanghelidj, F MD. *Your Body's Many Cries for Water: You Are Not Sick, You Are Thirsty!* [Falls Church, VA: Global Health Solutions, 1995]

Bensky, Dan; Clavey, Steven; and Stöger, Erich with Andrew Gamble. *Chinese Herbal Medicine: Materia Medica* [Seattle: Eastland Press, 3rd edition, 2004]

Boik, John. *Natural Compounds in Cancer Therapy* [Princeton, MN: Oregon Medical Press, 2001]

Bone, Kerry. *Clinical Applications of Ayurvedic and Chinese Herbs* [Queensland, Australia: Phytotherapy Press, 1996]

Boukraâ, Laïd, editor. *Honey in Traditional and Modern Medicine* [Boca Raton, FL: CRC Press, 2014]

Callanan, Maggie RN and Kelley, Patricia RN. *Final Gifts: Understanding the Special Awareness, Needs, and Communications of the Dying* [New York: Bantam Books, 1997]

Cech, Richo. *Making Plant Medicine* [Williams, OR: Horizon Herbs, 2000]

Chen, John K OMD, LAc and Chen, Tina T LAc. *Chinese Medical Herbology and Pharmacology* [City of Industry, CA: The Art of Medicine Press, 2004]

Coberly, Margaret PhD, RN. *Sacred Passage: How to Provide Fearless, Compassionate Care for the Dying* [Boston: Shambhala Publications, 2002]

Connelly, Dianne M LAc . *All Sickness is Homesickness* [Columbia, MD: Centre for Traditional Acupuncture, 1986]

Cooksley, Valerie Gennari RN. *Seaweed: Nature's Secret to Balancing Your Metabolism, Fighting Disease, and Revitalizing Body & Soul* [New York: Steward, Tabori, and Chang, 2007].

Dass, Ram with Stephen Levine. *Grist for the Mill* [New York: Bantam Books, 1976]

Dev, Sukh PhD. *Prime Ayurvedic Plant Drugs* [Tunbridge Wells, UK: Anshan Limited, 2006]

Eden, Donna with David Feinstein. *Energy Medicine* [New York: Jeremy P. Tarcher/Putnam, 1998]

Evans, WC. *Trease and Evans' Pharmacognosy* [London: WB Saunders Company Ltd., 1999, 14th edition]

Felter, Harvey Wickes MD. *The Eclectic Materia Medica, Pharmacology and Therapeutics* [1922]

Flaws, Bob. *The Book of Jook: Chinese Medicinal Porridges* [Boulder, CO: Blue Poppy Press, 2001]

Foster, Steven and Chongxi, Yue. *Herbal Emissaries: Bringing Chinese Herbs to the West* [Rochester, VT: Healing Arts Press, 1992]

Frawley, David OMD. *Ayurveda and the Mind: The Healing of Consciousness* [Twin Lakes, WI: Lotus Press, 1996]

Frawley, David OMD and Lad, Vasant MSc. *The Yoga of Herbs: An Ayurvedic Guide to Herbal Medicine* [Twin Lakes, WI: Lotus Press, 1986]

Fulder, Stephen. *The Tao of Medicine: Ginseng and Other Chinese Herbs for Inner Equilibrium and Immune Power* [Rochester, VT: Healing Arts Press, 1980]

Ganora, Lisa. *Herbal Constituents: Foundations of Phytochemistry* [Louisville, CO: Herbalchem Press, 2009]

Gardner, Zoë and McGuffin, Michael, editors. *Botanical Safety Handbook, 2nd edition* [Boca Raton, FL: CRC Press, 2013]

Gaynor, Mitchell L MD. *The Healing Power of Sound: Recovery from Life-Threatening Illness Using Sound, Voice, and Music* [Boston: Shambala Publications, 1999].

Goldstein, Joseph and Kornfield, Jack. *Seeking the Heart of Wisdom: The Path of Insight Meditation* [Boston: Shambala Publications, 1987]

Gorter, Robert MD PhD and Peper, Erik PhD. *Fighting Cancer: A Nontoxic Approach to Treatment* [Berkeley, CA: North Atlantic Books, 2011].

Hanson, Bryan A PhD. *Understanding Medicinal Plants: Their Chemistry and Therapeutic Action* [Binghamton, NY: Haworth Herbal Press, 2005].

Heinrich, Michael; Barnes, Joanne; Gibbons, Simon; Williamson, Elizabeth M. *Fundamentals of Pharmacognosy and Phytotherapy* [Edinburgh: Churchill Livingstone, 2004]

Hobbs, Christopher. *Foundations of Health: The Liver and Digestive Herbal* [Capitola, CA: Botanica Press, 1992]

Hobbs, Christopher. *The Ginsengs* [Santa Cruz, CA: Botanica Press, 1996]

Hobbs, Christopher. *Medicinal Mushrooms: An Exploration of Tradition, Healing, & Culture* [Santa Cruz, CA: Botanica Press, second edition, 1995]

Hobbs, Christopher. *Stress and Natural Healing: Herbal Medicine and Natural Therapies* [Loveland, CO: Interweave Press, 1997]

Hoffman, David. *Medical Herbalism: The Science and Practice of Herbal Medicine* [Rochester, VT: Healing Arts Press, 2003]

Kaminski, Patricia and Katz, Richard. *Flower Essence Repertory: A Comprehensive Guide to North American and English Flower Essences for Emotional and Spiritual Well-Being* [Nevada City, CA: The Flower Essence Society, Earth-Spirit, Inc., 1994].

Kaminski, Patricia. *Flowers that Heal: How to Use Flower Essences* [Dublin, Ireland: Newleaf, 1998]

Katz, Sandor Ellix. *Wild Fermentation: The Flavor, Nutrition, and Craft of Live-Culture Foods* [White River Junction, VT: Chelsea Green Publishing Co., 2003]

Kornfield, Jack. *After the Ecstasy, the Laundry: How the Heart Grows Wise on the Spiritual Path* [New York: Bantam Books, 2000]

Kuhn, Merrily A RN and Winston, David RH(AGH). *Herbal Therapy and Supplements: A Scientific and Traditional Approach* [Philadelphia, PA: Lippincott, 2nd edition 2008]

Lahans, Tai LAc. *Integrating Conventional and Chinese Medicine in Cancer Care: A Clinical Guide* [Philadelphia, PA: Churchill Livingstone/Elsevier, 2007].

Levine, Stephen. *Healing into Life and Death* [New York: Doubleday, 1987]

Levine, Stephen. *Who Dies? An Investigation of Conscious Living and Conscious Dying* [New York: Doubleday, 1982]

Maciocia, Giovanni. *The Foundations of Chinese Medicine* [London: Churchill Livingstone, 1989]

Margulis, Lynn. *Symbiotic Planet: A New View of Evolution* [New York: Basic Books, 1998]

Maté, Gabor MD. *When the Body Says No: Understanding the Stress-Disease Connection* [Hoboken, NJ: John Wiley & Sons, 2003].

McKinney, Neil ND. *Naturopathic Oncology* [Vancouver, BC: Liaison Press, 2012, 2nd edition]

Mills, Simon FNIMH and Bone, Kerry FNIMH. *Principles and Practices of Phytotherapy* [London: Churchill Livingstone, 2000]

Mojay, Gabriel. *Aromatherapy for Healing the Spirit*. [Rochester, VT: Healing Arts Press, 1997]

Murray, Michael ND. *Encyclopedia of Nutritional Supplements* [Rocklin, CA: Prima Publishing, 1996]

Murray, Michael ND, et al. *How to Prevent and Treat Cancer with Natural Medicine*[New York: Riverhead Books, 2002]

Pengelly, Andrew. *The Constituents of Medicinal Plants* [Merriwa, NSW: Sunflower Herbals, 1997, 2nd edition]

Phytochemical Database, USDA-ARS-NGRL [Beltsville Agricultural Research Center, Beltsville, MD, September 1999]

Pizzorno, Joseph ND. *Total Wellness: Improve Your Health by Understanding the Body's Healing Systems* [Rocklin, CA: Prima Publishing, 1996]

Pizzorno, Joseph ND and Murray, Michael ND. *Textbook of Natural Medicine 4th edition*. [St. Louis, MO: Elsevier/Churchill Livingstone, 2013]

Powell, Martin. *Medicinal Mushrooms: A Clinical Guide* [East Sussex, UK: Mycology Press, 2010]

Price, Shirley and Price, Len, editors. *Aromatherapy for Health Professionals* [Edinburgh: Churchill Livingstone/Elsevier, 2102, 4th edition]

Rinpoche, Sogyal. *The Tibetan Book of Living and Dying* [San Francisco: HarperSanFrancisco, 1992]

Rogers, Robert RH(AGH). *The Fungal Pharmacy: The Complete Guide to Medicinal Mushrooms and Lichens of North America* [Berkeley, CA: North Atlantic Books, 2011]

Sachs, Jessica Snyder. *Good Germs, Bad Germs: Health and Survival in a Bacterial World* [New York: Hill and Wang, 2007]

Singh, Narendra and Hoette, Yamuna with Ralph Miller. *Tulsi: The Mother Medicine of Nature* [Lucknow, India: International Institute of Herbal Medicine, 2002]

Skenderi, Gazmend. *Herbal Vade Mecum* [Rutherford, NJ: Herbacy Press, 2003]

Stamets, Paul with C Dusty Wu Yao. *MycoMedicinals* [Olympia, WA: MycoMedia Productions, 2002, 3rd edition]

Stargrove, MB ND, LAc, Treasure, J MNIMH, McKee, DL MD. *Herb, Nutrient, and Drug Interactions* [St. Louis, MO: Mosby/Elsevier, 2008]

Suzuki, Shunryu. *Zen Mind, Beginner's Mind* [New York: John Weatherhill, 1983]

Teeguarden, Ron. *Chinese Tonic Herbs* [Tokyo: Japan Publications, 1984]

Tisserand, Robert and Balacs, Tony. *Essential Oil Safety: A Guide for Healthcare Professionals* [Edinburgh: Churchill Livingstone, 1998]

USDA National Nutrient Database for Standard Reference.

Van Bentheim, Tineke *et al. Caring for the Sick at Home* [Edinburgh: Floris Books, 1987; Hudson, NY: Anthroposophic Press, 1987]

Walters, Richard. *Options: The Alternative Cancer Therapy Book* [Garden City Park, NY: Avery Publishing Group, 1993]

Willard, Terry. *Reishi Mushroom: Herb of Spiritual Potency and Medical Wonder* [Issaquah, WA: Sylvan Press, 1990]

Williams, JE OMD. *Prolonging Health.* [Charlottesville, VA: Hampton Roads Publishing Co. Inc., 2003]

Williamson, Elizabeth M. *Major Herbs of Ayurveda.* [London: Churchill Livingstone, 2002]

Winston, David RH(AGH), and Maimes, Steven. *Adaptogens: Herbs for Strength, Stamina, and Stress Relief* [Rochester, VT: Healing Arts Press, 2007]

Winston, David RH(AGH). *Herbal Therapeutics* [Broadway, NJ: Herbal Therapeutics Research Library, 8th edition, 2003]

Yance Jr, Donald R CN, RH(AGH). *Adaptogens in Medical Herbalism: Elite Herbs and Natural Compounds for Mastering Stress, Aging, and Chronic Disease* [Rochester, VT: Healing Arts Press, 2013].

Yance Jr, Donald R CN, RH(AGH). *Herbal Medicine, Healing and Cancer.* [Chicago: Keats Publishing, 1999]

— Index —

A

Abdominal bloating, 136
Abdominal massage, 77
Acetosella vulgaris, see Sheep sorrel
Achillea millefolium, see Yarrow
Activated charcoal, 62, 82, 88, 91, 272
Acupuncture, 59, 65, 94, 97, 101, 105, 106 125, 137, 139
Adaptogens
    - adaptogenic plants, 32, 45, 56, 96, **167-172**, 244, 249-250, **253-258**
    - defined, 167
    - in foods [recipes], 173-174
Aduki beans, **104**, 109
Aesculus hippocastanum, see Horsechestnut
Agar-agar, **49**, 266
Agrimony [*Agrimonia eupatorium*], 99
Agropyron repens, see Couchgrass
Alaria esculenta, see Wakame
Alchemilla vulgaris, see Lady's mantle
Alder, red [*Alnus rubra*], **78**, 89
Alfalfa [*Medicago sativa*], 51,53,137,173
Alginates, **103**, **143**, 159, 236, 269
Alkathymol, 69
Alnus rubra, see Red alder
Aloe vera [*Aloe vera*], 69, 83, 86, 101, 108, 124, 143, 270, 275
Alpha-lipoic acid, **93**, 270
Althea officinalis, see Marshmallow
American ginseng [*Panax quinquifolius*], 23, 103, **168**, **254**, 268
Amla [*Emblica officinalis*], **77**, 102, 103, 108, 109, 140
Anal fissures, **79**, 81
Anemia, 38, **52**, 60, 141, 169, 172, 254
Andrographis [*Andrographis paniculata*], 75
Angelica sinensis, see Dong quai
Anise [*Pimpella anisum*], 82
Anointing body, 40, 188
Antibiotics, 63, **90**, 98, 107, 133, 136, 197, 216, 218, 225, **228**, 246, 302
Anxiety, 17, 21, 28, **40**, 41, 42, 43, 44, 59, 61, 74, 82, 96, 100, **113**, 129, **167-174**, **175-184**, 202, 205, **233-236**, 242, **245-258**
Apium graveolens, see Celery
Appetite, 49, 109, 137, 165, 168, 181, 254, 278
    - loss of, 53-57, 75, 82, 91, 146, 149, 172, 176, 177, 272
Apple cider vinegar, 72, 148, 283
Arctium spp., see Burdock

Arctostaphylos uva-ursi, see Uva ursi
Arnica montana homeopathic 136, 261, 272, 273
Aromas, 24, 33, 35, 58, 62, 120, 126,
Aromatherapy, 40, 58, 62, 87, 126, 175, 213-214, **250**
Arrowroot powder, 39, 110
Artemisia absinthium, see Wormwood
Asian ginseng [*Panax ginseng*], 23, 103, **168**, 169, **254**, 266, 268
Astragalus [*Astragalus membranaceus*], 39, 51 **52**, 53, 84, 89, 91, 96, 103, 132, 140, 142, 147, 148, 150, 159, **169**, 173, 174, 243, 244, 266, 267
Astringent plants, 16, 39, 54, 62, 66, **67**, 70, 71, 72, 73, 74, 78, **80**, 81, 87, 88, 89, 90, 93, 95, 99, 100, 101, 105, 165, 166, 169, 171, 172, 174, 176, 177, 180, 181, 182, 183, 253, 256, 257, **278**
Atractylodis [*A. lancea*], 53
Avens [*Geum macrophyllum*] 67, 74, 80, 81, 101
Avocado, **55**, 85, 108, **155**, 158
Avocado/cacao pudding, 155
Azadirachta indica, see Neem

B

B-vitamins, 39, 52, 93, 94, 256, 261, 270
B_{12} Vitamin, 52, 54, 93, 153, 236
Bacopa [*Bacopa monnieri*], 108, 236, 250, 253, **256**, 258, 270, 272
Bacteria
    - beneficial, 63, 67, 69, 71, 75, 79, 88, 90, 92, 98, 133, 136, 137, 138, 142, 145, 163, 164, **221-232**, 244
    - drug-resistant, 75, **90-92**, 124, 228
Baked yam w/ tahini, 148
Baking soda, 72, 77, 88, 95, 274
    - bath, 87, 144
    - mouth rinse, 60, 67, 72
Baptisia homeopathic, **40**, 90, 212
Barley broth, 147
Basil, holy [*Ocimum sanctum*], 41, **171**, **177**, **257**, 266, 267, 269, 270, 272
Bay laurel [*Laurus nobilis*], 213
Bed arrangement, 35
Bedsores, 37
Beets, 56, 151, **155**, 266
Belladonna homeopathic, 90, 96, 272
Bentonite clay 75, 88, 95, 143, 261
Berberis spp., see Oregon grape

Compress, eye, **83**, 165
Compresses, 39, 72, 73, 80, 81, 83, 87, 88, 96, 101, 102, 165
Compression, 106
Congee [rice porridge], 50, **150**
Conjunctivitis, **83**, 176
Consistency, **32-34**, 43
Coptis [*Coptis* spp.], 89
Constipation, 15, 46, 48, 61, **76-79**, 80, 101, 136, 240, 82
Convalescence, 145-146
Coriolus versicolor, see Turkey Tail
Cornsilk [*Zea mays*], **99**, 266
Corydalis [*Corydalis ambigua aka C. yanhusuo*], **89**, **97**, 261, 269
Couchgrass [*Agropyron repens*], 99
Crampbark [*Viburnum opulus*], 79
Croton lechleri, see Dragon's blood
Cruciferous vegetables, 156, 163
Crystal bowls, 42, 202, 203
Cultured foods, 63, **71**, 88, 90, 98, 133, 136, 137, 146, 162
Curcuma longa, see Turmeric
Custard, curried egg, 151

D

D, Vitamin, 57, 151, 270
D-Mannose, **98**, 138, 262, 270
DGL [deglycyrrhizinated licorice], 69, **171**, 261, 267, 268, 270
Dandelion [*Taraxacum officinale*], 27, 44, 53, 54, 71, 78, **79**, 82, 86, 88, 90, 98, 104, 106, 133, 147, 159, 162, **164**, 166, 173, 213, 219, 230, 231, 236, 243, 244, 266, 267
Death, preparing for, 187-188
Deglycyrrhizinated licorice [DGL], see above
Depression, 40, 42, 165, 169, 170, 172, 177, 179, 181, 182, 183, 205, 218, **233-236**, 250, 254, 256, 257
Detoxification, 43, 45, 61, 63, 87, 104, 127, 130, 142, 143, 156, 162, 163, 165, 172, 181, 214, 215, 222, 223, 225, 236, 240, 244, 256, 267, 268, 272
Diaper rash balm, 74, 261, 271
Diarrhea, 40, **74-76**, 80, 91, 92, 137, 140, 166, 176, 177, 182, 218, 286
Digestive enzymes, 44, 46, 52, 54, 82, 109
Digital music device, 122, 123, 135
Dizziness, 52, **60-61**, 141, 145, 216, 218, 258
Dong quai [*Angelica sinensis*], 53, 270
Dragon's blood [*Croton lechleri*], 74, **95**, 266
Drugs, see Medication
Dry brushing, **106**, **214**, 275
Dry mouth, 57, **65-68**, 271
Dulse [*Palmaria* spp.], 58, 143, 148, 149, 236

E

E, Vitamin, 33, 74, 81, 85, 86, 95, **102**, 132, 134, 136, 138, 264
Ear plugs, 121, 276
Echinacea spp., 39, 84, 89, 91, 96, 176, 212, 243, 266
Eclipta [*Eclipta alba*], 108, 109
Eggs—55, **57**, 94, 109, 130, 146, 147, **151-153**
-    curried egg custard, 151
-    shiitake egg custard, 152
-    Mediterranean egg salad, 151
-    quiche, no wheat/dairy, 152-153

Eggwhite protein, 51, 137, 146, 159, 160, 262
Elecampane [*Inula helenium*], 75, 90, 98
Electrolytes, 16, 46, 48, 49, 74, 75, 85, **215-220**
Ellettaria cardamomum, see Cardamom
Emblica officinalis, see Amla
Emoto, Masaru, 210
Enemas, 13, 76, 78, **79**, 276
Energy awareness, 14, 17, 24, 32, **34**, 35, 37, 43, 47, 61, 107, 125, 130, 131, 133, 140, 157, 161, 167, 217, 303
Energy work practices, 11, 12, 13, 24, 27, 30, 34, **35-36**, 37, 42, 43, 47, 60, 62, 96, 106, 107, 132, 133, 135, 137, 139, 144, 302
Enteral feeding strategies, 56, 68, **157-158**
Environmental influences, 19, 24, **34-35**, 42, 43, 47, 48, 83, 128, 165, 188, 189, **202**, **209-210**, 213, 217, 221, 224, 225, 226, 228, **230**, 242, 246, 256, 284
Enzymes, digestive, 44, 46, 52, **54**, 68, 82, 95, 96, **104**, 109, **136**, 160, 267, 268, 269, 273
Epsom salts, 25, 42, 45, 271, 276
Eschscholtzia californica, see California poppy
Essiac tea, 164, **240**, 262, 266
Eucalyptus essential oil [*E. globulus*], 62, 74, 91
Eyes—
-    dry, 85
-    eyewash, **84**, 110, 276
-    infected, **83-84**, 176
Eye mask, 121, 275

F

Fasting, 115, 125, 135, 163
Fatigue, 23, **46-47**, 52, 141, 146, 168, 169, 170, 172, 205, 216, 218, 236, 254, 255, 256, 270
Feeding tubes, **157-158**, 160
Fennel seed [*Foeniculum vulgare*], 44, 59, **78**, 79, 82, 142
Fenugreek [*Trigonella foenum-graecum*], 79
Fiber, 46, 55, 76, 159
Flatulence, 49, 59, 74, **81-83**, 165, 179, 181, 182, 278

- supplement, 78
Magnolia [*Magnolia officinalis*], 41, 84, 267
Mahonia nervosa, see Oregon grape
Maitake [*Grifola frondosa*], 132, 133, 142, 147, 156, 245, 274
Mallow [*Malva neglecta*], **65**, 68, 80, 86, 99, 142
Manuka honey, 88, **229**, 263, 268, 271
Marjoram [*Origanum majorana*], 67, 74
Marshmallow [*Althea officinalis*], **65**, 68, 80, 86, 99, 142
Marrow Plus, **53**, 141, 263, 268
Massage, 25, **35-37**, 39, 42, 43, 47, 61, 62, 76, 77, 92, 93, 96, 98, 104, 105, 106, 108, 125, 137, 145, 175, 202, 214, 271, 281
Medicago sativa, see Alfalfa
Medical fundraising, 125, 134, **185-186**
Medical records, 120, 121, **124-125**, 276
Medication—46, 58, 64, 79, 83, 86, 87, 89, 92, 96, 97, 98, 99, 104, 107, 108, 120, 121, 124, 125, 126, 132, 136, 142, 143, 145, 161, 162, 165, 168, 170, 172, 178, 182, 183, 216, 218, 225, 228, 233, 244, 254, 257, 281, 303
- chaser [to improve taste], 58
- in suppositories, 64
Medical marijuana [*Cannabis* spp.], 41, 45, 47, 54, 60, 75, 91, **97**, 229, 232, 285
Melaleuca alternifolia, see Tea tree
Melaleuca viridiflora, see Niaoli
Melancholy, **40-41**, 46, 90
Melissa officinalis, see Lemon balm
Memory, 16, 43, 54, 168, 169, 171, 172, 177, 181, 182, 193, 211, **245-258**
Mentha piperita, see Peppermint
Microbiota, 91, 145, 163, 225, 228
Milk thistle [*Silybum marianum*], 136, 138, **142**, 162, **165**, 172, 236, 244, 266
Millet, 24
Miso, 24, **49**, **50**, 55, 57, 63, 69, 71, 74, 75, 88, 93, 94, 137, 138, 143, 146, 147, 148, 154, 162, 230, 267, 275
Modified citrus pectin [MCP], 135, 137, **143**, 263, 267, 270, 286
Montropa uniflora, see Indian Pipe
Moosh, **51**, 55
Mouth—
- dry, 57, 64, **65-66**, 68, 271
- *Herpes* eruptions, 41, **72-74**, **93-96**, 178, 179, 182, 272
- mucus, **67**, 68
- raw, 68-71
- rinses, 60, 63, 65, 66, 67, 68, 69, 70, 71, 72
- sores, 68-71
MRSA, 75, **90**, **228-229**
Mucositis, 68-71
Mucus, thick, 67

Music—35, 36, 40, 42, 44, 98, 127, 130, 197, 202-205, 209, 210, 235, 275
- before surgery, 134, 135
- for pain management, 98
- recommended listening, 202-205
- to ease sleep/restfulness, 24, 25, 34, 42, 43, 44
Myrrh [*Commifora myrrha*], 39, 66, 72, 74, **90**, 91, 263

N

Nat Mur homeopathic, 104
Natto, 137, 138, 162, 230, 273
Nausea, 15, 36, 40, 41, 45, 47, 48, 49, 54, **58-60**, 61, 64, 75, 91, 97, 119, 136, 142, 166, 176, 181, 275, 277
Neem [*Azadirachta indica*], 87, **89**, 138, 263, 272
Neti pots, 263, 271
Nettles, see Stinging nettles
Nerve pain [neuropathy], 11, 37, **92-93**, 100, 105, 165, 177, 180, 181, 182, 255, 271
Nervine herbs—23, 41, 84, 95, 100, 165, 168, 170, 171, **175-184**
- congenial combinations, 184
- selecting among, 175-183
Nettles, see *Stinging nettles*
Networking, 185-186
News fast, 210
Niaoli essential oil [*Melaleuca viridiflora*], 103, 138
Nigella sativa, see Black seed/black cumin
Non-steroidal anti-inflammatory drugs [NSAID], 98, 107, 162, 225
Nori [*Porphyra* spp.], 143
Nuts and nut butters—
- during *Herpes* outbreaks, 73
- for weight gain, 55

O

Oak [*Quercus* spp.], 67, 74, 80
Oatmeal—
- as food, 51
- colloidal, 87
- in bath, 87, 271

Ocimum sanctum, see Holy basil
Odors, body, 61-63
Oral health—**64-74**, 121, 263, 274
- chapped lips, 64
- dental hygiene, 33, 43, 63, **66-68**
- dry mouth, 65-66
- *Herpes* eruptions, 72-74

S

U

Ubiquinol [CoQ$_{10}$], 46, **140**, 270
Ulmus rubra, U. fulva, see Slippery elm
Urinary tract infection, **98-99**, 138, 165, 177
Urtica dioica, see Stinging nettles
Usnea [*Usnea barbata*], 71, 75, 84, 89, 91, 266
Uva ursi [*Arctostaphylos uva-ursi*], 99

V

Valerian [*Valeriana officinalis, V.* spp.], 23, 33,
  45, 79, 132, 134, 175, **183**
Vancomycin-resistant *Enterococcus* [VRE], 229
Vegetable broth, **49**, 50, 104, **147**, 148
Vegetable juice, **50**, 51, 56, 57, 63, 68, 76, 93,
  94, 103, **105**, 133, 137, 141, 148, 159, 172,
  213, 270. Also see Herbal juices.
Vegetable puree, 50, **148**, **149**
Vervain [*Verbena officinalis*], 86, 96, 175, **183**,
  184, 243
Vibrational hygiene, 43, 47, 133, **209-210**
Viburnum opulus, see Crampbark
Visualization, 122, **128**, 144, 200, 204, 205, 302,
  304
Vitamin B complex, 39, 52, 93, 94, 256, 261,
  270
Vitamin B$_{12}$, 52, 54, 93, 153, 236
Vitamin C, 39, 67, 70, 76, 78, 81, 84, 88, 94,
  102, 136, 138, 140, 148, 155, 158, 164
Vitamin D, 57, 151, 270
Vitamin E, 74, 81, **85**, 86, 95, 102, 132, **134**,
  136, 138, 264
Voluntary toxins, 162, 244

Volunteer helpers, 25, 31, 125, 126, 186, 188,
  191
Vomiting, 40, **58-60**, 67, 80, 110, 218, 277, 279.
  Also see Nausea.
VRE [vancomycin-resistant *Enterococci*], 229

W

Waiting for test results, 113-115
Wakame [*Alaria esculenta*], 143, 147, 154, 236
Wasabi, 156, 266, 270
"Watch and Wait", 117-118
Water, in overall health, 25, 42, 43, 45, 46, **48-
  49**, 60, 62, 76, 201, 209, 211, 213, **215-220**,
  221, 223, 225, 226, 240, 242, 243, 244, 246

Weight loss, undesired, 11, 38, 40, 52, **53-57**, 69,
  124, 133, 140, 146, 147-156, 172, 302
Western coltsfoot [*Petasites palmatus; P.
  frigidus*], 79, 267
Whey protein, 63, 69, 76, 93, 94, 103, 109, 137,
  146, 159, 160, 264, 270
Wormwood [*Artemisia absinthium*], 75, 82, 267
Wound healing, 38, 39, 43, 57, 62, 63, 68, 69,
  70, 73, 74, 80, 85, 87, 88, 89, 90, 91, 93, 94,
  95, 99, 100, 101, 102, 103, 105, 107, 133,
  136, 137, 138, 146, 166, 170, 171, 177, 182,
  184, 229, 232, 256, 257, 271, **284**, 286
Wrist bands for nausea, **59**, 275

Y

Yams, 49, 84, 148
Yams, baked, 148
Yantra, 42, 126, 205
Yarrow [*Achillea millefolium*], 29, 30, 54, 74,
  80, 81, 96, **99**, 101, 108, 135, **166**, 176, 214
Yeast infections, 55, **71-72**, 75, 99, 136, 267
Yeast, nutritional, 58, 68, 73, 85
Yeast, *Saccharomyces boulardii*, 75, **92**, 263,
  269, 270, 285
Yellow dock [*Rumex crispus*], **53**, 54, **78**, 86,
  219, 240, 243, 266
Yoga, 24, 42, 44, 47, 61, 101, 106, 115, 125,
  127, 130, 134, 202, 214, 249, 252, 258, **275**
Yogurt, 56, 63, 69, 71, 72, 88, 102, 137, 138,
  142, 146, 163, 230

Z

Zanthoxylum clava-herculis, see Prickly ash
Zea mays [cornsilk], **99**, 266
Zinc, 54, 55, **57**, 58, 63, 64, 67, 68, 73, 74, 81,
  84, 88, 94, 109, 124, 136, 151, 264, 269, 270
Zinc oxide cream, 74, 81, 124, 261, 271
Zingiber officinale, see Ginger

Entering the River

"Contemplate all energies without fear or disgust;
find their essence, for that is the stone that turns everything to gold."

— **Milarepa, Tibetan saint, 2nd century CE**

The first time I walked into the part of the oncology clinic where the pharmaceutical infusions were administered, it was as part of my introductory tour of the facilities. I was with two friends who had accompanied me to the initial appointment with my oncologist where we had laid out the treatment protocol.

As the nurse who was now guiding us pointed out the 'pod' setup of the infusion clinic—six groupings of four chairs each, facing inward—I found myself barely able to take it all in. Within each pod were very ill-looking people resting in reclining lounge chairs connected by tubing to bags of fluid suspended from metal IV-trees above their heads. Their faces looked dusky and generally somber, their life force dimmed. Many of them were older than myself.

In that moment of first exposure to the large treatment room, I flashed into a sense of surreality. My mind felt clearly that I did not belong here, that I was much healthier than these other folks. The thought flashed through my mind like lightning: 'What am I doing here?' I felt aversion. Then following, just as quickly, the realization that I, too, was sick; I, too, was in need of this medicine. I was engaged in the same struggle to live as those I saw in the chairs. I stood there, on my own edema-swollen legs, half-listening to the details the nurse was explaining—feeling the strong focus to silently breathe in the naked truth of my situation and allow it to fully penetrate. There was a lot to take in.

Appreciation for Life Practices

I had been clear from the first understanding of my diagnosis and the nature of the cancer process underway in my body that choosing to undergo the chemotherapy protocol was a choice for staying in the body. The deleterious impact of the lymphoma was progressing rapidly. Without the pharmaceutical interventions, the cancer would kill me—and soon.

I was equally clear that I would use all that I knew to complement the oncologist's recommended protocol: plant medicine [herbs, foods], nutritional supplementation, meditation/visualization, energy medicine practices, sound healing, journaling, dreamwork, and so on. These practices were already part of my normal life repertoire and so it was a matter of intensifying my focus and attention, of more regularly engaging some activities that had fallen from routine. I felt extremely grateful for being so well-equipped with life-enriching tools.

As part of this gratitude, I also came to realize that I was 'a healthy person dealing with cancer.' I had not 'failed' in my efforts in some way. The spheres of functional activity within major organ systems of my body were essentially healthy even though cancer process had gotten a foothold. My life force was markedly dimmed. Yet I had the best possible chance of turning this around and restoring order and harmony within my bodymind system. One of my intentions became using this situation to enhance my healthfulness and refine my vibration to levels even beyond what I had known previously.

This is not to say that I was attached to staying in the body at this point. I saw my situation in a multifaceted way, as a very immediate opportunity: to affirm the blessing and love of this lifetime; to discover and resolve unhealed material within my bodymind; to rest in peace and fulfillment as much as possible; to aim toward restored harmony within the many layers of being, whether or not the physical body was to recover from the current disequilibrium. Healing was not dependent on external outcomes—I understood deep healing as available in all moments and conditions.

Machete Woman

As much as I deepened my inner looking and practices to more gracefully surrender to whatever outcome life had in store, I was also called to make an unambiguous decision about my preference for either life or death at a juncture about a month into the journey. Although I had welcomed pharmaceutical therapeutics from the outset of diagnosis, it was at the moment of the first chemotherapy session that my clearness was tested.

My friend and I arrived at the infusion clinic at the appointed hour on the scheduled day. I was eager and grateful that the day had finally arrived, as it had been more than a month of various scans and tests since I had first said Yes to this treatment path—and my health status and comfort level had declined considerably during that intervening time. I had been able to stabilize my weight through concerted herbal and nutritional efforts—and the nourishing acts of lovingkindness of friends—but the lymphoma mass had been growing rapidly and there were significant consequences to its presence. I was more than ready to see if the chemotherapy would, indeed, change my experience.

As part of it, I was severely dehydrated, both because the abdominal mass made eating and drinking difficult at this point and because of deleterious intravenous antibiotics administered the previous day as a routine aspect of surgical insertion of a mediport [central venous catheter] in my chest wall in preparation for the therapeutic infusions.
As I stood standing at the clinic check-in counter, the staff informed me that my treatment had been postponed until the following week—that the health insurance

company had not yet approved my protocol, which was a standard treatment approach to the process present in my body. I heard these words in a state of utter disbelief. It already had felt like an interminable period of Herculean effort to sustain myself while waiting for this treatment to begin.

This delay simply did not work for me. I stood there, breathing intently to work strong energy arising. The whole of my being flowed tears and crystal clarity. The aspect of my beingness I name 'Machete Woman'—the woman who stands tall to speak truth to power—rose up through my feet. Her clear voice cried out. 'No, I will not accept that. I have an aggressive cancer growing inside of me. I will not die waiting for permission from an insurance company to live!'

The moment echoed with the strength of all the life force moving through me. Even as my body trembled, my feet felt rooted in the earth more securely than in many weeks. Machete Woman was clear—she was claiming life unequivocally. She would not be moved. She wished to live.

The clarity of Machete Woman—who flashes her blade only as needed—was met by the clear hearts of the staff at the infusion clinic. A small circle gathered around me in support. Eventually recognizing the whole of my situation, a solution was perceived which allowed my treatments to begin that very day.

Within the course of the following hours, it became unmistakably clear how what at first had seemed like obstacle and impediment was, truly, at its heart, a blessed opportunity. A challenge at the threshold. The grace of the moment had revealed itself layer by layer— and the morning's initially distressing circumstance was recognized as an agent for shift, a vehicle for carrying me to a heightened level of care and divine embrace. It was yet another teaching to simply trust the process as perfection.

Aversion into Opportunity

Experiencing keenly felt gratitude for the blessing of the medical staff and drugs that were available allowed me to transform my initial aversion to the chemotherapy clinic scene into appreciation. Facing the truth of that initial response without turning away became an opportunity to meet my situation clearly and wholeheartedly. How could I embrace the truth of the moment with the fullness of my being?

Staying open to all that was occurring in the clinic became a powerful aspect of relating to my experience in general. It took me deeper into the truth of common humanity, suffering and mortality, and sharpened my attention even further to the preciousness of each moment of aliveness, each soul encounter, each touch of lovingkindness. Some of us might make it out of the clinic alive, so to speak, but certainly not all. And, all of us— both 'patients' and compassionate helpers—would inevitably take our leave of this human lifetime at some point along the way.

The common currency was kindness and presence—as we each brought our most vulnerable, unvarnished selves to the shared space. All colors of emotion and attitude filled the clinic. Yet, interweaving all, a sense of heartfulness was pervasive. Each person quite naked, both witnessing and being witnessed.

Allopathic cancer therapies might be called a paradoxical medicine: taking a recipient to the fine edge between life and death in hopes of restoring health. I chose to embrace this paradox rather than meet it with fear or resistance, as the whole of nature reflects the truth of Death subsumed by Life.

Though the treatments could be challenging to receive and their mental and physical reverberations profound, these substances were working within my body to support the life within it. That is the way that I conceived it. I knew in my core that the more I could open to these drastic treatments the better they would work. And I equally knew that my elaboration of their activities through my attitude, visualizations and other efforts could support me greatly on this path toward renewed and improved well-being.

So the infusion clinic became a temple for me, the site of an intense two days of healing ministrations every three weeks for six cycles. I would bring the whole of myself there for purification and renewal of harmony on all levels of my being.

The foundation was to understand my time there as sacred. To support that, I renamed the treatments 'alchemical,' as in substantive transmutation; refinement of the mundane into the precious. I saw them as sacraments connecting me with infinite potential—divine healing elixirs aiding my own most heartfelt efforts at clearing my system of what was not serving my most vibrant bodymind wellness.

The infusion clinic itself became 'The Al-Chemo Lounge'; the treatments acquired the added potency of the image and intention I applied to each as it was administered. These visualizations were refined over the months of treatment, as my healing intentions evolved. Overall, I imagined these elixirs as not only benign but as actively permeating my bodymind with divine intelligence. I welcomed them as benediction.

This is not to suggest that I never felt apprehension at the prospect of these powerful substances entering the body I had long regarded as worthy of all efforts toward wholesomeness. At the cusp of voluntarily receiving such strong chemicals before the first infusion session, I was highly anxious. What would it feel like once they began dripping into my system?

But in the hospital setting where, eventually and perfectly, I received the first round of treatment, I already strongly felt the presence of Spirit nurturing my understanding. When it came time to experience the particular agent I felt the greatest fear toward, I did my best to incline my heart and mind toward gratefulness. The meditation that blossomed while receiving this elixir freed me in a way that reverberates still. The joke was on me if I believed these substances were anything separate from the divine whole!

And so it was that these agents that I would hear demonized over and over again during subsequent days in the clinic where the remainder of my treatments were administered, became for me powerful allies I could work with—originating from the same source and substance as all the green teachers I blessed and cherished. I understood that whatever the medical outcome, radiant truth heals the schisms that mind creates.

To be among the first to learn when *Deep, Grateful Bow*
is available for purchase,

Join my notification list

www.caroltrasatto.com

or via info@caroltrasatto.com

Acknowledgements

When I sit to reflect on where to shine the light of my gratefulness, the scene before me is vast. So many beautiful beings have crossed my path—or I theirs—in a way that has influenced my thinking, my ways of perceiving, my capacity to love and to serve. I am truly grateful for all the magic that has infused my life and offered me gifts that I could then cultivate in my own fashion before passing on to others.

Yet, there are a few individuals whom I must note by name. My parents Ann Masciantonio Trasatto and Nicholas Trasatto have supported me with a steady love throughout our journey together, although at times they may have had wondered at the path their daughter had been drawn to follow.

There are many teachers to honor, as in all things. My gratitude and love forever extends to the many fine herbalists I have sat with in circle—especially my core teacher David Winston as well as Jeannine Vannais, the late Billie Potts, Susun Weed, Donald Yance, Jonathan Treasure. The other good plant kinfolk from whom I have learned and shared nature love are too numerous to mention, but my gratitude flows to each of them as well. For many of us, still and always, the greenworld itself remains our wisest teacher. Of course, any errors contained herein must fall to my own shoulders.

I want to thank also those dear friends and family who have encouraged me over the years to share my work and passion more widely through my writing. My deepest gratitude to Susan Bush, Gray Crawford, Rosie Finn, Barbara Fogel, Laurie Guzoto, Lynda Heiner, Jennifer Johnson, Sally Jones, Dodie Jordan, Kerri Ward Merrill, the late Jacinta McKoy, Sara Moore-Heinz, Deb Petersen, Tobi Perrin, the late Joni Pohlig, Marie Poland, Sara Rivers, Claire Small, Jordan Taylor, Shari Trnka, Clydette Whitener, Jana Wiley, the Witley family [Vonda, Gary, Skye and Kaia]—and last but definitely not least my brother Steven Trasatto, my sister-in-law Doris Trasatto, my late aunt Alice Delkic and my uncle Feriz Delkic. There is so much to say to each of you beauties; please accept my infinite love and gratitude.

This effort is addressed to every client and friend who, over the years, has asked for my assistance in puzzling out a helping repertoire for themselves or a loved one. Thank you for the blessing of your asking and for your openness to tread a path perhaps unfamiliar. Your stories, queries, and feedback helped me orient this manual and motivated my efforts in bringing it to fruition.

May this offering serve to give ease

and may it support our witness for each other

within the infinite heart of compassion.

May Spirit guide us ever on.

About the Author

I have been studying and practicing the plant arts for almost four decades now, and it remains as inspiring and fulfilling a path as ever. Through my own healing journey and through maintaining a holistic wellness counseling practice for more than 20 years, I carry well-grounded confidence in the power of skillful plant medicine to help liberate the mind and body toward deep, profound healing. What that healing looks like is as particular and individual as we each are.

Since my first opening to the numinous world of the green, I was blessed to realize that the more intimate we become with our plant allies, the more our capacity for wonder and aliveness expands—opening our hearts and understanding to the sacred nature of all.

To my being, it follows that the practice of a truly holistic herbal medicine be inherently inclusive. A conscious, honoring relationship with the plants we live among is the heart and soul of traditional healing practices; and respectful stewardship of local habitat is the very foundation of health.

Years into recovering from cancer process and treatment myself, I am so grateful to embody the precious blessing of This Great Life and feel more motivated than ever to help folks recognize the indivisible connection between human health and the health of all beings and all the elements from which we sustain our forms.

Among my two-legged teachers, I particularly honor David Winston, Jeanine Vannais, the late Billie Potts, the writings of Susun Weed—and the many practicing herbalists with whom I have had the pleasure of sharing life-long learning. The insights of Donald Yance and Jonathan Treasure have been particularly key in informing my approach to life-threatening disease. And, as always, the plant spirits, the energies of place, and inner clarity remain the primary guides and teachers.

In addition to working on writing projects, I teach as well as offer private tutorials and consultations. I offer in-person classes as well as online instruction. For almost 18 years, Rosie Finn—my dear friend and brilliant astrologer—and I published and presented a monthly journal and talk, *Plants & Planets* [1998–2016], which featured my articles on plant medicine and holistic well-being. I have also been blessed to work at Radiance Herbs & Massage in Olympia, WA since 1992 as community herbalist, educator, and lead herb and supplement buyer.

To stay in touch and be informed about my classes, publications, and free offerings, email me at info@caroltrasatto.com to become part of my community.

I would love to hear from you.

Blessings on your journey!

CONSCIOUS CAREGIVING

CPSIA information can be obtained
at www.ICGtesting.com
Printed in the USA
LVHW10*0038230818
587864LV00009B/67/P

9 780999 578704